W9-CBC-376

Women's Edge
HEALTH ENHANCEMENT GUIDE™

Food Smart

Savory Strategies to Defy Disease

By Susan G. Berg
and the Editors of
PREVENTION Health Books for Women™

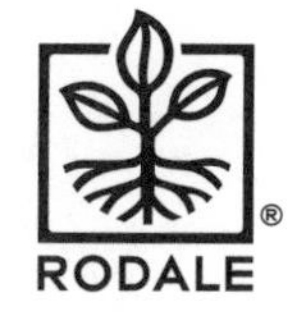

Notice

This book is intended as a reference volume only, not as a medical manual. The information given here is designed to help you make informed decisions about your health. It is not intended as a substitute for any treatment that may have been prescribed by your doctor. If you suspect that you have a medical problem, we urge you to seek competent medical help.

Printed in the United States of America on acid-free ♾, recycled paper ♻

The risk assessment for osteoporosis on page 89 was reprinted with permission from the National Osteoporosis Foundation, 1150 17th Street, NW, Suite 500, Washington, DC 20036.

"How Happy Is Your Diet?" on page 129 was excerpted from *The Duke University Medical Center Book of Diet and Fitness* by Michael Hamilton, M.D., Ronette L. Kolotkin, Ph.D., Dianne F. Cogburn, R.D., D.T. Moore, and Kathryn Watterson. © 1990 by Engel and Engel, Inc. Reprinted with permission of Engel and Engel, Inc., and the Duke University Diet and Fitness Center, Durham, North Carolina.

Library of Congress Cataloging-in-Publication Data

Berg, Susan G.
Food smart : savory strategies to defy disease / by Susan G. Berg and the editors of Prevention Health Books for Women.
p. cm. — (Women's edge health enhancement guide)
Includes index.
ISBN 0–87596–481–8 hardcover
1. Women—Health and hygiene. 2. Women—Diseases—Prevention. I. Prevention Health Books for Women. II. Title. III. Series.
RA778.B474 1998
613.2'082—dc21 97–35545

Distributed to the book trade by St. Martin's Press

8 10 9 hardcover

Visit us on the Web at www.rodalebooks.com, or call us toll-free at (800) 848-4735.

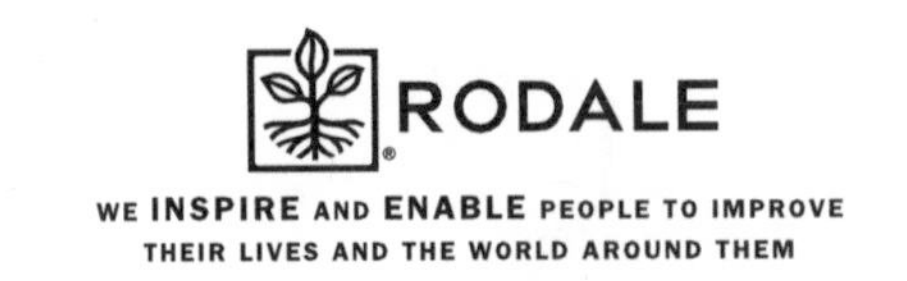

Food Smart Editorial Staff

Rodale Health and Fitness Books

Contents

Part One
What a Woman Needs

Part Two
Eating Healthy Every Day

Part Three
Eating for the Health of It

Board of Advisors for Rodale Women's Health Books

Part One

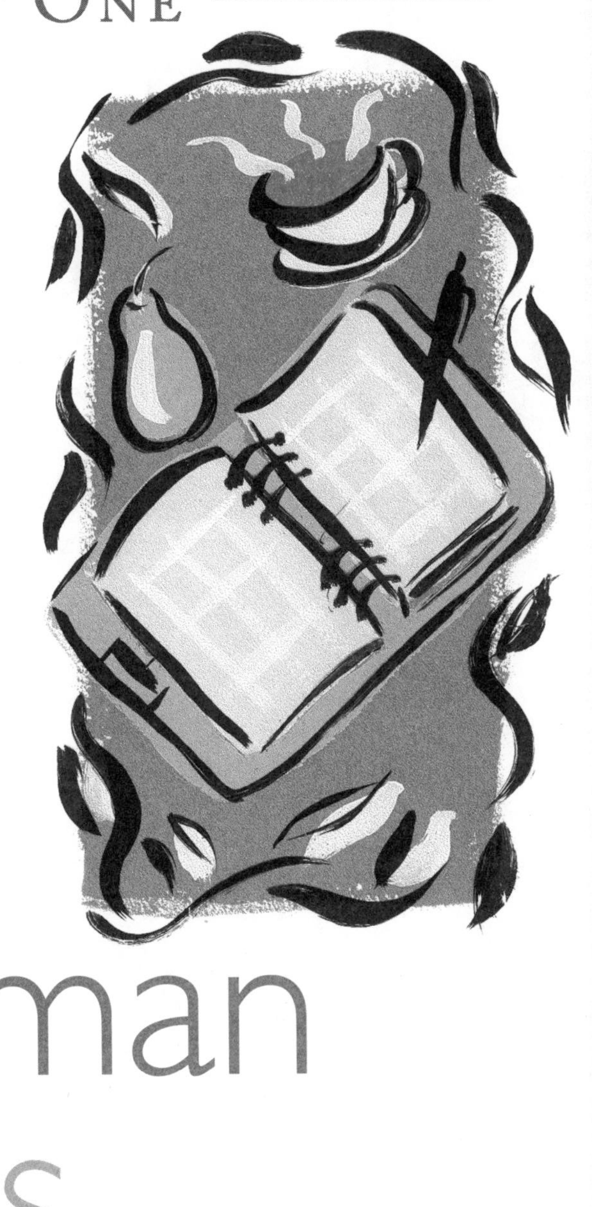

What a Woman Needs

Eat Smart for Life
20 Good Reasons to Make It a Habit

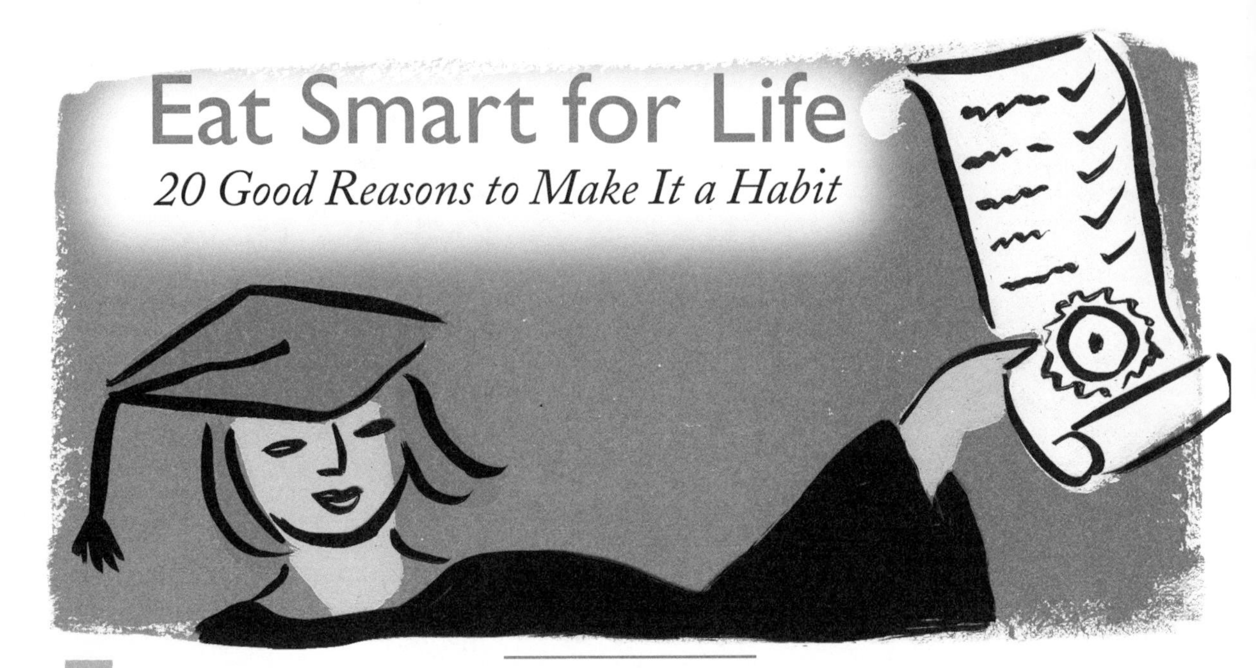

Eating the right foods can do wonders for your body. And the fact that you're a woman makes it all the more important.

Why? Because your body undergoes extraordinary changes over the course of your lifetime—much more so than a man's. "Women menstruate, they bear children, they go through menopause," notes Joanne Curran-Celentano, R.D., Ph.D., associate professor of nutritional sciences at the University of New Hampshire in Durham. "Each one of these events puts tremendous nutritional demands on your body."

What's more, women live longer than men. That in itself puts us at greater risk than men for chronic illness. The good news is that you can cut that risk, often dramatically, simply by eating healthfully.

If nutrition is such a big deal, why has your doctor rarely mentioned it—if ever? Because for years the medical community didn't give it much value. In fact, surprisingly few physicians received any training in it at all. But thankfully, that has changed.

"We now recognize that women have very unique health needs and that nutrition can influence those needs—for better or for worse," says Susan Calvert Finn, R.D., Ph.D., past president of the American Dietetic Association and chair of its Nutrition and Health Campaign for Women. "Eating right is perhaps the single most important element of a woman's health."

Those Incredible Edibles

Since women's nutrition is a relatively new field of study, scientists have barely scratched the surface in understanding the relationship between food and health. But what they've discovered so far is impressive. For example, here are 20 great things that eating right can do for your health.

Keep heart disease away. Heart disease ranks as the number one cause of death among women in the United States. Many experts attribute this dubious distinction to a much-too-high intake of dietary fat. But they also believe that foods such as olive oil, soy, garlic, and grape juice can cut your odds of developing heart disease by nearly 25 percent.

Lower cholesterol. You probably already know that a high-fat diet can send your cholesterol level through the roof. But now there's evidence that certain foods—especially fiber-rich beans and pectin-rich fruits such as grapefruit—can help keep your cholesterol low and your arteries clear.

Reduce high blood pressure. About 1 of every 10 women between the ages of 35 and 44 has high blood pressure. A quartet of nutrients that you can easily get from foods—calcium, magnesium, potassium, and vitamin C—may be the nutritional tools that your body needs to help whip your blood pressure reading into shape.

Outsmart cancer. One-fourth of all breast cancers might be prevented if women cut down on dietary fat and filled up on fruits, vegetables, and whole grains. And aggressive dietary changes can reduce your risk of ovarian cancer by half.

Derail diabetes. Up to two-thirds of people with Type II (non-insulin-dependent) diabetes may very well be able to manage it simply by eating right and exercising regularly.

Beef up your bones. As many as one in two women will suffer an osteoporosis-related fracture in her lifetime. You can cut your own risk in half just by making sure that you're getting enough bone-building calcium in your diet.

Eliminate weight gain. A low-fat, low-calorie eating plan that includes lots of grains and produce is

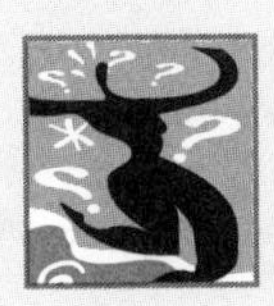

WOMEN ASK WHY

Why can't I just take a multivitamin every day to get all the nutrients I need?

Simply put, not all the nutrients you need are found in multivitamins. A perfect example is calcium, a mineral. While calcium is often added to multivitamins, the amount is usually only a fraction of the Daily Value because calcium isn't easily compacted like some vitamins or minerals. You would need a pill about three times larger than an average multivitamin to get all that you need.

Also, calcium is just one of the nutrients your body would miss if you relied too much on a supplement for good nutrition. Your body needs lots of other things that a vitamin pill just can't deliver—like complex carbohydrates, protein, and fiber.

Multivitamins can't provide more than a few phytonutrients, hundreds of naturally occurring chemical compounds that we can get from fruits and vegetables. A well-known example of phytonutrients is the carotenoids. There are about 600 different carotenoids, many of which protect against disease, particularly cancer and heart disease. But only beta-carotene is commonly found in supplements.

The other concern with relying solely on a multivitamin is bioavailability—your body's ability to absorb and use nutrients. Vitamins and minerals need to be extracted from foods or made synthetically to be used as supplements. This sometimes makes them more difficult for your body to absorb. For example, the form of iron found in multivitamins isn't as easily absorbed by your body as the iron found in food.

Being food smart means getting the nutrients you need from a healthy, well-rounded diet. So taking a multivitamin is a good idea only if you take it as nutritional insurance.

Expert Consulted
Abby Bloch, R.D., Ph.D.
Coordinator of clinical nutrition research
Memorial Sloan-Kettering Hospital
New York City

your best bet for saying bye-bye to extra baggage. You have a very good reason to do so: Overweight has been linked to serious health problems such as heart disease and certain types of cancer.

Turn back the clock. Many of the physical changes that occur as you get older—sagging skin, poor muscle tone, and reduced immunity—can be traced to cellular damage by renegade molecules called free radicals. By eating foods rich in antioxidants—vitamins C and E and beta-carotene—you can help slow the aging process and protect yourself against age-related disease.

Enhance immunity. Your body needs food to keep your immune system in good working order. It uses the nutrients as raw material to manufacture and repair cells.

Banish fatigue. Complex carbohydrates such as whole grains, beans, and vegetables can help keep your energy level on an even keel. Just as important, they supply the nutrients your body needs most when it's run-down.

Defuse stress. Many experts believe that prolonged stress depletes your internal supplies of key nutrients such as calcium and zinc. There's also preliminary evidence that vitamin C can help protect your body against the effects of stress.

Influence your emotions. Your body uses substances in food to produce neurotransmitters, brain chemicals that can dramatically affect your mood. So what you eat can lift your spirits or bring you down.

Boost your brainpower. You can turbocharge your alertness, concentration, and memory by munching on a little bit of low-fat protein. Protein supports the production of neurotransmitters that keep you mentally sharp.

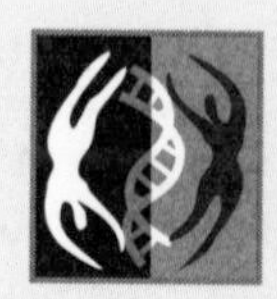

Woman to Woman

Daughter's Crisis Changed Mom's Health

Since childhood, Carol Politi, an administrative associate at a Pennsylvania bank, and her identical twin sister had allergies and skin problems. During adulthood, they were plagued with respiratory problems and exhaustion. But it wasn't until a health crisis hit her five-year-old daughter that Carol made drastic changes to her family's eating habits. The effects on her own health were positively astounding. Here's her story.

A fat-loving, cigarette-smoking couch potato—that's the type of person someone might think would have high cholesterol. So when my lively, petite, five-year-old was diagnosed with dangerously high cholesterol, I was understandably shocked. Even though my twin sister and I have been plagued with high cholesterol and other health problems all our lives, I never thought such a problem could hit my child—and at such a young age. My motherly instincts to do everything to protect her health were jolted into action.

The first thing I did was throw away any junk foods in our house. They were quickly followed by the eggs, the hamburgers, and the ice cream. To get my daughter to eat right, I knew the whole family's diet had to change. I started serving lots of fish, chicken, and pasta. Vegetables and fruits, never big in our household, became the house staples. I

Protect reproductive health. Like every other system in your body, your reproductive system depends on good nutrition to function properly. In fact, researchers now suspect that several aspects of reproduction—from fertility to delivering a healthy baby to nursing—may have a nutritional component.

Tame premenstrual symptoms. Both vitamin B_6 and calcium have shown potential for easing the irritability, insomnia, bloating, headache, edginess, constipation, fatigue, and breast tenderness that often accompany premenstrual syndrome.

Minimize the symptoms of menopause. Women in Japan experience fewer menopausal started making my own low-fat cookies and chips so my children could still snack on something salty or sweet. Occasionally, we would allow ourselves a fast-food meal or a slice of iced cake.

Thankfully, the dietary changes had an immediate positive effect on Christina's cholesterol. But after three months, I also discovered something more: a remarkable change in my own health. After lifelong bouts with upper respiratory problems from allergies, I hadn't had a sniffle. My skin, usually cracked and dry or itchy with rashes, was smooth and clear. My cholesterol dropped from 244 to 190. And, while I wasn't looking, 25 pounds just melted off me. At some point, my energy level soared. I tackled the responsibilities of my job and family with newfound stamina.

It has been two years since I pruned the fat from my diet, and I've never been healthier. I've missed 3 days of work over this period, a far cry from my record 25 days during one allergy season. Interestingly, I have a built-in measure of success: my identical twin sister. She continued to eat fat-laden foods during my two-year transformation, and her allergies and skin problems persisted. Fortunately, she's found inspiration in my story, and she's beginning to make healthy lifestyle changes. I'll be there every step of the way to help. They say that there are two sides to every story. I'm counting on these two stories to come out the same.

symptoms and side effects than women in the United States. And now researchers think that they know why. Japanese cuisine relies heavily on soy foods, and soy foods contain phytoestrogens, plant compounds that act much like the female hormone estrogen in the body.

Protect your skin. Eating healthfully can help prevent acne, canker sores, hives, and other minor skin eruptions. There's evidence, too, that chowing down on lots of fruits and vegetables can make you less likely to develop skin cancer.

Prevent anemia. Anemia, a condition usually characterized by extreme fatigue, results from a shortage of iron in the blood. You can replenish your iron stores by eating foods rich in the mineral, such as lean meats and kidney beans.

Vanquish varicose veins. A high-fiber diet, combined with regular exercise, can make you less likely to develop varicose veins. Fiber prevents constipation and weight gain, both of which can lead to varicose veins.

Protect your teeth. Calcium, your body's main bone-builder, also plays a role in mouth maintenance. Your teeth need the mineral to stay healthy and strong. Vitamin C and folate also chip in, feeding the gums of the teeth and helping to ward off infection.

Good Health by the Plateful

You'll reap all of these benefits—and countless more—when you eat the *Food Smart* way. In the pages that follow, we lay out for you a comprehensive nutrition strategy that you can customize to fit your needs and lifestyle. You'll get expert advice on virtually every aspect of shaping and maintaining a healthy diet—from navigating a salad bar to cooking with herbs and spices, from reading food labels to timing your meals, from ordering Chinese takeout to curing a craving for chocolate.

Yes, you'll probably have to make some adjustments in your current eating habits. But we promise that they're painless. In fact, as you make the switch to the *Food Smart* plan, you may find that you can eat more than ever and still be fit and healthy!

So get set to dig in. You're going to love what good nutrition can do for you.

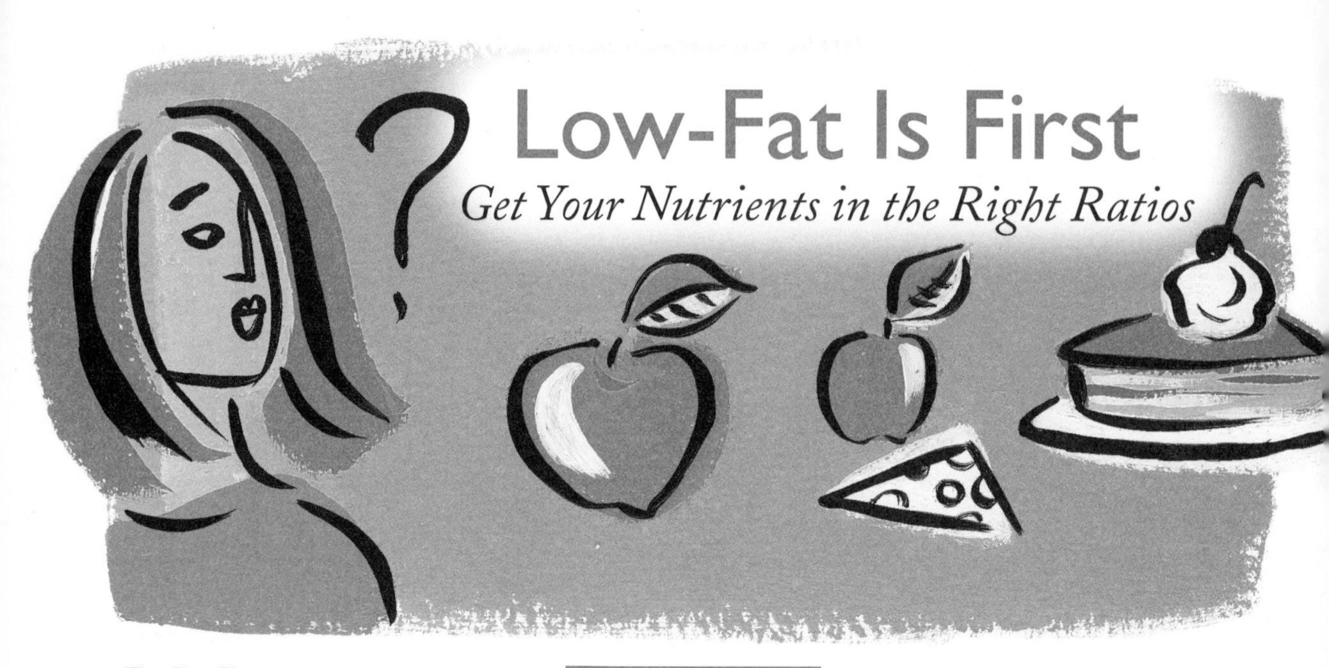

Low-Fat Is First

Get Your Nutrients in the Right Ratios

When you get right down to it, food is energy, pure and simple. It fuels your body by supplying it with calories to burn. You can consume and burn those calories in one of three forms: carbohydrates, protein, or fat.

Ideally, we women should get about 60 to 65 percent of our calories from carbohydrates, about 10 percent from protein, and the remaining 25 to 30 percent from fat. This is close to the nutritional profile that studies around the world have linked to lower rates of heart disease and cancer. In reality, we're falling quite short of this mark.

By one estimate, the typical woman consumes just 20 to 25 percent of calories from carbohydrates—less than half the recommended amount. That means, of course, that she's making up the difference by overdoing it on protein and fat. And how! Statistics suggest that we're eating roughly twice as much protein as we should, with fat tipping the scales at 34 percent of calories.

Certainly, these days we're much more fat-conscious than we used to be, and that's good. Eating low-fat *is* important. "But women have to remember that their diets are about more than just fat," says Doris Derelian, R.D., Ph.D., a former president of the American Dietetic Association. They're about balance—getting healthful amounts of not only fat but carbohydrates and protein, too.

Carbs: The Tiger in Your Tank

Of all three nutrients, carbohydrates are your body's fuel of choice. They easily break down to a form that your body then uses to keep its systems running smoothly and efficiently. They also team up with protein, forming compounds that are essential for combating infections, lubricating joints, and maintaining healthy skin, bones, and nails.

Actually, there are two kinds of carbohydrates, and your body utilizes them in slightly different ways. Simple carbohydrates consist of tiny, single or double molecules of sugar. They have familiar names, like glucose, fructose, and lactose. These carbs are already in their most basic form, which means that they are absorbed into the bloodstream quite quickly. There they circulate as glucose, or blood sugar, until getting snapped up by cells and converted into energy.

Simple carbohydrates also join together to form complex carbohydrates. Complex carbs are found almost exclusively in plant foods such as grains, beans, fruits, and vegetables. When you eat complex carbohydrates, your digestive system has to break them down into their simple form before they can be absorbed into your bloodstream and used as fuel. This "production time" makes for a steadier, longer-lasting energy source than simple carbs provide.

In fact, there's evidence to suggest that your body burns more calories digesting complex carbohydrates than digesting protein or fat. Research has shown that vegetarians have higher metabolic rates than meat-eaters, and scientists attribute the difference to the vegetarians' high-carbohydrate diets.

As mentioned earlier, complex carbohydrates should comprise at least 60 percent of your total daily calorie intake, nutritionists advise. For example, if you're following a 2,000-calorie-a-day eating plan, you should get about 1,200 of those calories as carbs. That translates to about 300 grams of carbohydrate per day.

We women consume far fewer complex carbohydrates than we should—and far fewer than we used to. At the beginning of the twentieth century, carbohydrate consumption in the United States hovered around a much healthier

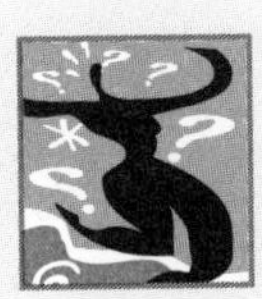

WOMEN ASK WHY

Why do women need fewer calories than men of the same size and weight?

The truth is that a woman could need *more* calories than a man of the same height and weight—it all depends on her activity level. But all things being equal, a woman can't compete with a man when it comes to calorie intake. You can blame it on hormones.

Women naturally have a lower basal metabolic rate (BMR)—the rate at which we burn calories and fat. Although the female hormone estrogen increases the metabolic rate slightly, the rate is only one-third the speed imposed by the male sex hormone testosterone.

Men, in general, have higher metabolisms than women because of testosterone, which increases the body's ability to build lean muscle—and lean muscle metabolizes calories quickly. Women have more essential body fat to enable us to bear children and nurture our infants. Our lack of testosterone means that we also have less lean muscle.

We can, however, tinker with fate a little by exercising. Regular aerobic exercise stokes your metabolism, meaning that a fairly active female can eat considerably more than a sedentary female—and, in some cases, a sedentary male.

Your body stores unused, or excess, calories, and excess calories from fat are easily stored. So if you're overweight, eating a low-fat diet is also a smart idea. In addition to this, eating small amounts of food will prevent your insulin levels from fluctuating so much during the day. This is important since insulin promotes the storage of fat.

But exercise is the real key to eating success. Reset your BMR through regular exercise, and you'll be able to get away with eating just as much as almost any Joe.

Expert Consulted
Michele Trankina, Ph.D.
Nutritional physiologist
Professor of biological sciences
St. Mary's University
San Antonio

70 percent of calories. Ironically, as we got wealthier, our eating habits got worse, as meats and sweets, which were symbols of affluence, became more affordable, says Maria Linder, Ph.D., professor of biochemistry at California State University, Fullerton.

So what can you do to get your carbohydrate intake on track? Give these tips a try.

Stay whole. Whole-grain foods such as brown rice, whole-wheat bread, and oatmeal are better carbohydrate choices than refined-grain foods, says Nan Kathryn Fuchs, Ph.D., a nutritionist in Sebastopol, California, and nutrition editor of *Women's Health Letter*. Refined grains such as enriched white flour and white rice are missing some B-complex vitamins, nutrients that are essential to carbohydrate metabolism. They also don't have fiber, and fiber ensures that your body absorbs carbohydrates at a slow, steady pace.

Read the fine print. Check the label on whole-wheat bread to make sure that whole-wheat flour, not just wheat flour, tops the ingredient list, Dr. Fuchs advises. You can't go by the color of the bread as a guarantee of its "whole-graininess." Some manufacturers add coloring to their breads and other baked goods to make them look browner and more wholesome.

Woman to Woman

She Shed Pounds by Eating More

Susan Carlson, a convention center sales manager in Newport, Rhode Island, lost 72 pounds and dropped from size 18 to sizes 6 to 8 in two years when she discovered low-fat eating. It changed her life for good. In fact, she's thinner now than she was in her twenties. This is her story.

My mom was the Shake 'n Bake queen. I grew up eating a lot of processed foods—often my lunch was a bologna sandwich on white bread, rounded out with chips and Twinkies, all washed down with whole milk. I began putting on weight in high school, and by the time I was pregnant with my son at the age of 31, I had swelled to 196 pounds. I remember standing on the scale and praying that it wouldn't go over 200.

Then I moved in with my grandmother. Stuck with a baby in the house, surrounded by my grandmother's custard pies, I ate and ate and ate. I wore maternity clothes for a month after my son was born, never dressing up. I went shopping and nothing fit me. I still weighed 181 pounds and was spiraling into depression. I wanted to get out of the house and go back to work, but not looking the way I did. Finally, I got fed up and went on my first diet. I knew I needed help, so I joined a commercial weight-loss program and lost my first 32 pounds.

That motivated me enough to join a gym. It killed me at first, and I clung to the back wall at the aerobics class—but I did it, three to five times a week. The more people I met, the easier it became for me to go, and I lost some more weight.

By then I also knew that if my weight loss was going to continue, I'd have to change my diet. I dropped out of the weight-loss program and switched to low-fat—permanently.

Pair off pasta. Spaghetti, macaroni, noodles, and other types of pasta are usually made from white flour, so they're not as good a carbohydrate source as whole grains. You can improve their nutritional profile, though, by topping them with carb-rich veggies, Dr. Fuchs suggests. For example, try adding lightly steamed broccoli or escarole, red and green peppers, onions, garlic, mushrooms, zucchini, or any vegetable you like to traditional red sauce.

Foil the fat. Croissants, biscuits, many crackers, potato and corn chips, french fries, and processed macaroni and cheese contain more

Now, nearly 10 years later, I usually weigh between 124 and 134 pounds and am eating more than ever before. I feel great! I always have fruit in my house, and I focus my meals on healthy fruits, vegetables, and whole grains. And I drink plenty of water—about 1½ liters a day (about two quarts).

I eat breakfast every day. When I was fat, I never ate breakfast—I couldn't stomach the thought of it. Now I eat either oatmeal, Kashi cereal with strawberries, or whole-wheat toast with a slice of cheese. I usually have an apple in the morning at work, which satisfies my urge to eat something crunchy.

My biggest meal of the day, though, is lunch. My grandmother used to say, "Eat like a queen in the morning, a king at noon, and a pauper at night." Since I work in a hotel, there's a lot of high-fat food around, so I often bring my lunch, usually a turkey sandwich on whole-wheat or eight-grain bread with mustard, plus a salad, fruit, and steamed broccoli. Around 3:00 P.M., I have an apple or some fresh melon.

My dinners are very light. Often I have half a bagel with a little cream cheese and fresh tomato on top. Two other favorites are a baked potato and salsa or angel hair pasta with sauce. I don't cook big dinners, and I think that helps.

Overall, I eat low-fat the natural way. I don't eat fat-free fake food with chemical ingredients I can't pronounce. I eat the real thing, but less of it. For example, I love cheese, but when I tried the fat-free kind and found it tasted terrible, I thought, "I can't do this."

My new life is very hectic. Staying busy has helped keep the weight off. Before I got into shape, I was sluggish all of the time. Hundreds of aerobics classes, thousands of low-fat meals, and about 70 fewer pounds later, I have energy to spare—I wish I had known then what I know now.

calories from fat than from carbohydrates. The same goes for packaged rice pilaf dishes, potatoes au gratin, and some breakfast cereals—especially granola. If you must eat these foods, reserve them for an occasional treat, Dr. Fuchs recommends.

Protein: Too Much of a Good Thing?

You might think of protein as the Swiss Army knife of nutrients. Your body uses it to carry out an astounding array of tasks. Indeed, every single cell in your body contains protein. It plays an indispensable role in building and repairing body tissues, digesting food, and fighting infections. It supports the manufacture of chemical messengers in your brain and, in the process, makes you more mentally alert. In a pinch, it can be converted to fuel.

Chemically, proteins consist of varying combinations of about 20 amino acids. Your body can produce most of these amino acids, but there are nine essential ones that it can get only from the foods you eat. Lysine falls into this category. Your body needs it in order to absorb calcium, the mineral that keeps your bones strong.

Red meats and dairy products were once considered superior protein sources because most of these foods contain all of the essential amino acids—in other words, they're complete proteins. Their downside, of course, is that they also contain large amounts of heart-unhealthy saturated fat.

Plant foods such as grains, beans, fruits, and vegetables are incomplete proteins, meaning that individually, they don't supply all of the essential amino acids. You can make them complete, though, by combining them.

Even better, it's not necessary to eat these complementary foods at the same time to reap the benefits of a complete protein. Thanks to the rather leisurely pace of the digestive process, the oatmeal you eat for breakfast combines with the baked beans you eat for lunch, the sunflower seeds you have for a snack, and the rice you eat for dinner to create a high-quality protein that has all of the essential amino acids.

The Daily Value for protein is 50 grams. If you're pregnant or nursing, you need 60 to 65 grams per day. But you shouldn't worry too much about not getting enough protein. Studies indicate that most women get more than enough.

When you eat more protein than your body can use, the excess is stored as body fat. It can also interfere with the absorption of some minerals, such as calcium.

You can get all the protein you need without fear of overdoing it. Just heed this advice from the experts.

Minimize meat. Change the way you look at your dinner plate. Relegate meat to a bit part and let grains, beans, fruits, and vegetables take over the starring role. This dietary recasting supplies a sufficient amount of protein while sparing you unwanted saturated fat and cholesterol. "If we would stop planning our meals around meat and start planning them around plant foods, we'd be much better off," says Elizabeth Somer, R.D., author of *Nutrition for Women* and *Food and Mood*.

Visit your local fishmonger. Broiled, baked, or poached, fish is a standout source of protein that just happens to be low in saturated fat. As a bonus, fish such as salmon, mackerel, and tuna contain omega-3 fatty acids, which may help protect you against heart disease.

Love those legumes. Nutrition-wise, dried beans and peas in all their different colors and shapes have plenty going for them. Of course, they contain generous amounts of protein: One-half cup of kidney beans, for example, has more protein than either a whole egg or two tablespoons of chunky peanut butter.

Celebrate soy. Tofu, tempeh, and other soy foods offer abundant supplies of plant protein. Technically, soy is a legume. But it merits special mention because it is also rich in phytoestrogens, chemical compounds that may reduce your risk of breast cancer. Soy foods are so versatile that you can use them as healthy substitutes for high-fat ingredients in everything from meat loaf to cheesecake.

Fat: Get the Facts

You probably already know all the bad stuff about fat: how it clogs your arteries and sets the stage for heart disease, how it magnifies your risk of certain types of cancer, how it even ups your odds of gallstones and osteoporosis-related fractures. With a rap sheet like that, fat doesn't figure to be the kind of dietary company you'd want to keep. Yet it's absolutely essential to your good health.

"We spend a lot of time trying to get rid of the fat in our diets," says Michele Trankina, Ph.D., nutritional physiologist and professor of biological sciences at St. Mary's University in San Antonio. "In reality, our bodies need a certain percentage of the nutrient to function properly."

Fat is an internal transportation system, moving the fat-soluble vitamins A, D, E, and K to their job sites within your body. It surrounds vital organs such as your heart and kidneys, protecting them from injury. It maintains body temperature, insulates nerves, and supports the production of compounds that regulate blood pressure, blood clotting, and inflammation.

Your body also uses fat to store calories until they're needed for energy. In fact, of all three nutrients, fat is the most efficient at this task. It can hold nine calories per gram, compared with protein and carbohydrates' four.

There are actually three types of fat found in foods. Of the trio, monounsaturated and polyunsaturated fat are considered the healthiest. Studies have shown that vegetable oils rich in monounsaturates (such as canola and olive oils) and polyunsaturates (such as corn and soybean oils) can help lower your total cholesterol count. And, as mentioned, omega-3 fatty acids, polyunsaturated fats found in some types of fish, have similar heart-healthy effects.

On the other hand, high amounts of saturated fat—the kind found in meat and dairy products—have been linked to an increased risk of heart disease and colon cancer.

So just how low should you go with your fat consumption? Many experts recommend 25 percent of calories from fat. Based on our sample 2,000-calorie-a-day eating plan, no more than 500 calories should come from fat. And since there are 9 calories in one gram of fat, you'd want to limit yourself to about 55 grams of fat a day.

As many of us know firsthand, excess dietary fat can all too easily turn into excess stored fat. Your body hoards all excess fat, stashing it in fatty tissue. Then when your body needs to supplement its energy supply, it turns to these fat stores.

Thankfully, managing your fat intake doesn't require perpetual number crunching. The following strategies take the hassle out of low-fat living.

Think in thirds. The American Heart Association has devised the Rule of Thirds: One-third of daily fat grams from monounsaturates, up to one-third from polyunsaturates, and no more than one-third from saturates. If you eat 2,000 calories and 55 grams of fat a day, no more than 18 grams (one-third of fat grams) should come from saturated fat.

Don't Get Caught in the Fat Trap

This morning you opened a package of your favorite fat-free fig bars. Now, just eight hours later, it's all but empty. But you're not too worried. After all, they're fat-free.

Fat-free, yes. Calorie-free, no. While you may not have consumed a smidgen of fat, you've already downed a whopping 1,200 calories—almost an entire day's allotment spent on your fig-bar fling. You're caught in the fat trap.

With all the emphasis on fat these days, and with so many nonfat and low-fat products available, many of us have gotten the impression that we no longer need to watch our calorie intakes. But calories do still count. And it takes just 3,500 of them—or roughly three packages of those fat-free fig bars—to add another pound on you.

So the next time you're tempted to eat the whole thing, refer to these figures for a jolt back to calorie reality.

Snack	Calories per Serving	Calories per Package
Fat-free caramel corn cakes	50	700
Fat-free chocolate cookie cakes	50	600
Fat-free fig bars	100	1,200
Low-fat tortilla chips	110	880
Pretzel chips	110	880
Reduced-fat mini cheese crackers	120	600
Reduced-fat mini chocolate chip cookies	130	910

Oust the obvious. Scan your diet for easy ways to trim fat. For example, you can bake, steam, broil, or microwave your foods rather than frying them, says Elaine Kvitka-Nevins, R.D., a nutrition consultant in Scottsdale, Arizona. Spread your morning toast with all-fruit preserves instead of butter. Switch from full-fat ice cream to low-fat or nonfat ice cream or frozen yogurt. "There are a million ways to cut your fat intake," she says.

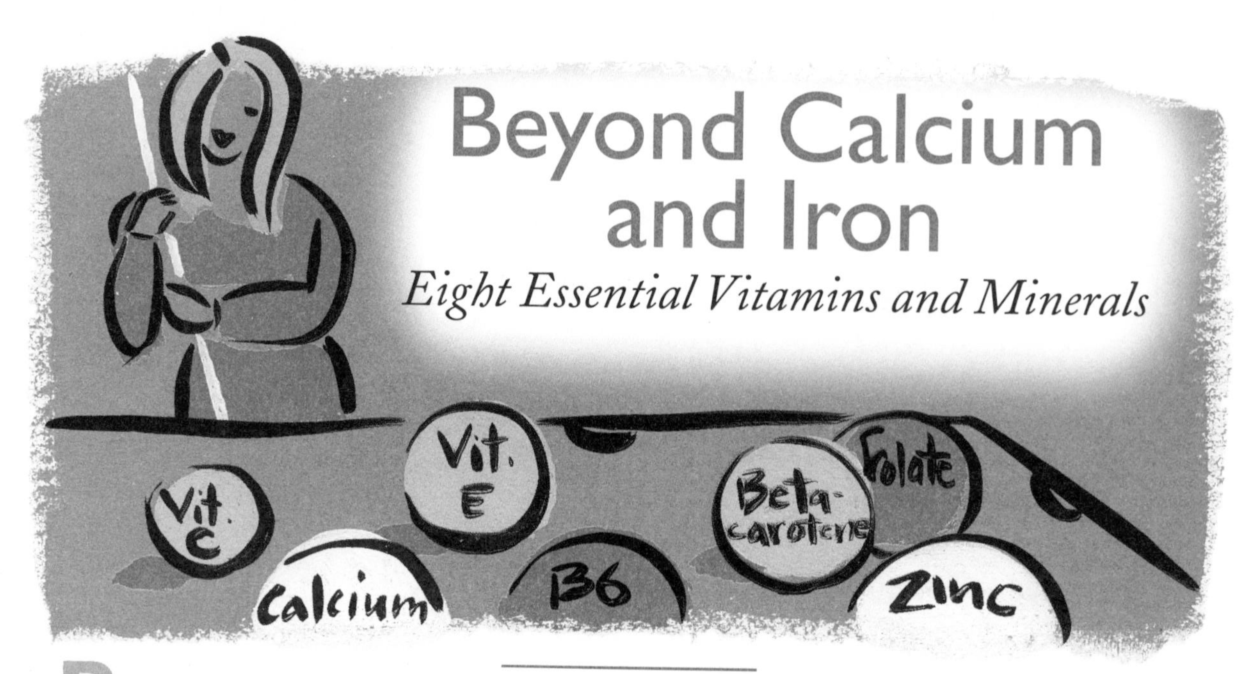

Beyond Calcium and Iron

Eight Essential Vitamins and Minerals

Pick a fruit. Any fresh, ripe fruit will do—cantaloupe or cherries, papaya or peach. Now take a bite. Suddenly your mouth is awash with flavor as the juices drench every square millimeter of your tongue. Ambrosial bursts tantalize your palate as you chew. *Mmmm*...delicious.

Your tastebuds thank you for this gustatory indulgence. And the rest of your body seconds the motion.

Of course, your tastebuds are only interested in the sensuous pleasure that eating provides. The rest of your body has much more at stake. It relies on food for vitamins and minerals, substances you need to survive and thrive.

Feed Your Body Right

Your body uses about two dozen vitamins and minerals every day just to support routine bodily functions, explains Cheryl Rock, Ph.D., professor of nutrition at the University of Michigan in Ann Arbor. Two of these nutrients—vitamin D and vitamin K—it can make itself. The rest must come from foods.

Unfortunately, women aren't very good at getting their daily share of essential nutrients. The problem, in part, stems from our low calorie intakes. We eat roughly 1,800 calories a day, and if we're trying to lose weight, we may eat even less. By comparison, when dietitians at Utah State University in Logan tried to design a menu that supplied adequate amounts of all the vitamins and minerals that women need, they couldn't get the calorie count below 2,200.

What's more, our bodies require more of certain nutrients than men's do simply because we're women. For example, both pregnancy and menopause—uniquely female life events—can boost a woman's daily calcium quota by as much as 50 percent. Yet most of us don't get nearly enough of the mineral to begin with.

In fact, calcium is one of eight nutrients that we need in our diets, says Margo Woods, D.Sc., who teaches nutrition at Tufts University School of Medicine in Boston. The other seven? Well, you've probably already guessed iron. Then there are the antioxidants—beta-carotene and vitamins C and E—plus folate, vitamin B_6, and zinc.

How Much Is Enough?

Take a look at the nutrition information on any packaged food, and you'll see the abbreviation DV. It stands for Daily Value, a federal government label guideline for how much of a certain nutrient you should be getting each day. There are DVs established for 25 vitamins and minerals as well as for other nutrients, including carbohydrates, protein, and fat.

What the label doesn't tell you is that the DVs do not reflect a woman's unique nutritional needs. The recommended intakes for the various vitamins and minerals are, for the most part, based on the nutrient requirements of a 15- to 18-year-old male.

Far more useful for women are the Recommended Dietary Allowances, or RDAs. (The exceptions are folate, vitamin E, and calcium, for which the DVs are considered better guidelines.) The RDAs take into account gender, age, and whether you are pregnant or nursing. Currently, RDAs are established for 11 vitamins and seven minerals plus protein. And they're updated periodically, as research turns up new information about how much of a nutrient is required to correct a deficiency and how much is normally consumed by people in good health.

Still, some experts contend that even the RDAs don't make the grade as dietary standards. First, while the RDAs will pretty much guarantee that you will keep deficiency at bay, they aren't a measure of how much you need for optimum health. Second, the RDAs are set to meet the needs of *healthy* people; people trying to fight disease likely need more.

Take vitamin C as an example. The RDA for women is 60 milligrams (which, incidentally, is the same as the DV). Yet many studies of the nutrient show that vitamin C does the most

DO YOU NEED SUPPLEMENTS?

Experts agree that the best way for women to get their vitamins and minerals is by eating right. But sometimes specific health or lifestyle issues make it difficult to get the nutrients your body requires through diet alone. In those instances, you may want to consider taking a supplement to pick up the slack.

Use the following questions as a guide to determine where you might be falling short, nutrient-wise. Before you begin a supplement program, though, it's a good idea to talk to your doctor or a qualified nutrition expert.

Do you smoke cigarettes or have you recently quit? Smoking appears to deplete vitamin C stores.

Are you at high risk for heart disease? Vitamin E may help keep your heart healthy.

Do you consume dairy products such as skim milk, low-fat or nonfat yogurt, and low-fat cheese? These are some of the best sources of bone-building calcium. If they're not on your menu, you may not be getting enough of the mineral.

Do you eat meat? If you don't eat at least three three-ounce servings of red meat a week, you might benefit from an iron supplement.

Do you plan to get pregnant? Folate is essential for fetal development. Without it, your baby is at risk for a birth defect like spina bifida.

Have you passed through menopause? Folate is important for you, too—it can reduce your risk of heart disease and cervical cancer.

good—functioning as an antihistamine, boosting immunity, and protecting against cancer—in daily doses of at least a few hundred milligrams.

To reap all the health benefits that vitamins and minerals offer, you may have to go beyond the RDAs (while remaining within safe limits).

The New Phyto Foods

They have names that only an etymologist could love, like *isothiocyanates* and *monoterpenes*. But if current research pans out, they may also have the most potent healing powers this side of vitamin C.

"They" are phytochemicals—literally, plant chemicals. Found in plentiful supply in vegetables, fruits, legumes, and whole grains, these compounds have shown potential as defenders against heart disease, cancer, and a host of other serious health problems.

Plants use phytochemicals to safeguard themselves against bugs, bacteria, viruses, and other natural enemies. When you eat those plants as foods, you get the same protective benefits—not against aphids and leaf spot, of course, but against human ailments.

Scientists have yet to pinpoint how the various phytochemicals work. So far, they know that many of these com-

Phytochemical	**Best Food Sources**
Allylic sulfides	Onions, garlic
Carotenoids	Carrots, broccoli, cantaloupe, greens, tomatoes
Flavonoids	Onions, kale, endive, citrus fruits, apples, broccoli, cranberries, red wine, grape juice
Indoles and isothiocyanates	Broccoli, cauliflower, cabbage, mustard greens
Isoflavones	Soybeans, chickpeas, lentils, kidney beans
Lignans	Flaxseed
Monoterpenes	Citrus fruits, cherries
Phenolic compounds	Almost all fruits, vegetables, cereal grains, green and black teas
Saponins	Soybeans, chickpeas, spinach, tomatoes, potatoes, nuts, oats

The Essential Eight

For many women, just meeting the minimum daily requirement is a tall order—never mind getting extra. To help make it easier, here's a rundown of the eight nutrients that you need most, along with their recommended daily intakes and best food sources. Where appropriate, we've asked several experts to recommend protective amounts that may help ward off disease.

Calcium: The Best for Your Bones

By now you probably know that calcium reigns as your body's champion bone-builder. The mineral joins forces with phosphorus to form hard, crystal-like substances that provide the framework for a strong skeleton.

Around age 40, you begin to lose calcium from your bones faster than it can be replaced. This process speeds up at menopause as production of estrogen—a hormone that helps your bones absorb calcium—shifts into low gear.

That's why now is the time to take steps to preserve the bone you already have, says Gail Frank, R.D., Dr.P.H., professor of nutrition at California State University, Long Beach. That means getting enough calcium in your diet before menopause begins. Yet statistics show that most women get only half of the 1,000 milligrams of calcium a day recommended

pounds function as antioxidants, disarming destructive free radicals and preventing the renegade molecules from doing damage in your body. There's also evidence that phytochemicals neutralize toxic chemicals and flush them out of your system before they have a chance to make you sick. And phytos may help keep certain hormones—most notably, the female hormone estrogen—at healthy levels.

The different types of phytochemicals number in the thousands, so as you might imagine, researchers have just begun to scratch the surface in understanding what these nutrients can do. For now, your best bet is to eat a variety of plant foods. That way, you can be sure you're getting a healthy mix of phytos in your diet.

Here's a sampling of the phytochemicals that have been isolated so far, along with where you can find them and what they can do for you.

Benefits
Raise beneficial HDL cholesterol; lower triglyceride (blood fat) levels; prevent heart disease; stimulate enzymes that suppress tumor growth
Act as antioxidants; prevent heart disease and certain cancers
Act as antioxidants; prevent blood clots and heart disease
Stimulate cancer-preventing enzymes; block estrogen activity in cells
Block estrogen activity in cells; prevent certain cancers
Act as antioxidants; block estrogen activity in cells; may prevent certain cancers
Prevent cancer by blocking certain cancer-causing compounds
Act as antioxidants; activate cancer-fighting enzymes
Bind with and flush out cholesterol; stimulate immunity; prevent heart disease and certain cancers

by the National Institutes of Health.

In the Netherlands, a team of scientists evaluating 33 studies of a total of 4,000 18- to 50-year-old women concluded that those who consume 1,000 milligrams of calcium a day retain 1 percent more bone in their hips and backs every year than those who don't get that much. So a 40-year-old woman who starts defending her current calcium stores now may have preserved 20 percent more of her bone density by the time she reaches age 60. This could make the difference between a sturdy skeleton and a brittle one.

Calcium can do more for you than keep your bones strong. One study of almost 35,000 women concluded that those with the highest calcium intakes have half the risk of heart disease–related death of those with the lowest calcium intakes. There's also evidence that the mineral can minimize premenstrual and menstrual symptoms such as breast tenderness, cramps, and backaches, and can cut your chances of developing kidney stones.

Calcium is also proving to be a major player in healthy pregnancies. Moms-to-be who get between 1,500 and 2,000 milligrams of the mineral a day may protect themselves from both high blood pressure and preeclampsia, a serious complication often related to high blood pressure that can cause bleeding, stroke, and, in rare cases, even death. Among 2,459 healthy women, those who matched these high calcium intakes reduced their risk of high blood pressure by 70 percent and preeclampsia by 62 percent.

Calcium is at its best only when it's working with co-nutrient vitamin D. Without D to guide it, calcium can't break through the intestinal wall to get where it wants to go. Fortunately, your body makes plenty of D on its own—with a little help from Old Sol. Sunlight is a natural source of D. Because vitamin D is toxic in large amounts, it should never be taken in supplemental form.

How much you need: The National Institutes of Health recommends that women between the ages of 25 and 50 get 1,000 milligrams of calcium a day. This matches the DV but exceeds the RDA by 200 milligrams. Experts say you may need as much as 1,200 to 1,500 milligrams a day for maximum health benefits. As for vitamin D, you should aim for the RDA for women of 5 micrograms, or 200 international units (IU).

Where to get it: Fortified skim milk can supply healthy doses of both calcium and vitamin D. An eight-ounce glass contains 302 milligrams of calcium. (You'll need to check the label for the vitamin D content. Milk is often fortified with 100 IU per cup.) Other good food sources of calcium include nonfat yogurt, nonfat or low-fat cheese, canned salmon with bones, calcium-fortified orange juice, and frozen collard greens.

Put a Little Meat on Your Bones

Fifty years or so ago, few women would have even dared to serve their families a meal without a slab of sirloin or a hunk of ham. But these days, it seems, we're going meatless—or almost meatless—in droves. In one survey of 500 women, 25 percent reported that they eat meat only occasionally, while another 10 percent said they seldom, if ever, touch the stuff.

Some women forsake foods from animal sources for religious or ethical reasons. But for most of us, the prime motivator is not ideology but biology. We believe that a vegetarian or semivegetarian lifestyle is key to good health.

Indeed, an array of studies have linked vegetarianism to a reduced risk of atherosclerosis (clogging of the arteries) and high blood pressure, both major contributors to heart disease. Other preliminary research suggests that a meatless diet may protect against cancer, prevent osteoporosis, and minimize menopausal symptoms such as hot flashes, insomnia, and weight gain.

The downside is that, when you cut back on or cut out meat, you give up a top-notch source of certain essential nutrients. Take iron, a mineral that 40 percent of women chronically run low on. You won't find a better food source of it than red meat, says Elizabeth Somer, R.D., author of *Nutrition for Women* and *Food and Mood*. She points out that your body can absorb up to three times as much iron from meat as from plant foods such as vegetables, fruits, legumes, and grains.

If you're pregnant or nursing, a low-meat or no-meat diet can put both you and your baby at risk for a nutrient deficiency. You need to be especially diligent about getting all the vitamins and minerals you need.

Experts like Somer recommend that all women eat a token amount of meat every day—maybe a couple of ounces

Iron: The Mineral for Mettle

True or false: Women must take supplements of iron to make up for what's lost during menstruation.

True...and false.

Yes, you lose iron every month via your period. But many experts agree that few women need supplements to replenish what's lost. In general, we get plenty of iron in our diets. Those who stand the greatest chance of running low are women who have heavy periods and female athletes who train vigorously.

Still, roughly 20 percent of all women don't get as much iron as they should. "I would say that women need to be a little more thoughtful mixed into chili or a stir-fry. If you're willing to compromise, you can reap the nutritional benefits of meat while controlling intake of fat. But if you'd really rather go without, experts say you should pay particular attention to your intakes of the following nutrients.

Iron. Many plant foods have an abundance of iron. The problem is that it's nonheme iron, the kind that isn't absorbed into your bloodstream all that easily. Still, nutritionists say, you can protect yourself against a deficiency by consuming lots of whole grains, beans, and leafy green vegetables. If you do think you're running low, try eating iron-rich foods with vitamin C–rich foods. Vitamin C can help your body hang on to more iron.

Vitamin B_{12}. Vegans—vegetarians who eschew not only meat, fish, and poultry but also eggs and dairy products—are at considerable risk for running low on vitamin B_{12}, since it's almost exclusively available in foods from animal sources. An ongoing shortage of the nutrient can lead to pernicious anemia, a form of the disease that is sometimes fatal.

You can get this B vitamin by consuming lots of B_{12}-fortified foods such as breakfast cereals and B_{12}-fortified soy milk or by taking a B_{12} supplement. The Daily Value for the vitamin is six micrograms.

Calcium. Vegetarians who don't consume dairy products also need to keep an eye on their calcium intakes. "It's theoretically possible to get enough of the mineral from plant foods, but it's not practical for most people," says Connie Weaver, Ph.D., professor of foods and nutrition at Purdue University in West Lafayette, Indiana. She recommends getting as much calcium as you can from foods—particularly dark, leafy greens and nuts—and making up the difference with a calcium supplement. You may also want to try a calcium-fortified beverage such as soy milk or orange juice.

than men about iron, in the same way that women should be a little more cautious about their calcium intakes because of osteoporosis," says Adria Sherman, Ph.D., professor and chair of the department of nutritional sciences at Rutgers University in New Brunswick, New Jersey.

Iron's primary responsibility in your body is the formation of hemoglobin, the substance that helps your red blood cells transport oxygen from your lungs to the rest of your body. The mineral also helps prepare your immune system's infection-fighters for battle and supports the production of collagen to build your body's tissues.

When you don't get enough iron or your body's stores run low, the red blood cells can't move oxygen as they should. This can lead to fatigue, pallor, and listlessness, which are all hallmarks of iron-deficiency anemia, Dr. Sherman says.

How much you need: The RDA of iron for premenopausal women is 15 milligrams a day. That's roughly one-third more than you'll need at menopause. (The DV is 18 milligrams.)

Where to get it: Foods supply two kinds of iron. Heme iron, found primarily in meats, is better absorbed than nonheme iron, found primarily in plant foods such as potatoes and kale. But you can improve the absorption rate by pairing off a nonheme iron source with a vitamin C source.

Let's say you're having a bowl of Cream of Wheat for breakfast. The cereal provides a generous eight milligrams of iron—but it's all nonheme. So to make sure that more of the iron gets absorbed, just add a glass of vitamin C–rich orange juice to your meal.

If you prefer meat as your iron source, be sure to choose a lean cut such as bottom or top round. Even chicken breast and turkey breast can boost your intake. Or you can add a little ham to baked beans to enhance the absorption of iron from the beans.

Beta-Carotene: Color Yourself Healthy

Technically, beta-carotene is not a vitamin. It is a member of the carotenoid family, a group of compounds that give red, orange, and yellow fruits and vegetables their vibrant hues. So why mention it here? Because your body converts beta-carotene into vitamin A on an as-needed basis.

Vitamin A has a major role to play in the development and maintenance of your immune system. Without it, you'd become more vulnerable to a host of infectious diseases ranging from measles to AIDS. Vitamin A also protects your vision and supports bodily processes such as growth and cell differentiation.

But too much vitamin A is not a good thing. In large amounts, it can poison your system and produce severe symptoms, including anemia and an enlarged liver and spleen. These problems are more likely to be caused by supplements than by foods. Still, most experts recommend that you get your vitamin A from beta-carotene, since you essentially can't overdose on the nutrient.

Over the past few years, preliminary studies have shown that eating lots of beta-carotene–rich fruits and vegetables can greatly reduce your risk of heart disease, cancer, and stroke.

For example, among 87,000 participants in the Harvard University Nurses' Health Study—considered a landmark study in the women's health field—women who ate 15 to 21 milligrams of beta-carotene a day were 22 percent less likely to have heart attacks than women who ate less than 6 milligrams a day. Those with high beta-carotene intakes also had a 40 percent lower risk of stroke.

Another study showed that eating foods rich in beta-carotene cut women's odds of developing breast cancer after menopause by more than half. The women's risk dropped off sharply with a daily beta-carotene intake of about four milligrams—the amount in a little less than one-third of a carrot.

REAL-LIFE SCENARIO

Diet Soda Has Her at Risk

Elizabeth, age 43, considers herself a healthy eater, and she has for years. She eats a bagel with jam for breakfast, a salad or turkey sandwich for lunch, and pasta or fish—no red meat!—with plenty of vegetables for dinner. She snacks a lot, too—on sunflower seeds, raisins, pretzels, and fruit. Her fave is low-fat frozen yogurt. She draws the line at liquids, however. Nothing with calories passes her lips—ever. Her drink of choice is diet cola, which she buys by the case. As she approaches menopause, she wonders, "Am I getting adequate nutrients?"

Although we have no idea what kind of portions Elizabeth is eating, it sounds like she eats a well-balanced diet that includes a variety of foods. Thanks to her polite refusal of any beverages beyond water and diet soda, however, her diet is sorely lacking in calcium—a mineral crucial to a woman approaching menopause and its accompanying risk of osteoporosis.

While a serving of frozen yogurt provides her with a small amount of calcium (about what's in a glass of skim milk), that single serving of dairy isn't enough. What's more, carbonated beverages, including diet colas, contain phosphoric acid, which is more bad news for her bones. Studies have found that one or two diet colas a day contain enough phosphoric acid to interfere with calcium absorption. This could spell bad news for Elizabeth. Unless she cuts down on colas and includes more dairy products in her diet, Elizabeth could be setting herself up for osteoporosis. Since it appears that she has already put herself at risk, she may want to look into taking a calcium supplement.

Something else Elizabeth may want to reconsider is her avoidance of red meat. It may be that she has eliminated meat for a reason unrelated to nutrition, but if eating healthy is her motivation, she should opt for an occasional slice of lean red meat. Many women cut out red meat because they're watching their cholesterol intake, but today you can buy leaner cuts without even having to ask the butcher to prepare something special. Red meat provides several important nutrients, including iron, zinc, B vitamins, and other minerals. Meat is also the best source of iron and one of the few sources of heme iron, the kind our bodies absorb best.

Overall, Elizabeth does a great job of eating nutritious, low-fat foods. But she should take a second look at what she's missing when she forgoes red meat and milk. Her iron may be sufficient, but there's no doubt that she's going to need to bump up her calcium intake a few notches in order to hold off the risk of osteoporosis.

Expert Consulted
Annette Pederson, R.D.
Dietitian and health educator
Diabetes Care and Education Center
Robinson Memorial Hospital
Ravenna, Ohio

Beta-carotene also plays a role in protecting against cervical dysplasia, a condition involving the development of abnormal cells in the cervix that can progress to cancer. There's evidence that women who don't get enough beta-carotene in their diets are more likely to have cervical dysplasia.

Scientists attribute beta-carotene's preventive powers to the fact that it's an antioxidant. This means that it works primarily by neutralizing free radicals, harmful molecules that damage healthy molecules by robbing them of electrons (a process known as oxidation). Free radicals occur naturally in your body as by-products of day-to-day functions. But their numbers grow dramatically in the presence of external factors such as air pollution, cigarette smoke, and excessive sun exposure.

What about reports that beta-carotene may actually increase your chances of developing heart disease and lung cancer? Many experts are quick to point out that the Finnish study responsible for these findings used beta-carotene supplements rather than foods. For the most part, they believe that food sources of the nutrient are perfectly safe.

You have good reason to choose beta-carotene–rich foods over supplements. These foods contain other members of the carotenoid clan, including alpha-carotene, lycopene, zeaxanthin, and lutein. Preliminary research suggests that these compounds have disease-fighting potential as well. In fact, they may turn out to be even more potent than beta-carotene itself.

How much you need: No RDA or DV has been established for beta-carotene. But to meet the RDA of vitamin A for women, which is 800 micrograms retinol equivalents (the DV is 5,000 IU), you'd have to take in about 5 milligrams of beta-carotene a day. Some experts recommend a much higher dosage—15 to 20 milligrams (25,000 to 33,000 IU)—to obtain beta-carotene's disease-fighting effects.

Where to get it: The best sources of beta-carotene have deep, rich colors. Check out red, orange, and yellow produce such as carrots, cantaloupe, and sweet potatoes and dark green, leafy vegetables such as turnip greens, beet greens, spinach, and parsley.

Folate: Not Just Baby Food

When you look in the mirror, you can thank folate for what you see. This B vitamin helps to make you...*you*. It works with about 20 different enzymes to construct DNA, the material that contains your very own genetic code.

Scientists say that folate plays a significant role in the health of developing babies. Study after study has shown that the vitamin can protect against life-threatening defects of the brain and spine, such as spina bifida. These problems, known as neural tube defects, occur during the first two weeks of pregnancy—long before most women realize that they've conceived. That's why it's so important for all women of childbearing age to make sure that they're getting enough of the nutrient in their diets.

"Fifty to 70 percent (of neural tube defects) could be prevented if women got enough folate," says Joanne Curran-Celentano, R.D., Ph.D., associate professor of nutritional sciences at the University of New Hampshire in Durham.

But according to one survey, a startling 90 percent of women of reproductive age don't know that folate can protect the health of unborn babies. And 85 percent are unaware of the U.S. Public Health Service recommendation that all women capable of bearing children get 400 micrograms of folate every day. Most of us get only half of that amount.

Even if pregnancy isn't in the picture, you shouldn't shirk folate. The vitamin is essential to your good health, too. For starters, it helps to keep your cardiovascular system in tip-top shape by clearing it of homocysteine, a bad-guy amino acid that research has linked to heart disease and stroke. Apparently, folate speeds the metabolism of homocysteine into a less harmful substance, so it can't do your arteries any harm.

One review of all the published studies on the subject concluded that increasing folate intake to 400 micrograms a day could prevent as many as 50,000 heart disease–related deaths every year. This means the average woman's heart disease risk could drop by more than 6 percent.

Folate may also help protect against cervical cancer. In a study at the University of Alabama in Birmingham, researchers found that women with high folate levels in their cervical cells were two to five times less likely than women with low folate levels to develop dysplasia when exposed to risk factors such as cigarette smoke, human papillomavirus, and contraceptives.

If you take oral contraceptives, be aware that they can deplete your body's stores of folate and the other B vitamins, according to Chris Rosenbloom, R.D., Ph.D., associate professor in the department of nutrition and dietetics at Georgia State University in Atlanta and a spokesperson for the American Dietetic Association.

How much you need: The U.S. Public Health Service advises—and many experts agree—that you should try for at least 400 micrograms a day. (The DV is 0.4 milligram, or 400 micrograms; the RDA for women is 180 micrograms.) "But your body can use only about 50 percent of the folate that you consume," says Shirley A. A. Beresford, Ph.D., an epidemiologist at the University of Washington in Seattle. "So to get 400 micrograms of folate a day, you'd have to take in roughly 800 micrograms." A multivitamin can help you hit the mark.

Where to get it: Recognizing the importance of folate in the diet, the Food and Drug Administration requires that certain grain-based foods manufactured in the United States—including pastas, cereals, and breads—be fortified with folate. Read the labels of the products you choose to find out their folate contents. The amount of fortification can vary from food to food.

Almost any legume provides a nice amount of

folate. One-half cup of lentils, for example, contains a hefty 179 micrograms of the nutrient. In the produce aisle and the frozen food section, check out asparagus, broccoli, okra, and spinach.

Vitamin B_6: All Systems Go

It may not have the name recognition of nutritional big guns like beta-carotene, calcium, and vitamin C. Yet vitamin B_6 performs a number of essential tasks within your body.

Among the B vitamins, B_6 stands out as a major player in keeping your immune system strong. It helps transform food into energy and assists in the creation of neurotransmitters, the chemicals that enable brain cells to communicate with one another.

The list of conditions for which vitamin B_6 is gaining acceptance as a possible treatment continues to grow. Preliminary research suggests that it has the potential to protect against atherosclerosis and ease premenstrual symptoms. It also appears to improve your chances of conception.

Scientists cannot yet explain why, but B_6 also has the ability to stop the chronic wrist pain that characterizes carpal tunnel syndrome.

How much you need: The RDA of vitamin B_6 for women is 1.6 milligrams; the DV is 2 milligrams. That's not a whole lot, yet most women's diets come up short. For the therapeutic effects of the nutrient to kick in, you'd have to go

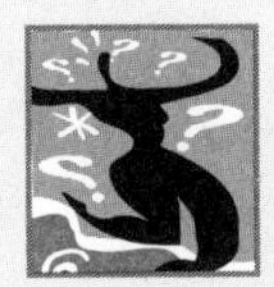

Women Ask Why

If they're equally important, why do I need 1,000 milligrams of calcium but only 15 milligrams of iron every day?

Don't doubt that calcium and iron are equally important. In the short run, a lack of iron can lead to anemia; in the long run, a lack of calcium can lead to osteoporosis. You can see that it's difficult to say which is worse! The fact is that both calcium and iron are essential to a woman's body. The difference between the two is that you need a relatively large amount of calcium to get its benefits, while you need only a little iron for it to do its job effectively.

The chief function of calcium is to keep our bones strong. We need a big supply—1.5 to 2 percent of our body weight—to get the job done right. Iron's job is to transport oxygen through our blood. While this is also an important job, it only takes a minute amount—less than a teaspoon—to work effectively (which is why iron is known as a trace mineral).

The problem is that many women don't get the right amounts of either of these minerals. One reason is because women tend to shy away from meats and dairy foods, and the main sources of both calcium and iron are found in animal products. Vegetarians, obviously, are at greater risk for low stores of iron.

If you don't eat dairy products, you should consider alternative food sources of calcium and/or calcium supplements. You may also need to take a multivitamin/mineral supplement. And for better absorption, be sure to take iron separately from calcium. Ask your doctor or a registered dietitian which nutrition strategies would work best for you.

Expert Consulted
Janet Hunt, R.D., Ph.D.
Research nutritionist
U. S. Department of Agriculture
Human Nutrition Research Center
Grand Forks, North Dakota

even higher—perhaps as high as 10 milligrams, according to experts.

Where to get it: Almost any kind of fish can beef up your B_6 intake. For example, a three-ounce serving of Atlantic mackerel supplies 0.4 milligram of the nutrient, or 20 percent of the DV. And rainbow trout supplies 17 percent of the DV. Or have a banana: One four-ounce fruit gives you 0.7 milligram of B_6.

Vitamin C: A Most Prolific Protector

Call vitamin C the can-do nutrient. No other vitamin or mineral possesses C's ability to defend your body against an astounding array of illnesses, from the common cold to breast cancer.

Like beta-carotene and vitamin E, vitamin C is an antioxidant. It works by defusing those molecular time bombs known as free radicals, paving the way to good health. In studies of the relationship between vitamin C and cholesterol, for example, scientists have found that people with high levels of vitamin C in their blood have less chance of developing heart disease. In particular, women with high levels of vitamin C also have high levels of HDL cholesterol, the good kind that helps to keep your arteries clean.

Further, when researchers in Spain compared women who had breast cancer with women who didn't, they discovered that the breast cancer patients consumed fewer vitamin C–rich foods—namely, fruits and vegetables—in their diets.

There's evidence that vitamin C may even play a vital role in your body's bone-building process. When scientists examined the bone densities and eating habits of 775 postmenopausal women, they found that those with the sturdiest skeletons were getting daily doses of vitamin C along with their calcium. Even more noteworthy, for every 100 milligrams of C that these women ate, their bone densities were almost 2 percent higher, compared with the women who ate less vitamin C. Two percent may not sound like much, but every bit of bone that's spared puts one more step between you and the debilitation that osteoporosis can bring.

That's not all. Other research has linked vitamin C to a lower risk of chronic pulmonary disease—an umbrella term for respiratory diseases such as asthma, bronchitis, and emphysema—and to dramatically reduced progression of arthritis. The nutrient may also help protect the eyes, nerves, and kidneys from diabetes-related damage.

As for colds...well, contrary to popular belief, vitamin C can't stop you from getting one. But if you do get one, vitamin C has been proven to help chase it away. Pump yourself with vitamin C, and you can help make sure that your cold doesn't hang around for long and that its symptoms are less severe.

How much you need: When it comes to vitamin C, the experts say, "Fill 'er up!" Most recommend consuming 100 to 500 milligrams of the nutrient a day—roughly 1½ to 8 times the RDA for women, which is 60 milligrams.

Where to get it: Oranges are practically synonymous with vitamin C. Indeed, just one 4½-ounce fruit contains 70 milligrams of the nutrient—well above the RDA. But why not treat your tastebuds to other superior sources? Check out guava (165 milligrams), kiwifruit (75 milligrams), papaya (94 milligrams), and strawberries (85 milligrams) as well as broccoli (58 milligrams) and sweet red peppers (95 milligrams).

Vitamin E: Eat to Your Heart's Content

Like its antioxidant amigos vitamin C and beta-carotene, vitamin E neutralizes those disease-provoking free radicals that are floating around your system. The nutrient appears to play a prominent role in protecting you against the dastardly duo of heart disease and cancer.

Indeed, compelling research has reinforced the link between a high vitamin E intake and a healthy heart. Postmenopausal women who got lots of vitamin E from foods such as nuts and margarine had half the risk of a fatal heart attack over a period of seven years, compared with women who consumed only small amounts.

Meanwhile, a study involving more than 600 women suggests that vitamin E may protect against cancer. The most dramatic protective effects occurred in women with family histories of breast cancer. Those who got the most vitamin E from foods managed to cut their chances of developing the disease by an impressive 80 percent, compared with other women. And among the women without family histories of breast cancer, consuming lots of vitamin E–rich foods produced a 40 percent dip in risk. The association between high vitamin E intake and reduced risk of breast cancer appeared strongest in premenopausal women.

There's also evidence that E can fend off respiratory problems and bolster your immune system's ability to combat infectious diseases.

How much you need: The "high-intake" women in the breast cancer study were getting roughly 10 IU of the nutrient a day—less than the RDA of 12 IU (eight milligrams alpha-tocopherol equivalents). Still, to get the most benefit from vitamin E, your daily intake should hover between 100 and 400 IU, experts advise. This exceeds even the DV of 30 IU.

Where to get it: The bad news about vitamin E is that it's found primarily in high-fat vegetable oils and nuts. The good news is that you may not need all that much to experience its protective effects. For example, the women in the heart study with high intakes of vitamin E were actually eating only a few servings of nuts and margarine over the course of a week. Likewise, the high-intake women in the breast cancer study were getting less than the RDA.

Use high-fat vitamin E sources sparingly. Among oils, choose olive and peanut. Both have decent amounts of E, and more important, most of their fat is the heart-healthy unsaturated kind. Wheat germ also has a generous amount of vitamin E: One-quarter cup, toasted, supplies roughly 40 percent of the RDA. Try sprinkling it on nonfat frozen yogurt and adding it to casseroles and baked goods.

Zinc: Don't "Cell" Yourself Short

Zinc specializes in cell production. When your body needs new cells—for healing, growth, or pregnancy—zinc works overtime to keep up with demand, according to Dr. Sherman.

Suppose, for example, you've been infected with a virus. Before your body can take on the foreign invader, zinc joins forces with compounds called zinc-dependent enzymes to build new immune system cells to fight the infection.

Zinc's ability to replicate quickly comes in handy when you have a cut or wound. The mineral supports the production of collagen, the connective tissue that helps such injuries heal.

Zinc may also help to counteract the stay-away-from-me feelings that often accompany premenstrual syndrome. At least one study has found that zinc levels drop around the time of the month that premenstrual symptoms set in. This has led researchers to speculate that running low on the nutrient can unbalance the emotions, leading to mood swings.

How much you need: The RDA of zinc for women is 12 milligrams; the DV is 15 milligrams. Next to calcium, zinc is the mineral most often lacking in women's diets.

Where to get it: Just six medium steamed oysters provide 76 milligrams of zinc—a whopping 500 percent of the RDA. Lean meats and poultry are also excellent sources. Some whole-grain breads, cereals, and pasta contain decent amounts, as does nonfat yogurt.

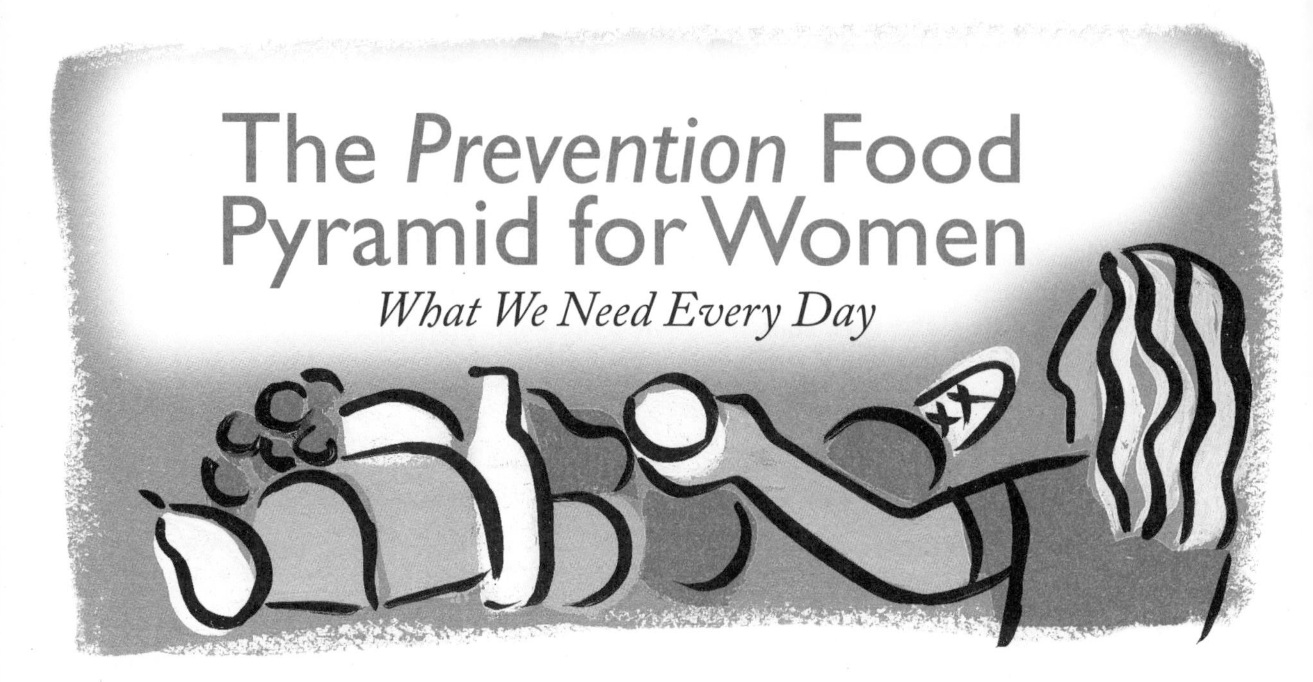

The *Prevention* Food Pyramid for Women

What We Need Every Day

You're a little rusty on the state capitals. And you'd be hard-pressed to explain the difference between an isosceles and an equilateral triangle. But we'd wager that at least one bit of grade school learning remains indelibly imprinted on your memory: the Four Food Groups.

Those were the days when meat was the main attraction in almost every meal, and veggies and fruits made only cameo appearances at the dinner table. That all changed in the early 1990s, when the U.S. Department of Agriculture officially concluded that the Basic Four no longer served the nutrition needs of the general population. And so they went back to the drawing board to come up with new, more realistic standards for what people should be eating.

Their efforts led to the creation of the Food Guide Pyramid, which has since become as familiar an icon as the Four Food Groups once were. (According to a survey conducted by *Parade* magazine, 63 percent of Americans say they're familiar with the pyramid.) It has changed the way many of us look at our dinner plates. Grains, fruits, and vegetables have been given top priority, since they offer the most nutrients for the least amount of fat. Meats and dairy products, meanwhile, have been downsized from mainstays to virtual blips.

The Food Guide Pyramid is built on reams of scientific research into what constitutes a healthy diet. The question is, for whom?

Taking It Personally

"The Food Guide Pyramid presents a very broad view of good nutrition. It was purposely designed that way, so it would apply to the general population," says Joanne Curran-Celentano, R.D., Ph.D., associate professor of nutritional sciences at the University of New Hampshire in Durham. But in trying to be all things to all people, she explains, the pyramid ends up overlooking some very specific—and very important—nutrition needs among women.

For example, you may have noticed that each food group in the pyramid lists a range of servings—a generous 6 to 11 for the grains that make up the pyramid's base. The low number applies to someone who requires just 1,600 calories a day, most likely a sedentary woman. The high number, on the other hand, is for someone who eats 2,800 calories a day, most likely an active man. How do you know where you fit in?

The pyramid also doesn't explain which foods supply the vitamins and minerals that women need most. "If you don't know of any other sources of calcium besides dairy products, for instance, you can take in way too many calories trying to meet the recommended daily intake of 1,000 milligrams," Dr. Curran-Celentano explains.

"There's no question that the Food Guide Pyramid is an improvement over the Four Food Groups and that it points us in the right direction for nutritional health," she adds. "But I think for it to be really useful for women, it should be redesigned with their specific nutrition needs in mind."

Making a Good Thing Better

Okay, we confess: We were hoping she'd say that. We, too, feel that it's about time for us women to have our own nutrition guidelines that focus specifically and exclusively on what our bodies require to function at their best. So in collaboration with Dr. Curran-Celentano, we've created the first-ever *Prevention* Food Pyramid for Women.

True, the shape is familiar. But inside we've made some very important changes that can help you eat better and smarter. By using the pyramid as a guide in making your daily food choices, you can be sure that you're getting the necessary mix of nutrients and the right number of calories to maintain a healthy weight. Best of all, you don't have to worry about counting grams of fat, because the right amount is built into the serving sizes and numbers.

The Food Pyramid for Women is based on 1,800 calories a day. Compared with the original Food Guide Pyramid, this figure more closely aligns with what the typical moderately active woman between the ages of 35 and 50 consumes, Dr. Curran-Celentano explains.

Tied into the number of calories is what Dr. Curran-Celentano calls nutrient density. Women have to get more vitamins and minerals in fewer calories than men. This means that the foods you choose must supply lots of nutrients. So in the fruit and vegetable group, we've broken out the essentials—such as calcium, folate, and the carotenoids—and listed some of their best food sources.

Above all, the pyramid stresses variety, which Dr. Curran-Celentano feels is absolutely necessary for meeting all your nutrition needs. "There are women who say, 'I really like orange juice, so I'll just drink that to cover my fruit and vegetable servings for the day,'" she explains. "You may be getting enough servings, but you're not getting the mix of nutrients that other fruits and vegetables can provide." Besides, she adds, variety makes healthy eating interesting and fun.

"In a way, the pyramid is emancipating," Dr. Curran-Celentano says. "It lets you see that filling your meals with good, wholesome foods is actually very easy to do. And it gives you lots of choices, so you can have what you like." When you compare your current eating habits with the pyramid's recommendations, you may very well discover that you're not doing so badly after all. And if you are coming up short on certain key nutrients, consuming more of the right foods may be enough to put you over the top.

Navigating the Pyramid

The Food Pyramid for Women is tailored to accommodate a woman's specific nutrition needs. You can customize it even further, based on your calorie intake.

The *Prevention* Food Pyramid for Women

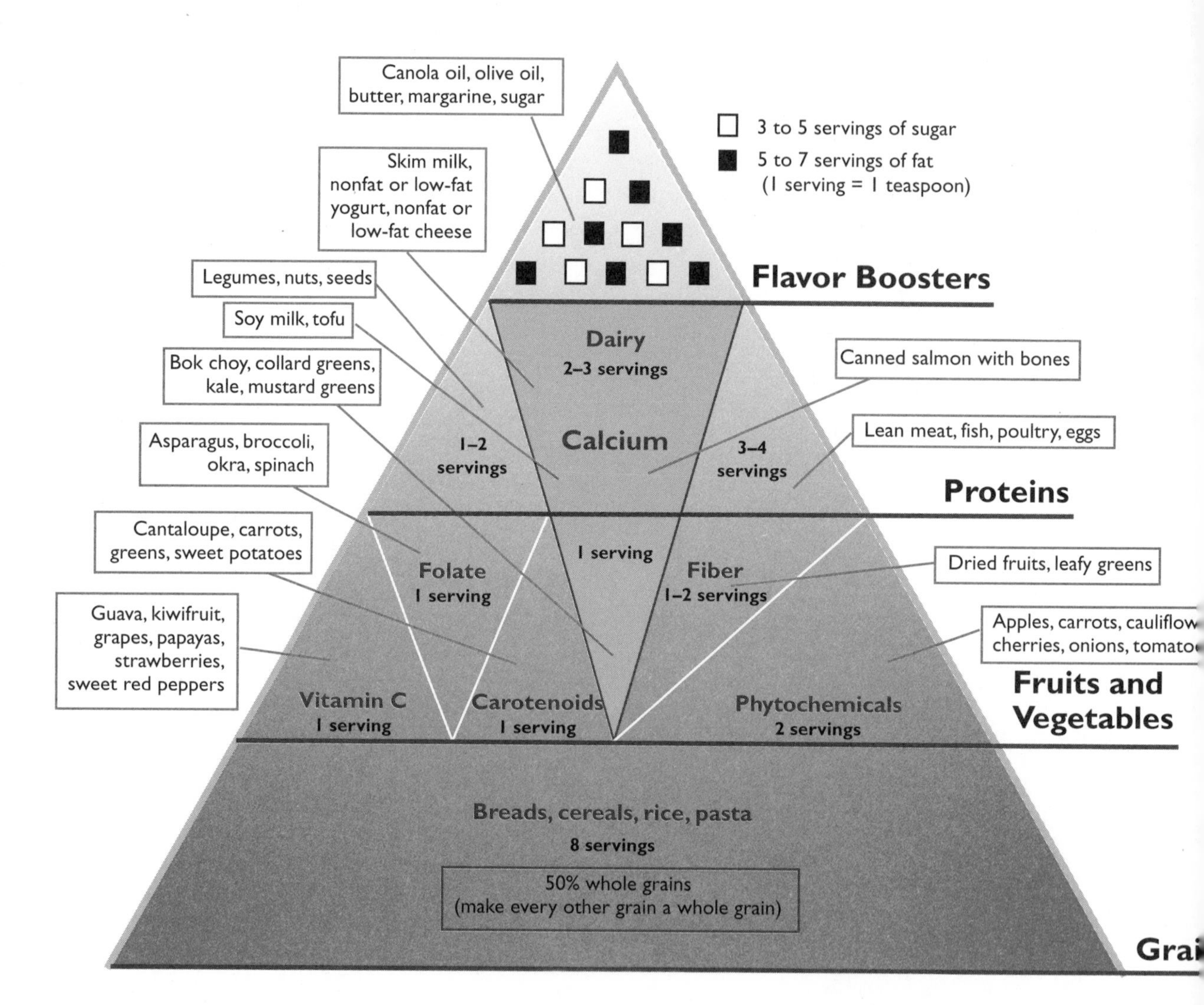

The Prevention *Food Pyramid for Women makes good nutrition a breeze. You can see at a glance the kinds of foods you should consume, and in what proportions, to get all the nutrients your body needs on a daily basis. You don't have to worry about counting calories or fat grams. To plan your meals and snacks, simply follow the serving recommendations. Using the pyramid as your guide guarantees that you're eating for optimum health.*

As mentioned earlier, most women consume about 1,800 calories a day. But you may need more or less than that, depending on your lifestyle and other factors. An active woman may require as many as 2,200 calories a day to fuel her body properly. But for someone who's sedentary or trying to lose weight, 1,600 calories a day may do the job.

You could use one of those mathematical formulas you find in your doctor's office to figure out what your calorie intake should be. Their downside, according to Dr. Curran-Celentano, is that they don't account for individual factors, such as your basal metabolism, that influence how many calories your body requires. (Your metabolism is your body's calorie-burning mechanism.) A better method is to simply go by what feels right and comfortable to you.

For this plan to work, of course, you must be attuned to your appetite and your eating pattern. "Often women don't pay that much attention to their food choices and to portion sizes, so they underestimate how much they're eating," Dr. Curran-Celentano explains. "They look at the pyramid and think, 'Wow! That's a lot of food!' But in reality, it's probably less than they're eating now. It's just spread out to include more types of foods, and the variety is more health-supporting."

Once you know your ideal calorie intake, you can pick and choose foods from each tier of the pyramid, using the serving numbers as guides in planning your daily menus. Remember, if you eat the recommended number of servings from each food group, you'll get just the right mix of nutrients that your body requires for good health.

Of course, many foods are good sources of not one but several nutrients. Such foods should serve single duty in your diet—in other words, you should select a different food from each category in the pyramid, suggests Dr. Curran-Celentano. Orange juice, for instance, supplies vitamin C and folate and may be calcium-fortified as well. So if orange juice is your folate source for the day, then have some strawberries for your vitamin C and skim milk for your calcium. This strategy boosts your intake of all the nutrients, Dr. Curran-Celentano says.

Let's take a closer look at each tier of the pyramid, starting at the bottom and working our way up.

Grains

Grains supply carbohydrates, your body's fuel of choice. They also offer generous amounts of fiber, iron, and B vitamins. Whole grains have the most to offer, nutrition-wise. That's why Dr. Curran-Celentano recommends that every other grain you eat be a whole grain.

What about pasta? "Well, I think we've gone a bit overboard with it," Dr. Curran-Celentano says. "Certainly, pasta is a good source of carbohydrates, but that's about it." There are whole-grain pastas available, which would be better than the refined pastas that most people eat.

Servings: If you're following an 1,800-calorie eating plan, Dr. Curran-Celentano advises aiming for eight servings of grains a day. Women consuming 1,600 calories a day should go for six servings; 2,200 calories a day, nine servings. A serving equals half of a bagel, a slice of bread, ¾ cup dry, ready-to-eat cereal, ½ cup cooked rice or pasta, or 3 cups of air-popped popcorn.

Fruits and Vegetables

This tier of the pyramid actually consists of five subgroups, each one featuring an essential nutrient.

Vitamin C. Vitamin C from food is an antioxidant. That means it helps to neutralize free radicals, harmful molecules that travel around your body and steal electrons from healthy molecules to stabilize themselves (a process known as oxidation). By incapacitating free radicals, vitamin C helps to protect against serious health problems, including heart disease and cancer.

Servings: Everyone—regardless of calorie intake—should try to consume at least one serving of a vitamin C–rich food a day, Dr. Curran-Celentano says. A serving can be ½ cup of broccoli, strawberries, or sweet peppers or a six-ounce glass of orange, grapefruit, or tomato juice.

Folate. "This B vitamin has really come into its own in recent years," Dr. Curran-Celentano says. "Before we just thought of it in terms of keeping red blood cells healthy. But now we know it can do much more than that." It helps protect developing fetuses from neural tube defects, serious complications that affect the brain and spine. And it appears to lower a woman's risk of heart disease.

Servings: No matter what your calorie intake, Dr. Curran-Celentano suggests that you try for at least one serving of a folate-rich food a day. Suggestions include a six-ounce glass of orange juice, ½ cup of cooked asparagus or broccoli, or 1 cup of raw spinach.

Phytochemicals. These little-known compounds may turn out to be our most potent weapons against disease, if the latest research is any indication. The catch is that you can get them only from fruits, vegetables, and other plant sources—at least for now. So you'll do yourself a big favor by squeezing some phyto-rich foods into your daily menu.

Servings: Dr. Curran-Celentano recommends at least two servings of top-notch phytochemical sources a day for everyone, regardless of calorie intake. Among the best: ½ cup of tomatoes, ½ cup of cooked broccoli, and ½ cup of kale.

Carotenoids. Beta-carotene is probably the best known of the carotenoid clan. Your body converts many of these compounds—which are, incidentally, phytochemicals—to vitamin A, a nutrient that's essential for normal vision and a strong immune system. But the carotenoids are showing promise in their own right as potential protectors against heart disease and cancer.

Servings: One a day for everyone, Dr. Curran-Celentano says. Choose from six ounces of apricot nectar, one-quarter of a cantaloupe, or ½ cup of cooked carrots, sweet potatoes, or greens.

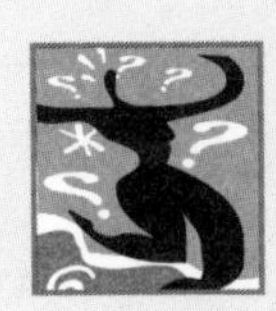

Women Ask Why

Why can French women eat all those rich sauces and pastries and stay so slim and healthy?

Although French cuisine is famous for its rich sauces and fattening desserts, the average French woman doesn't eat them everyday. In fact, she is much more likely to eat fruit for dessert than sweets.

Contrary to popular belief, the typical French meal really isn't high in fat. A meal might begin with soup made of pureed vegetables. Since the water content in soup is so high, it is filling but carries with it very few calories. By the time she reaches her entrée, the French woman is more easily satisfied with a smaller portion. So even if the dish (most likely fish or poultry) is laced with a heavy sauce, she's only eating a small portion. And sauces are added to accent food—not to drown it! The French love their bread—little fat in that—but they never eat it with butter. In fact, you'd be hard-pressed to find butter on a French dinner table.

Possibly just as significant as what the French eat is how they eat it. While Americans eat and work, eat and watch television, or even eat and drive, the French engross themselves in eating as a major event. They savor textures and subtle nuances of flavors and spices and are very much in tune with the pleasures and sensations of eating. A French meal is eaten very slowly and can sometimes last for hours, which aids in digestion.

Because they are so in touch with their food, they also know when to stop eating. Americans, on the other hand, are much less particular about the foods they eat and could practically polish off a bag of snacks before they even realize they're eating. Snacking isn't a part of the French lifestyle.

Take a lesson from the French. Instead of trying to ignore food, practice immersing yourself in the sensory experiences of eating. Eat slowly and focus on savoring each and every flavor. Don't deprive yourself of the desserts and rich sauces you love, but eat them sparingly.

Expert Consulted
Susan Ahlstrom Henderson, R.D.
Health sciences research associate
Human nutrition program
School of Public Health
The University of Michigan
Ann Arbor

Fiber. Technically, fiber doesn't qualify as a nutrient, because it passes through your body without getting absorbed. What it does is add bulk to the foods you eat, which helps you feel full on fewer calories while keeping your digestive system working smoothly. Fiber may also bind with cholesterol and bile acids and escort them out of your body.

Servings: Women who are consuming 1,800 calories a day should aim for one to two servings of fiber-rich fruits and vegetables a day, according to Dr. Curran-Celentano. Those following 1,600-calorie plans can get by with one serving, while those on the 2,200-calorie plan require at least two servings. Good choices include 1/4 cup of dried fruit, 1 cup of a leafy green, and 1/2 cup of any other vegetable.

Proteins

Your body uses protein to carry out a variety of tasks. It helps to build and maintain all of your muscles—including your heart muscle—and supports the production of hormones, blood cells, and immune cells. You should get half of your protein from animal sources and the other half from legumes and soy foods. Of course, if you're a vegetarian, you can get all of your protein from plant sources.

Dairy. In addition to protein, dairy products such as milk, cheese, and yogurt supply generous amounts of calcium, your body's premier bone-builder. Fortified milk may be your skeleton's best friend. It delivers calcium as well as vitamin D, which your body needs in order to absorb the mineral.

Servings: All women should consume two to three servings of nonfat or low-fat dairy products a day, states Dr. Curran-Celentano. Help yourself to 8 ounces of skim milk, one cup of nonfat or low-fat yogurt, 1½ ounces of nonfat or low-fat cheese, or 2 ounces of processed cheese. If you are lactose-intolerant or you avoid dairy products for other reasons, you can substitute one cup of fortified soy milk or 2 ounces of soy cheese, both of which are good sources of calcium.

Meats. Think of it as meats-plus: This protein category also includes poultry, fish, legumes, and soy products. Many of these foods supply healthy doses of iron and zinc, two essential nutrients that women routinely run low on. Iron, in particular, can be a problem for some women because the body's stores of the mineral are depleted every month during menstruation.

Soy is shaping up to be a real nutrition superstar, according to Dr. Curran-Celentano. Studies suggest that it may help to lower cholesterol and to boost bone density. It's also rich in phytoestrogens, phytochemicals that have the potential to protect against breast cancer. "I'd certainly recommend trying to eat soy foods at least several times a week," Dr. Curran-Celentano says.

Servings: Dr. Curran-Celentano recommends that all women consume up to six servings of these protein-rich foods every day. Of that number, one or two servings should come from nonmeat sources. One ounce of lean beef, chicken, or fish constitutes a serving, as does one egg, ½ cup of legumes, two tablespoons of peanut butter, or one ounce of tofu. By combining meat and nonmeat sources, you get more variety in your diet over the course of the day. That makes it easier to meet your body's nutrient needs.

Calcium

We've already mentioned that milk and other dairy products are top-notch sources of calcium. The fact is, you can get the mineral from a variety of foods, including fish, soy products, and produce. That explains why calcium holds the place of honor at the center of the pyramid, overlapping all three tiers. Your body uses the mineral for many tasks besides bone-building, including muscle function and heartbeat regulation. But the bottom line is that stocking up on calcium now can spare you the debilitating effects of bone loss later in life, Dr. Curran-Celentano says.

Servings: All women should eat at least one serving of a calcium-rich vegetable a day in addition to the two to three servings of dairy foods (or soy-based substitutes) mentioned earlier, recommends Dr. Curran-Celentano. So help yourself to ½ cup of broccoli or a dark, leafy green such as kale or bok choy. Other excellent nondairy sources of calcium include three ounces of canned salmon with bones, three ounces of tofu, six ounces of fortified soy milk, and six ounces of calcium-fortified orange juice.

Flavor Boosters

The Food Pyramid for Women allows for moderate amounts of fat and sugar—what Dr. Curran-Celentano refers to as flavor boosters. You'll find them at the very top of the pyramid. Both have their place in good nutrition: Sugar is a carbohydrate, while fats such as vegetable oils supply vitamin E, an antioxidant that preliminary research has linked to a reduced risk of heart disease. Including them in the pyramid also serves an important psychological purpose. "It's expected that you're going to eat a chocolate chip cookie once in a while, so the pyramid is designed to accommodate that," Dr. Curran-Celentano explains. "It's all part of eating healthfully." Still, she says, you don't want to add seven pats of butter to one food item and use up all your flavor boosters in one sitting. Spread them out all through the day.

Servings: If you're following an 1,800-calorie eating plan, you can have five to seven servings of fat per day, according to Dr. Curran-Celentano. A serving equals a teaspoon of a vegetable oil (preferably olive or canola oil) or a teaspoon of butter or margarine. As for sugar, the pyramid allows for three to five servings a day, with a serving being the equivalent of one teaspoon.

How does this work? Well, suppose you have reduced-fat milk rather than skim on your breakfast cereal. That means you should skip the pat of butter on your dinner roll.

Part Two

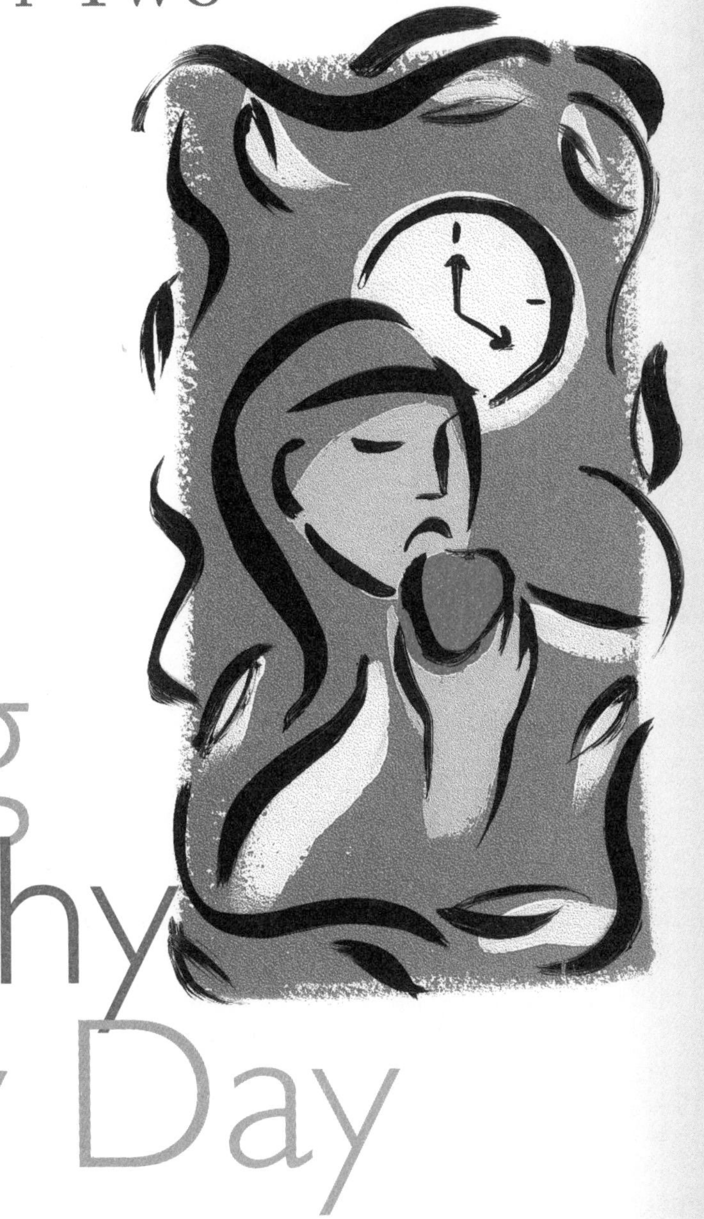

Eating Healthy Every Day

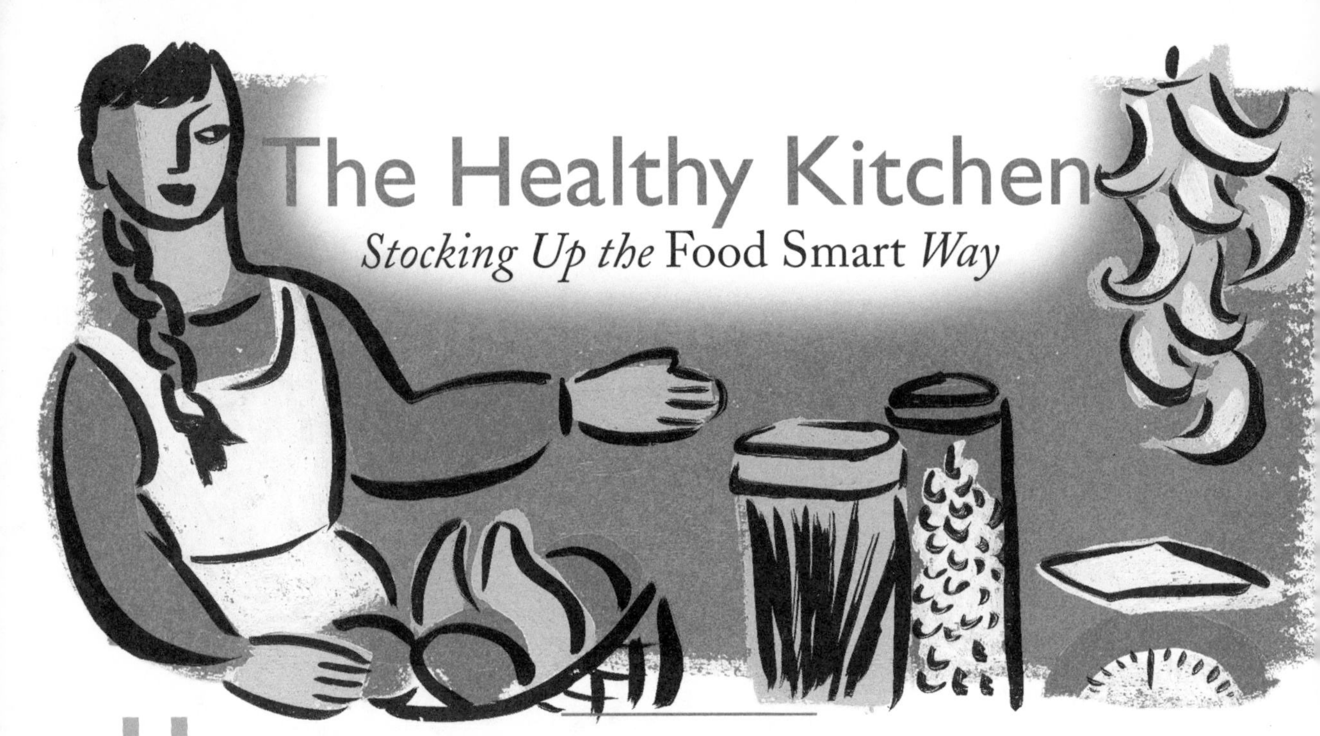

The Healthy Kitchen

Stocking Up the Food Smart *Way*

Healthy cooking has long had a reputation as a time-consuming, costly, complicated venture. The truth is that it doesn't require exotic ingredients or expensive equipment. For that matter, it doesn't require any special culinary skills. Even a novice can prepare nutritious meals quickly and easily.

The real trick to healthy cooking, nutritionists agree, is to heed the Boy Scout motto and be prepared. That means stocking up—filling your pantry and refrigerator with nutritious, versatile staples and outfitting your kitchen with quality, user-friendly gear. What you choose to have on hand really depends on your personal likes and dislikes as well as your lifestyle. And if you're feeding a family, you'll need to consider their preferences as well. The idea is to create an environment that encourages healthy cooking by putting all the essential supplies within reach.

First-Rate Fixin's

The following foods are recommended by nutritionists and chefs as healthy-cooking essentials. Consider this list a jumping-off point for stocking (or restocking) your own kitchen. As you try new recipes and develop healthier versions of old favorites, you'll come up with your own collection of can't-do-without ingredients. Keep in mind, too, that you don't necessarily want a lot of each item on hand. Buying in small quantities ensures that what you have is fresh.

Canned tomato puree. Tomatoes are brimming with lycopene, a nutritional newcomer that in studies appears to protect against cervical dysplasia as well as several different types of cancer. You can whip up a low-fat, nutrient-rich spaghetti sauce or pizza topping by blending tomato puree with garlic and spices. Just be sure the tomato product you choose is low in sodium.

Chili peppers. These potent peppers pack intense flavor, not to mention a healthy dose of vitamins A and C. "If you're not used to cooking with chili peppers, always remember to wear rubber gloves when cutting them," cautions award-winning chef Rick Bayless, author of *Rick Bayless's Mexican Kitchen*. "The oil contained in the membranes and the seed pods—not the seeds themselves—can irritate your skin."

Citrus fruits. The citric acid in oranges, lemons, limes, and grapefruit is a natural flavor enhancer that's especially adept at giving pizzazz to low-sodium dishes. Use the juices from these fruits liberally in everything from salad dressings and soups to stir-fries and desserts. They'll give you a burst of vitamin C to boot.

Grains. Quick-cooking varieties—including bulgur, couscous, millet, oats, and some types of barley and brown rice—can be ready in half an hour or less, so you can prepare them even when you're pressed for time. Cooked grains also freeze well.

Herbs and spices. No healthy kitchen should be without them! Use these seasonings instead of fat and salt when you cook. The flavor of fresh herbs is diminished with long cooking, so it's best to add them to a dish just before serving. Dried herbs benefit from longer cooking to rehydrate them and release their flavors. (For more information about herbs and spices, see The Spice Is Right on page 54.)

Legumes. Beans, peas, and lentils can't be beat for fiber content. They're also good sources of protein, which makes them ideal substitutes for meat in all types of dishes. Dried beans do take a long time to cook, but you can use

SMART COOKING

How you prepare a food can make all the difference in its healthfulness. Fish that is creamed or sautéed can cancel out all good intentions. Broccoli that is boiled loses a great deal of its superior nutritional edge. The following cooking methods help preserve a food's nutrients while keeping fat and calories to a minimum.

Baking. Meats, fish, and poultry retain their distinctive flavors when prepared in this manner. To prevent the food from drying out, cover it for at least part of the baking time.

Braising. This cooking method, in which food simmers in liquid in a moderately hot oven, works exceptionally well for tenderizing lean cuts of meat and dense vegetables such as potatoes and carrots. Any fat seeps out of the food into the cooking liquid, where you can skim it off.

Broiling. Use this cooking method to prepare lean meats, poultry, and fish. The food is placed on a broiler rack, which allows the fat to drain into the pan below.

Grilling. Broiling and grilling have similar benefits, nutrition-wise. The main difference: With the former, you place food under the heat source, but with the latter, the food cooks over the heat source.

Microwaving. Sure, it saves time. But microwaving also saves nutrients—not to mention flavor.

Poaching. With this cooking method, food simmers in liquid—such as water, broth, or juice—for a short period of time. It's ideal for preparing fish and boned poultry as well as fragile fruits such as pears.

Roasting. Like baking, roasting uses dry heat. You can help keep the food moist by basting it with broth, fruit juice, or low-fat marinade.

Steaming. The healthy alternative to boiling, steaming preserves nutrients because the food is cooked over water rather than in it.

Stir-frying. Any combination of vegetables becomes a meal in minutes with this quick cooking method. Try using water, defatted broth, or citrus juice instead of oil for an even healthier stir-fry.

canned beans in most recipes. Just be sure to rinse them well to wash away the thick liquid—and some of the excess sodium—that they're packed in. Among the most versatile legumes are black beans, chickpeas, kidney beans, lentils, lima beans, pea beans, pinto beans, and split peas.

Onion-family vegetables. This odoriferous clan includes garlic, leeks, scallions, shallots, chives—and, of course, onions. Use them liberally to add flavor to savory dishes of all types. Cooking onions slowly gives them a sweet, mild taste. Leeks are inherently mild, as are Vidalia, Walla Walla, and Maui onions. Roasting garlic tames its sharp flavor and softens it to a creamy consistency. If you grow chives, let them flower and sprinkle the flower petals over salads.

Pasta. Pasta cooks up quickly for a fast low-fat meal. Look for enriched pasta, which supplies healthy doses of a number of vitamins and minerals, most notably niacin and thiamin, both B vitamins. But you can easily destroy pasta's natural goodness by drowning it in a fatty cream sauce. Be sure to stick with a lighter topping—for example, one made from fresh tomatoes. Read labels when buying pasta; many types of fresh pasta have considerably more fat and cholesterol than dried.

Tofu. This soy product is rich in phytoestrogens—supernutrients that have been shown to minimize the physical effects of menopause and to reduce the risk of breast cancer. Tofu is also an excellent source of protein, so you can use it instead of meat. It does taste bland when served plain, but it readily takes on flavors from other ingredients. Freezing tofu and then thawing and crumbling it gives it the texture of ground meat.

Tortillas. You can wrap just about any filling in this low-fat Mexican bread for a quick and easy lunch or dinner. Or top it with low-sodium tomato sauce or salsa, sliced vegetables, and shredded low-fat cheese for a personal pizza. Corn tortillas are your best nutritional choice. One six-inch corn tortilla contains less than 0.5 gram of fat compared with over 2 grams for a six-inch flour tortilla.

Gearing Up

Of course, no healthy kitchen is complete without some essential tools. The key word here is *essential*: It's not necessary to buy one of each gadget on display in the housewares section of your local department store. You can prepare just about any meal with a carefully selected collection of small appliances, cookware, and utensils.

To get you started, here's a list of equipment that nutritionists and healthy chefs consider must-haves in the kitchen. They make healthy cooking a breeze by helping to reduce the fat content of foods while preserving their nutrition and flavor.

Egg separator. For years, eggs have gotten a bad rap because of their high cholesterol content. The fact is that all that cholesterol is concentrated in the yolk. The white, on the other hand, has no cholesterol, no fat, and hardly any calories. It's also an excellent source of protein. An egg separator makes it easy to strain the white from the yolk without breaking the yolk.

Electric spice grinder. Freshly ground spices have much more intense, robust flavors than preground varieties. An electric coffee grinder reserved for spices does the job in just seconds. It also comes in handy for mincing fresh herbs. Clean the grinder by adding torn white bread to it and processing; the bread will pick up the spice residue.

Fat separator. A fat separator looks something like a measuring cup, but it has a spout that starts at the bottom. It's great for defatting homemade stock. The fat floats to the top of the separator, so you can pour off the lean liquid underneath.

Hot-air popcorn popper. Popcorn is an ideal snack—provided it's not made in oil and coated with butter. A hot-air popper doesn't use oil, and the popcorn it produces has less fat, less sodium, and fewer calories than store-bought microwave popcorn.

Kitchen scale. A scale comes in handy when you're trying to figure out portion sizes. You want one that can weigh ounces.

Nonstick pots and pans. Cookware with a nonstick coating allows you to prepare foods with little or no added fat. Be aware that some nonstick coatings scratch easily—and once they're damaged, they lose effectiveness. For this reason, you should use only wood or plastic utensils when cooking. Some newer nonstick pots and pans have improved coatings that are guaranteed to last for at least 20 years. They also come in all shapes and sizes. The 10-inch and 12-inch skillets are the most versatile, so you may want to start your collection with them and add on as necessary.

Slow cooker. In a slow cooker, lean meats simmer in their own juices for a long period, so they become as tender as their fatty counterparts. This appliance is also ideal for preparing foods with long cooking times, such as soups, stews, and beans.

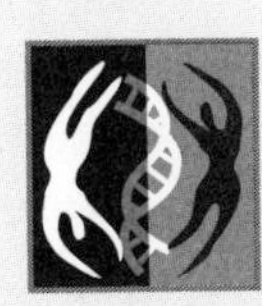

Woman to Woman

She Discovered a Love of Healthy Cooking

When she got married, Tammy Munson, an emergency services dispatcher in Jamestown, New York, didn't know how to make Jell-O. Now, 11 years later, she cooks healthy foods for fun and has converted her husband into a healthy eater with her culinary skills. Plus, she lost 143 pounds in the process! Here's her story.

When I first got married, I knew nothing about cooking. Rather than picking up a spatula, my husband and I dined on takeout. I wasn't thin to begin with, so eating what I wanted when I wanted began to take its toll. My diet ran amok, and a year after our wedding, my weight peaked at 253 pounds.

I realized that the only way I would regain control of my weight was to rein in my diet. I knew that I was going to have to learn about healthy cooking, so I started going to the library. I went every day. I spent so much time there that the librarians worried about me when I didn't show up!

I read every cookbook I could find. I was fascinated by what I was learning about healthy cooking—and how you could actually convert your favorite fatty foods into healthy foods. I started experimenting and found I loved cooking—and loved the food!

I've found that it's important to start with the right ingredients. My mother's idea of seasonings was simply salt and pepper, but now I love cooking with herbs and spices—fresh garlic, cilantro, rosemary. I swap applesauce or prunes for oil to greatly reduce the fat in baked goods.

Now I love fruits and vegetables, and I make my meals colorful with many varieties. I sauté vegetables in wine instead of oil. Wine adds so much flavor and no fat, and most of the alcohol cooks right off. In baking, I use phyllo dough for low-fat piecrusts and always skip the margarine when I make Rice Krispies treats. The marshmallows hold them together just fine. To make my cooking even more fun, I splurge on equipment.

Also, I don't taste when I'm cooking because once you start eating, it's hard to stop. I can "taste" a dish by its smell.

Steamer. Steaming isn't just for vegetables anymore. This versatile cooking method also produces great-tasting meats, poultry, and fish. It takes less time than boiling, and it does a better job of preserving a food's nutrients and flavor. You can choose a stainless steel or bamboo steamer to use with other cookware or a free-standing electric model.

Stove-top grill. Enjoy grilling year-round by bringing it indoors. This type of grill fits right over one or two burners on your stove. Use it to make meats, fish, and vegetables without extra fat or oil.

Wok. If you enjoy stir-fries, a wok is your cookware of choice. It cooks quickly, so foods retain their nutrients, but it requires only a small amount of oil. Choose one with a nonstick surface and a lid. And for the best heat conduction on American gas and electric ranges, buy a wok with a flat bottom.

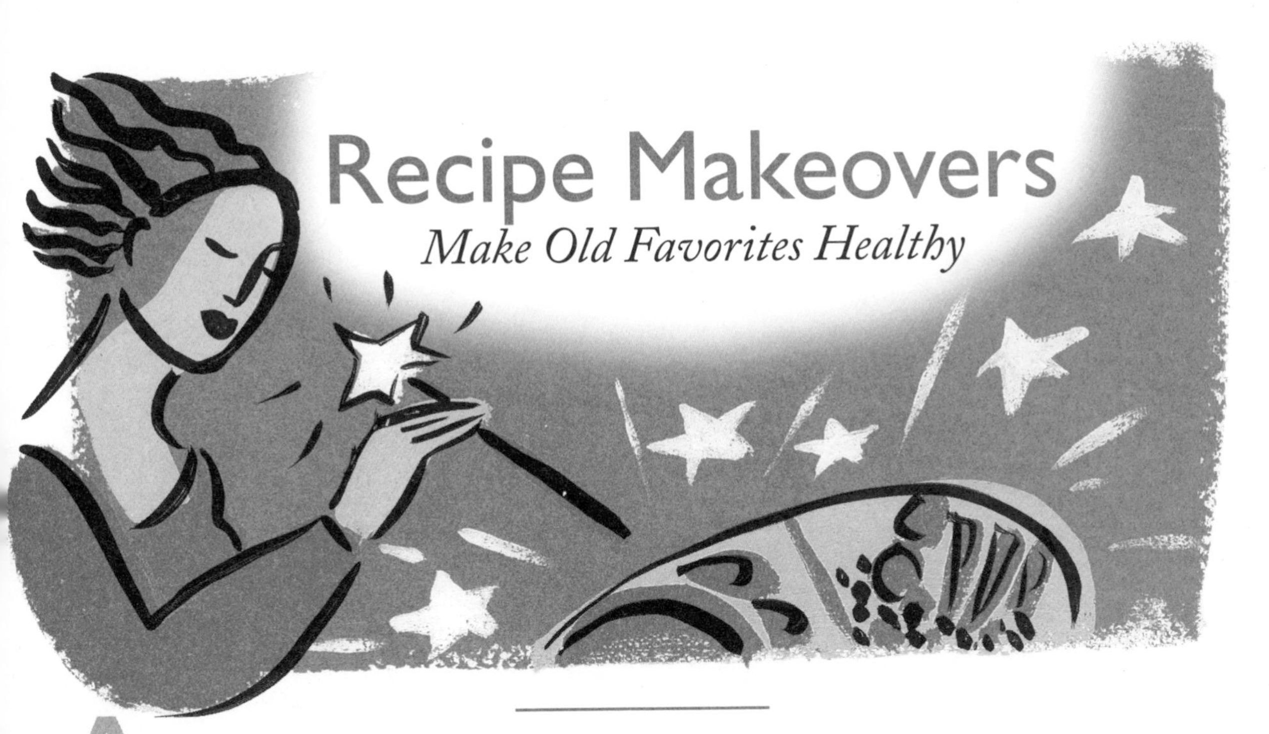

Recipe Makeovers

Make Old Favorites Healthy

A very famous French TV chef who shall remain anonymous once told a group of food writers that "low-fat food is an oxymoron."

"What's the point in eating food if you take all the fat out of it?" she trilled. "Fat *is* where you find the flavor."

Sorry, Chef, but we're about to prove you wrong. Low-fat food has suffered long enough from its reputation of being bland, boring, and tasteless. Great chefs all over the country are betting their reputations on creations brimming with flavor and devoid of fat.

So how do you make great-tasting food—the favorite foods you and your family love to eat—without all the fat? It really isn't all that hard. All you need to know is how to substitute a little of this for a little of that.

Look on the Light Side

Revamping a recipe to cut down on fat is not an exact science. You'll have to do some tinkering to find the "formula" that meets your standards for both fat content and taste. Your best bet is to make just one change to a recipe at a time, advises Evelyn Tribole, R.D., author of *Healthy Homestyle Cooking*. That way, if the dish doesn't turn out quite as you expected, it's much easier to troubleshoot. Be sure to take notes on your change and the result. If it turns out well, you can incorporate another fat-reducing change the next time you make it.

Here are some fat-paring pointers from the culinary pros to help you cook up your very own lean cuisine.

Know your fat facts. Oils are pure fat, so you should skimp on them as much as possible when you cook. But just as important as how much you use is which kind you use. Butter is high in saturated fat, which you should avoid. Instead use canola, olive, and peanut oils. These are high in monounsaturated fat, which is better for you.

Incidentally, when you use oil, don't pour it straight into the pan. Instead, put some into a spray bottle, then give the pan a squirt. "People do use less oil with a spray," notes Franca Alphin, R.D., nutrition director at the Duke Uni-

Smart Substitutes

A little culinary sleight of hand goes a long way in cutting the fat content of your favorite recipes—and saving them from mealtime extinction. By exchanging high-fat ingredients for leaner alternatives, like those listed below, you can keep on eating the foods you love. And just look at the fat grams you'll save!

Instead of...	Use...	And Cut the Fat by...
½ cup oil (for baking)	½ cup applesauce	109 g.
½ cup oil (for salad dressing)	½ cup unsweetened pineapple juice	109 g.
½ cup margarine or butter (for baking)	½ cup baby food prunes	92 g.
½ cup margarine or butter (for frosting)	½ cup marshmallow cream	92 g.
8 oz. cream cheese	8 oz. nonfat ricotta cheese	79 g.
1 cup cream	1 cup evaporated skim milk	60 g.
1 cup sour cream	1 cup nonfat yogurt	40 g.
4 oz. full-fat Cheddar cheese	4 oz. nonfat Cheddar cheese	38 g.
1 cup whole-milk ricotta cheese	1 cup 1 percent fat cottage cheese	30 g.
3 oz. 80 percent lean ground beef	3 oz. ground skinless turkey breast	17 g.
1 tbsp. full-fat mayonnaise	1 tbsp. nonfat mayonnaise	11 g.
1 cup whole milk	1 cup skim milk	8 g.
3 oz. canned oil-packed light tuna	3 oz. canned water-packed light tuna	6 g.
1 whole egg	2 egg whites	5 g.
1 oz. unsweetened baking chocolate	3 tbsp. cocoa powder plus 2 tsp. vegetable oil	4 g.

versity Diet and Fitness Center in Durham, North Carolina. "Remember, a second of spraying equals seven calories."

Skip the oil in sautés. Instead of sautéing vegetables in oil, switch to water, fruit juice, or nonfat vegetable, chicken, or beef broth. Besides cutting down on added fat, these cooking liquids do a better job than oil of playing up a food's natural flavors.

Rethink meat choices. "In most cases, you can substitute turkey for red meat in recipes without making any other changes," says Joanne D'Agostino, a low-fat cooking consultant in Easton, Pennsylvania. For example, ground skinless turkey breast works well in meat loaf, chili, and spaghetti sauce.

If you have a casserole recipe that calls for ground beef, try replacing half the beef with cooked brown rice, bulgur, couscous, or chopped beans. You'll reduce the fat content of the dish—and you'll get a healthy dose of fiber.

Whip up a dream cream. Recipes for soups and sauces often use cream, egg yolks, and other high-fat ingredients as thickeners. Make them healthier by substituting pureed cooked vegetables, such as carrots, potatoes, or cauliflower.

In a bisque soup, try using buttermilk, nonfat half-and-half, or evaporated skim milk instead of heavy cream. (Although its name makes it sound fatty, buttermilk is actually equal to 1 percent low-fat milk in terms of fat content.)

Bake better goodies. You can slim down cakes, muffins, and other sweet treats by replacing the shortening with fruit-based butter and oil replacement, which you'll find with the cooking oils in the supermarket. Applesauce, mashed bananas, or canned pumpkin can also be used to replace some of the fat. Start by cutting the amount of shortening in half and making up the difference with the fruit substitute. Continue reducing the amount of shortening and increasing the amount of fruit substitute until you find a proportion that produces a taste and texture you like.

Favorites with a Big Fat Difference

Now that you know the basics, you can transform virtually any food into a lean and luscious version of its former fat-laden self. To give you a head start, the country's top nutritionists and chefs have provided their healthy remakes of some popular dishes. Try your hand at these favorites—and discover just how easy revamping recipes can be.

Beef stroganoff. Canned cream of mushroom soup is a traditional ingredient in stroganoff. Replace it with a reduced-fat version of the soup. Or try this suggestion from Tribole. Mix an envelope of onion-mushroom soup mix with one cup of evaporated skim milk and one tablespoon of cornstarch. Bring to a boil, add the browned beef, then ladle the mixture over noodles.

Brownies. Slim down these treats by using unsweetened cocoa instead of semisweet chocolate and pureed prunes instead of butter, recommends Susan Purdy, author of *Have Your Cake and Eat It, Too*. "The prunes keep the brownies moist, and the overall fat content is about one-

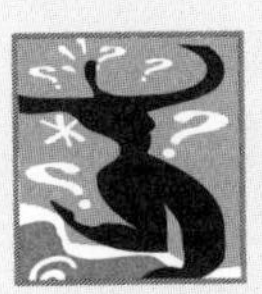

Women Ask Why

Why does butter make food taste so darn good?

If you think the answer is because it's 100 percent fat, think again. You wouldn't spread your English muffin with Crisco—and that's 100 percent fat, too! While there are obvious differences between butter and other fats, what exactly gives butter its universal appeal is unknown. But we do know that it has a lot to do with its "sense appeal."

First, of course, is our sense of taste. Then there's smell and touch—in this case, the way it feels in your mouth. Close your eyes and imagine the difference between butter and Crisco in terms of these senses. Melting butter adds to its allure. The smell as it browns in the pan and the image of it in your mouth is enough to make your mouth water.

Butter is so sensory-appealing that "buttery" has become a metaphor for heavenly taste. It's so strong, in fact, that we learn to detect it early on. Kids can tell the difference between icing made with Crisco and sugar and a true buttercream icing. Even though kids are notorious lovers of sweets, they often will choose a less sweet-tasting buttercream icing over a sugary one made with Crisco. This may explain why we can eat so much of those fat-free cakes and cookies. They just don't satisfy the way a buttery treat does.

If you truly love butter but are concerned about the artery-damaging saturated fat and high number of calories (102 per tablespoon), you can wean yourself away from it. It really only takes a little bit to satisfy your senses. Cut back a little at a time, and you'll eventually begin to savor other tastes in foods. There are plenty of people who will tell you that they never realized the taste treat they were missing until they stopped topping their bread with butter.

Expert Consulted
Beverly Cowart, Ph.D.
Director of the taste and smell clinic
Monell Chemical Senses Center
Philadelphia

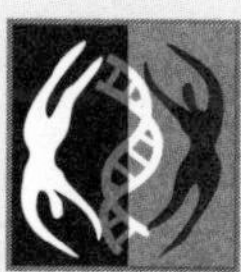

WOMAN TO WOMAN

Taste and Convenience Spell Success

Being the sole member of a family to make a major lifestyle change isn't easy. Debbie Ostrofsky, of Whitehall, Pennsylvania, made switching to a more nutritious diet a little easier on herself: She got her whole family to join in. Now they are all enjoying the benefits of a healthier lifestyle. And you can, too.

If someone had told me just two years ago that I would be able to eat more nutritiously—and persuade my family to eat more nutritiously—I'd have said they were crazy. But I did it. I stopped making french fries and started making healthier dishes, such as baked sweet potatoes. I also started to substitute ingredients in some of my old favorite recipes—using chicken instead of beef in tacos, making chicken patties instead of beef patties, and using skim milk instead of whole milk in all of my recipes, for example. And, to ease the transition for my family, I made an effort to make the dishes look appealing.

Surprisingly, my husband and kids actually preferred many of the new and made-over recipes to our old fare. We have theme suppers, and for Mexican night, my kids actually ask for the tacos made with chicken instead of beef.

I noticed that my four daughters and I tend to eat whatever is convenient. So my strategy was really pretty simple—make healthier foods more accessible than unhealthy ones.

For example, we used to drink a lot of soda at home. Now I've made water even more convenient by purchasing a home watercooler and having good-tasting, chilled water delivered.

We still have junk food in the house, but it's not as easy to reach. For instance, a bowl of fruit is always on the top shelf in the refrigerator. The kids see it before anything else, so that's what they grab. We also have candy bars in the refrigerator (my husband thinks they taste better cold), but they're hidden away in the produce drawer.

As I look back, getting my family to eat healthy food wasn't too hard. Basically, I lead by example and put the more nutritious foods in the forefront. And it has all been worth it. We have more energy now to enjoy fun physical activities together, like biking and walking.

fifth of the fat in a traditional brownie recipe," Purdy says. And by using nonstick spray to "grease" the pan, you'll save even more fat grams.

Burgers. Even extra-lean ground round—the "healthiest" choice—isn't so healthy after all: Just three ounces, broiled and well-drained, has almost 14 grams of fat. That doesn't mean you have to give up your beloved burgers. Just replace some of the ground beef with shredded vegetables (such as carrots, onions, and green peppers) or replace half with mashed pinto or black beans.

Cheesecake. Cottage cheese gives cheesecake a wonderfully smooth texture but without all the fat of cream cheese. Don't use it straight from the container, though: First drain it to remove excess liquid, then puree it in a food processor until it's the consistency of sour cream, Purdy says. She also suggests reducing the number of eggs you use. If your recipe calls for three whole eggs, for example, switch to one whole egg plus two egg whites.

Chocolate cake. Slice the fat from this favorite by using less butter or shortening—say, 2/3 cup instead of 1 cup, Purdy suggests. Then go one step further by replacing a small portion of the remaining butter or shortening with nonfat or low-fat plain yogurt.

Clam chowder. If you're accustomed to adding bacon to your chowder, try a couple of drops of liquid smoke instead, Tribole says.

She also suggests using low-fat (1 percent) milk instead of whole milk and evaporated skim milk instead of cream.

Fettuccine sauce. Traditional recipes for this favorite pasta topping usually call for butter, heavy cream, and Parmesan cheese. For a trim and tasty imitation, blend nonfat cream cheese, skim milk, and nonfat cottage cheese in a food processor for about four minutes, then warm the mixture, says Lynn Fischer, author of *Fabulous Fat-Free Cooking*. If you like, you can also add ¼ cup of very lean diced ham and 1 cup of peas.

French fries. Cut unpeeled potatoes—or sweet potatoes, for a new twist on an old favorite—into ½-inch-thick slices. Coat the slices with a mixture of low-sodium soy sauce and a few drops of dark sesame oil. Then grill or broil the "fries" until they turn crisp and golden.

French toast. Skip the whole eggs and dip your bread in egg substitute instead, Fischer suggests. And remember not to slather your French toast with butter—stick with a small amount of maple syrup.

Fried chicken. Remake a high-fat standby with this suggestion from Marilyn Cerino, R.D., nutrition consultant at the Benjamin Franklin Center for Health of Pennsylvania Hospital in Philadelphia. Dip boneless, skinless chicken breasts in a mixture of skim milk and egg whites, then roll them in either bread crumbs or seasoned flour. Coat a nonstick pan with nonstick spray, add one teaspoon of olive or canola oil, and flash-fry the chicken over medium-high heat for 30 seconds on each side to make it crispy. Then bake at 400°F for five minutes, or until the chicken is cooked through.

Lasagna. Lighten up this Italian classic by substituting a mixture of extra-lean ground beef and ground turkey breast for the usual high-fat sausage. Even better: Layer the noodles with roasted or grilled vegetables, such as eggplant or zucchini, says Julia Della Croce, author of *The Vegetarian Table*. And don't forget to use nonfat ricotta cheese rather than the full-fat variety.

Manicotti. For manicotti filling, process nonfat cottage cheese in a food processor for a few seconds. It works just as well as full-fat ricotta cheese, according to D'Agostino. You can make the filling even healthier by mixing the cottage cheese with frozen spinach that has been thawed and squeezed dry.

Meat loaf. Make your meat loaf with extra-lean ground beef and replace half the usual amount with a packaged soy meat substitute, Fischer says. Then add chopped onions, celery, carrots, mushrooms, green peppers, or the whites of hard-boiled eggs to keep the loaf moist. And if your recipe calls for whole eggs, use just the egg whites instead.

Muffins. Most muffin recipes call for oil. You can get away with half the amount by replacing half the oil with drained applesauce or pureed prunes, says Jeanne Jones, "Cook It Light" syndicated columnist and author of *Healthy Cooking for People Who Don't Have Time to Cook*. To eliminate the fat altogether, try fruit-based butter and oil replacement.

Pie. Phyllo dough makes a perfect piecrust, with a lot less fat than a regular crust, Cerino says. Cut three sheets of phyllo in half. Lay one piece across a nine-inch pie plate and press it into place. Fold any overhanging dough toward the center of the plate, crumpling it slightly to make it fit. Mist the phyllo with nonstick spray. Repeat this process with the remaining pieces. Then bake the crust at 375°F for four to six minutes, or until golden. Add fresh fruit, such as strawberries, just before serving, Cerino suggests.

Pizza. These days, many "gourmet" pizzas skip the cheese entirely, D'Agostino notes. You don't have to eliminate it from your homemade pies, though—just switch to a low-fat variety and use only about two ounces. And try replacing high-fat toppings such as sausage and pepperoni with grilled vegetables such as zucchini, peppers, and eggplant.

Potato salad. Slim down this summertime standby by switching to nonfat or low-fat mayonnaise and using just the whites of hard-boiled eggs rather than the whole eggs, Fischer says. You can also boost the salad's taste and texture by adding chopped Spanish onions, celery, dill pickles, and scallions.

Quiche. Quiche recipes traditionally call for a high-fat combination of milk, eggs, and cheese. You can reduce the fat content of this dish considerably by using skim milk, egg substitute (1/4 cup for each whole egg), and shredded low-fat cheese.

Sloppy joes. Extra-lean ground beef or ground turkey breast works just as well as regular ground round. You can spice up the flavor by combining 1/2 cup of chunky salsa with a can of tomato sauce.

Spaghetti. Skip the meat sauce and create your own flavorful low-fat spaghetti topping by combining chopped fresh tomatoes, basil, garlic, and a touch of balsamic vinegar. For a meaty texture, use crumbled-up soy burgers or veggie burgers instead of the usual ground beef.

Strawberry shortcake. If you bake your own shortcake, Purdy suggests replacing the butter with canola oil to eliminate the saturated fat; your tastebuds will never know the difference. Also, nonfat vanilla frozen yogurt makes an excellent substitute for whipped cream.

Stuffing. Holiday feasts just wouldn't be the same without stuffing. You can make it low-fat with this recipe from Tribole: Sauté chopped onions, celery, and mushrooms in a nonstick skillet that you've coated with nonstick spray. Combine the vegetables with unseasoned cornbread stuffing in a two-quart casserole, then add some defatted chicken broth to moisten the mixture. Bake at 350°F for 30 to 40 minutes.

Tuna noodle casserole. The tuna and noodles aren't so bad—it's the rest of the casserole that packs the fat. You can make yours lean by substituting evaporated skim milk for whole milk and using reduced-fat versions of the canned cream of mushroom soup and the cheese. Also, be sure to choose tuna that's packed in water rather than oil.

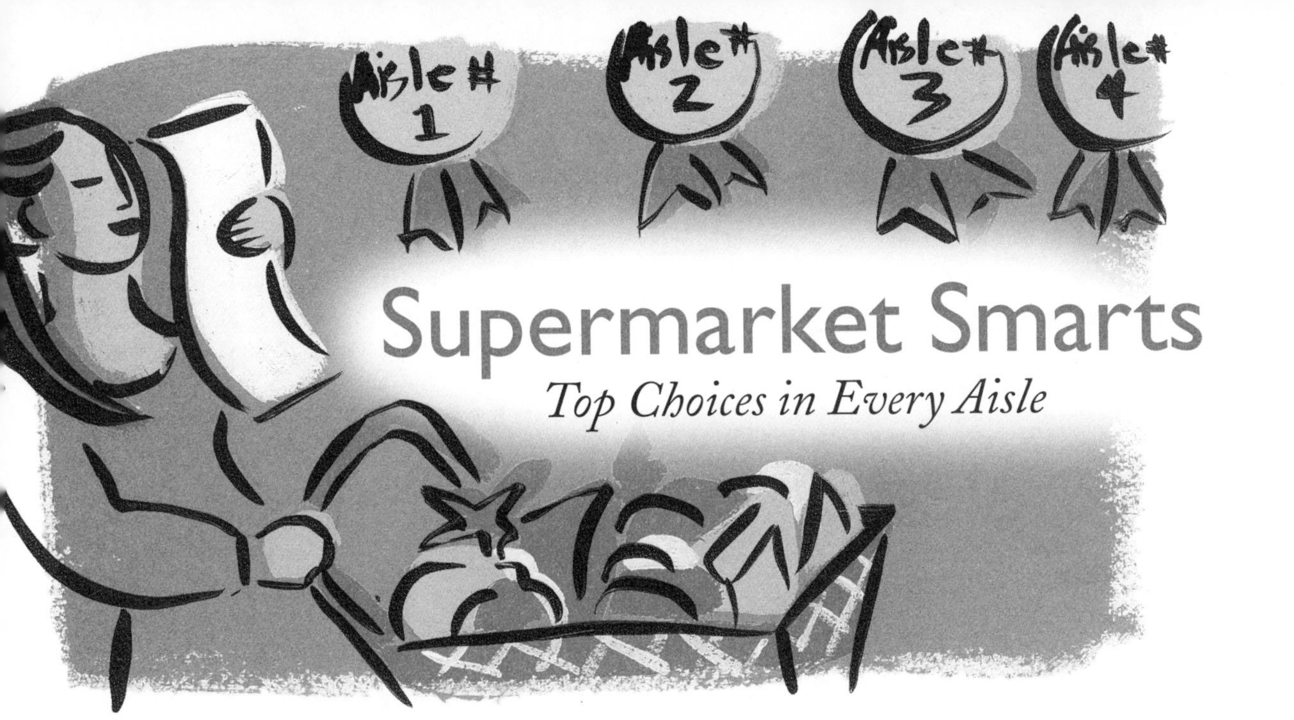

Supermarket Smarts

Top Choices in Every Aisle

The modern American supermarket is a cultural center, a form of entertainment, and a masterpiece in marketing.

—*The Tufts University Guide to Total Nutrition*

Oh, yeah. It's also where you buy food.

A foray into one of today's huge grocery stores can make you long for a time gone by, when you simply asked the man behind the counter for a box of cereal and he handed you one. Instead, you have to choose from among literally hundreds of brands, comparing cost, taste, and nutritional value. And that's just for one item. Keep in mind that the average supermarket carries about 30,000 different products, edible as well as nonedible. And every one of them is screaming, "Buy me!"

Short of moving to your own Green Acres and home-growing everything you need to feed yourself and your family, there's not much you can do to avoid the grocery gauntlet. You have to eat, which means you have to buy food. So how do you make your visits to the nearby mega-supermarket more pleasant and productive—and ensure that you arrive home with precisely those items that will do your body good?

You need a plan—an aisle-by-aisle shopping guide to help you bypass the bad stuff and fill your cart with good-for-you foods. "To eat healthy, you need to buy healthy," notes Bonnie Tandy Leblang, R.D., author of the nationally syndicated column "Supermarket Sampler" and six cookbooks, including *Beans: Seventy-Nine Recipes for Beans, Lentils, Peas, Peanuts, and Other Legumes*. "Smart supermarket shopping strategies are the key to eating well at home."

Shopping à la Cart

It would be nice to think that the supermarket you frequent shares your concerns about good nutrition. To some extent, it probably does. Many chain stores have instituted consumer education programs, posting signs and distributing pamphlets that detail the nutritional values of specific items.

Still, their bottom line is...well, the bottom

line. They want you to spend—and to leave the store with more items than the two or three you originally planned to buy. And so they invest literally billions of dollars in dizzying, dazzling displays designed to make the most of every selling opportunity.

You can outwit such temptations and stay true to your healthy eating habits by learning a few grocery ground rules. Here's what the experts recommend.

Don't be list-less. A shopping list is your most important navigational tool for getting around the supermarket. It keeps you focused, minimizes impulse buys, and ensures that you leave the store with exactly what you went in for.

If you seldom have time to write down what you need, create a master list of the items that you most often buy and photocopy it. Then you can simply check off items as they run low.

Clip carefully. Coupons undoubtedly appeal to your money-saving side. But nutrition-wise, they may not be a bargain. Be wary of those discounted items that don't support your healthy eating habits. If you come across a coupon for a new product that you think you'd like to try, take a good look at its nutrition label before buying. Look for low-fat items, which provide less than three grams of fat per serving, or items that provide at least 10 percent of the recommended amount of either vitamin A, vitamin C, iron, or calcium (or meet both criteria).

Fill your tank first. "Never, ever, ever shop on an empty stomach," notes Michele Tuttle, R.D., former director of consumer affairs for the Food Marketing Institute in Washington, D.C. "If you're hungry, you'll always buy things that you didn't intend to, and everything will always look more appealing."

This doesn't mean that you have to plan every shopping trip around breakfast, lunch, or dinner. Just munching on an apple or a banana can tide you over, suggests Debra Waterhouse, R.D., author of *Outsmarting the Female Fat Cell* and *Why Women Need Chocolate.*

Go it alone. It's best not to turn grocery shopping into a social event with a friend—or, for that matter, to take along your kids. Either way, you're more inclined to end up with unhealthy foods that you wouldn't otherwise buy.

Watch the clock. Shopping when you're pressed for time or when the supermarket is crowded sets the stage for hasty, unhealthy food decisions. Plan your supermarket runs for off-peak hours. Go on a weekday rather than a weekend, either early in the morning or late in the evening. (With so many chain stores now open 24 hours, you can shop at three o'clock in the morning, if you're so inclined.) Just allow yourself plenty of time, so you can read labels carefully and choose foods wisely.

Don't go for come-ons. Supermarkets strategically position every single product to maximize its "sell-ability." Nothing is left to chance—every item in the store has a reason for being placed in a certain aisle, on a certain shelf, and at a certain height. Among the techniques you should be wary of are end-of-aisle displays (sometimes called end caps), which showcase specially priced items; cross-merchandising displays, which pair complementary products like potato chips and soda; and checkout-lane displays, which encourage last-minute impulse purchases.

Skip the samples. You already know how full-fat Swiss cheese tastes, so just say no when someone asks you to make like a gustatory guinea pig. Passing up a 1½-ounce chunk of cheese means sparing yourself a whopping 160 calories and over 11 grams of fat.

Think small. Don't buy those gargantuan family-size and economy-size packages of food unless you really think you need that much. For one thing, you may end up throwing a lot of it away because of spoilage—which means that you really don't save any money on the purchase. For another, a series of studies at the University of Pennsylvania in Philadelphia has shown that people tend to use more of a food at a time if it comes in a larger package.

Don't ponder the possibilities. The phrase "just in case"—as in "just in case company drops by" or "just in case the kids want something sweet"—has scuttled many attempts at eating right. Shop with only you and your immediate family in mind, not some phantom guests who may or may not show up on your doorstep. And even if they do, you can serve them the same delicious, nutritious foods that you already have on hand.

Just the Facts, Ma'am

Compared with labels of five years ago, the ones we see these days present a veritable *Encyclopaedia Britannica* of nutrition information. An ingredients list and a Nutrition Facts chart graces nearly every packaged food as well as many fresh foods. They tell you not only what a particular product is made from but also how much of certain nutrients it contains. That way, you can decide whether that product has a place in your healthy diet.

Of course, you have to know how to interpret all those servings, percentages, and ten-syllable chemical names. Here's a short primer on what they mean and what to look for.

Serving size. According to the Food and Drug Administration, which regulates food labeling, the serving size reflects the portion that people *actually* eat. (This is different from the *Prevention* Food Pyramid for Women serving, which reflects the portion that women *should* eat for good health.) You have to ask yourself whether this amount of food seems realistic. If you think you consume more or less—if you have, say, four cookies instead of the serving size of two—then the rest of the figures in the Nutrition Facts chart won't hold up. In the case of the cookies, you'd be getting twice as much of everything listed in the chart.

Percent Daily Value. This column of the Nutrition Facts chart shows how a food helps you meet your daily nutrient needs. The percentages are calculated for a 2,000-calorie-a-day diet. If you're eating smaller portions and fewer total calories overall—as many women do—you'll be getting smaller amounts of the nutrients as well.

To quickly assess a food's nutritional value, use these rules of thumb from the American Dietetic Association. For total fat, cholesterol, and sodium, each Percent Daily Value should not exceed 100 percent—and the lower, the better. For fiber, vitamins A and C, calcium, and iron, higher Percent Daily Values are ideal. (In general, food labels list only these four vitamins and minerals plus fiber because people tend to not get enough of them.)

Calories and total fat. These figures come in handy if you're counting calories and fat grams. For example, if a food contains almost one-third of the fat grams in your daily budget, you'll want to keep that in mind for the rest of the day so that you don't go over your budget.

Saturated fat and cholesterol. A diet high in either of these nutrients may increase your risk of a serious health problem such as heart disease or cancer. So look for low numbers here. You shouldn't get more than 7 percent of your daily calories from saturated fat. For example, if you're eating 2,000 calories a day, no more than 140 calories should come from saturated fat. Count up the saturated fat listed on nutrient labels for everything you eat, and limit it to 15 grams a day. (A gram of fat has 9 calories.) As for cholesterol, the American Heart Association recommends consuming no more than 300 milligrams a day.

Sodium. Limit your daily intake of sodium to

under 2,400 milligrams per day. High-sodium diets have been linked to high blood pressure.

Dietary fiber. According to the National Cancer Institute, you need to consume between 20 and 30 grams of fiber every day for optimum health.

Ingredients. You'll find this list separate from the Nutrition Facts chart. Be sure to check it out. The ingredients appear in descending order by amount, from most to least. Look for foods with short lists rather than long ones. And make sure that any fat or oil is way down on the list.

THE REAL MEANING OF LITE

You're all set for your weekly run to the supermarket. You have your shopping list, your calculator, your secret decoder ring...what? No decoder ring? How will you ever read those food labels?

The terminology used on labels these days can seem impossible to decipher. But behind every low-this and reduced-that is a standardized definition developed by the Food and Drug Administration and the U.S. Department of Agriculture. Each definition sets forth specific nutritional criteria that a food must meet in order to feature that term on its label. If you know what the various terms mean, you can compare foods at a glance and choose the one that best meets your dietary needs.

Here's a sampling of some commonly used label lingo and the nutritional information that it represents.

Sugar-free: Contains less than 0.5 gram of sugar per serving.

Calorie-free: Contains fewer than five calories per serving.

Low-calorie: Contains 40 or fewer calories per serving.

Reduced-calorie: Contains 25 percent fewer calories than the regular product.

Fat-free: Contains less than 0.5 gram of fat per serving.

Low-fat: Contains three grams or less of fat per serving.

Reduced-fat: Contains no more than 75 percent of the fat found in regular versions or comparable food.

Light or lite: Contains one-third fewer calories or half the fat of the regular food.

Cholesterol-free: Contains less than two milligrams of cholesterol and two grams or less of saturated fat per serving.

Hello, Good Buys

You know the inside scoop on supermarket shopping strategies, and you've learned how to decipher label lingo. You're all set for a nutrition-savvy shopping spree.

To get your trip down the aisles off on the right foot, we asked Elizabeth A. Brown, R.D., nutritionist and weight-control specialist at the Lehigh Valley Hospital Center for Health Promotion and Disease Prevention in Allentown, Pennsylvania, to take you on a personal, guided tour of a typical grocery store. Here are her recommendations for what to buy and what to bypass.

Produce

You can't go wrong in this aisle—the bright colors tell you that these foods are loaded with vitamins and minerals. Don't be afraid to experiment with the many exotic fruits and vegetables you find here. Variety and balance are very important to good nutrition, as research continues to uncover "hidden" nutrients in an array of produce. Flavonoids are a good example: These little-known chemical compounds, found in abundance in kale, cranberries, onions, and in the white pulp of citrus fruit, may help reduce your risk of heart disease and cancer.

Best choices: Just about anything from the

Low-cholesterol: Contains 20 milligrams or less of cholesterol, 2 grams or less of saturated fat, and 13 grams or less of total fat per serving.

Reduced-cholesterol: Contains 75 percent or less of the cholesterol found in the regular food and two grams or less of saturated fat per serving.

Sodium-free: Contains less than five milligrams of sodium per serving.

Very low sodium: Contains less than 35 milligrams of sodium per serving.

Low-sodium: Contains 140 milligrams or less of sodium per serving.

Reduced-sodium: Contains no more than 75 percent of the sodium found in the regular food.

Extra-lean: Refers to meat, seafood, or poultry that has less than two grams of saturated fat, less than five grams of total fat, and less than 95 milligrams of cholesterol per three-ounce serving.

Lean: Refers to meat, seafood, or poultry that has 4.5 grams or less of saturated fat, less than 10 grams of total fat, and less than 95 milligrams of cholesterol per three-ounce serving.

High in: Supplies 20 percent or more of the Daily Value (DV) of a given nutrient per serving.

Good source of: Supplies 10 to 19 percent of the DV of a given nutrient per serving.

Fresh: Refers to a food that is raw, that has not been processed, frozen, or heated, and that contains no preservatives.

Freshly: Refers to a food that has been made recently; may be used with "baked."

produce aisle will do your body good. Choose dark green vegetables such as broccoli and kale for fiber and orange, red, and yellow produce such as carrots, cantaloupe, and sweet potatoes for beta-carotene. Kale has a lot of nutritional value, with healthy doses of vitamins A and C, but be aware that it has a very strong flavor. Other notable nutrient-rich selections include asparagus, oranges, papaya, and green peppers.

Deli

Proceed with caution! Most of what you see in the deli showcase serves up lots of fat and calories, and since the nutrition information is seldom posted for these items, it's hard to know exactly what you're getting. If you want to buy lunchmeat, fresh is a better choice than processed. Select only the leanest cuts. Avoid cured meats—they contain nitrites, food preservatives that have been linked to health problems ranging from migraines to cancer. And go easy on the prepared salads. They're usually made with full-fat ingredients.

Best choices: Chicken breast and turkey breast come up winners here. Both are low in fat and excellent sources of niacin and vitamin B_6. In fact, three ounces of chicken breast supplies 58 percent of the Daily Value (DV) of niacin for women. You get nice amounts of iron, too.

Breads/Baked Goods

Another dietary danger zone. You're especially vulnerable to impulse purchases in this department when you're tired or shopping on an empty stomach. At times like these, your body craves carbs, which makes high-fat, high-sugar treats seem especially attractive. Bypass the cakes and doughnuts and head for the whole-grain breads and other baked goods. Read the label for fiber and iron content, and choose items that are enriched and fortified.

Best choices: Bagels are a good source of iron and of the B vitamins niacin, riboflavin, and thiamin. Just watch the serving size. With some of the larger bagels, you could end up consuming a lot more calories than you think. Among breads, whole-grain types are versatile and supply two to three grams of fiber per slice. Be aware, though, that fiber content varies from one brand of whole-grain bread to the next—and some brands may not even have significant amounts of the nutrient. On the other hand, many "light" versions of breads and English muffins can pack three to six grams per serving. Read the label to be sure.

Dairy

Here you'll find the cream of the calcium crop. Milk, yogurt, and cheese all weigh in with generous amounts of the mineral. Unfortunately, the regular varieties also have generous amounts of fat. Select leaner alternatives when you can, such as nonfat or low-fat (1 percent) milk and nonfat or low-fat yogurt. Likewise, the healthiest choices in cheese are made from nonfat or low-fat milk and are not highly processed.

As for the margarine-versus-butter debate: Margarine seems better than butter, but it may not be as good as you think. It contains trans-fatty acids, which in your body act like heart-unhealthy saturated fat. Choose light margarine over regular. And if you don't like the taste of margarine—many people don't—it's okay to have a pat of butter once in a while. Either way, portion control is what counts. In fact, if you tend to be heavy-handed with margarine or butter when cooking, you may want to switch to a spray product to cut down on the amount you use.

Best choices: Yogurt supplies even more calcium than milk: A one-cup serving of the nonfat variety has 488 milligrams, or 49 percent of a woman's recommended daily intake. Look for a brand with active cultures, which may help prevent recurrent yeast infections. Be wary of brands sweetened with aspartame (NutraSweet). Not enough studies have been done to know what effects this ingredient may have on the body.

Pasta, Rice, and Beans

The *Prevention* Food Pyramid for Women says you should eat five one-ounce servings of protein-rich foods every day. Beans make

REAL-LIFE SCENARIO

She Lives on Convenience Foods

Like a lot of working women, Lisa rarely has the time (or desire) to cook. Still, she tries to eat right. A typical day starts with a breakfast bar and a glass of skim milk. Lunch is canned soup and a tuna sandwich—with low-fat mayo, of course. She even goes for the low-fat chips. After a good workout at the gym at night, she microwaves a frozen entrée—low-fat ravioli is her fav—and she always makes it a meal with a can of green vegetables and some nonfat frozen yogurt. Her TV snack is popcorn. She's proud to say that she hasn't gained an ounce in years, but she's worried that her diet of canned, frozen, and packaged foods may be leaving her nutritionally shortchanged.

Lisa has reason to be concerned. Filling up her shopping cart every week with packaged foods—especially canned goods—in lieu of fresh foods means that she's filling up on too much sodium and depriving herself of the vitamins and minerals that are leached out during processing.

Lisa would be much better off microwaving some fresh peas and carrots than cracking open can after can of veggies at mealtime. And it's just as easy to throw a couple of frozen spears of broccoli in a steamer as it is to open a can of beans. Fresh or frozen vegetables not only retain vitamins and minerals better but they're also much less salty than canned vegetables. As far as frozen entrées go, most packaged meals are also notoriously salty. And did Lisa say her favorite snack is popcorn? Talk about salt! Lisa needs to find a low-salt and low-fat variety.

The good news is that there are low-sodium varieties of all of Lisa's staple foods, but even if sodium wasn't a concern, Lisa's diet could still use some work. Besides occasionally substituting one frozen entrée for another, Lisa eats pretty much the same thing every day. For example, she is not getting nearly as many different kinds of fruits and vegetables as she needs. Vegetable soup is not the way to get variety in her diet.

Even though Lisa has little time to cook, it would take just a tad more effort to put variety in her diet. For example, she can pick up a bag of fresh salad greens already cut and packaged and substitute it for her canned soup at lunch. She should grab an apple in place of her potato chips or munch veggies—she can buy them already cut—or other high-fiber snacks throughout the day.

Lisa should also bite the bullet and cook dinner. Cooking healthy dinners can be simple and quick, and they'll go a long way in adding variety to her diet. If she keeps turning to her old favorites, however, Lisa should at least take a multivitamin to help make up for the lack of variety.

Expert Consulted
Debra Wein, R.D.
Sports nutritionist and exercise physiologist
University of Massachusetts
Co-founder of The Sensible Nutrition Connection
Boston

an excellent protein source, especially if you don't eat a lot of meat. So stock up on all varieties.

Pasta counts toward your daily grain quota of six to nine servings. Opt for dried whole-wheat varieties over fresh, since fresh is usually made with eggs and tends to have more cholesterol and fat. Whole-wheat varieties are also a great source of fiber.

Roll your cart right past those premixes and heavily prepared foods, like packaged pasta and rice dishes. Besides feeding you a hefty amount of fat, they offer little nutritional value.

Best choices: Beans, beans, beans. They pack a nutritional punch of protein, fiber, iron, and folate, and they're filling and versatile to boot. And don't forget rice. One-half cup of the brown variety, in particular, supplies some fiber and the B vitamins B_6, niacin, and thiamin in exchange for no cholesterol and just a smidgen of fat. You may also want to try bulgur. It has even more fiber than rice, no cholesterol, and practically no fat.

Cookies and Crackers

Crackers are an okay snack, as long as you pay attention to how many you're eating. Most people eat between 10 and 12 at a time, which exceeds the typical serving size. Cookies of any kind should be reserved for an occasional treat, since they're nutritionally empty.

Best choices: Look for whole-wheat crackers that contain no more than three grams of fat per serving. Also check out the animal crackers and graham crackers. All of these are cholesterol-free and low-fat, too.

Snack Foods

Pick up some popcorn for a filling snack that provides a bit of fiber. Just read the label to make sure it's low-fat. If it's something sweet you're after, opt for marshmallows, gummy candies, or jelly beans. None of these has any nutritional value, but they do have a lot less fat than most candies. Check out the ingredient list on the package. The shorter it is, the fewer additives the item contains.

Best choices: Besides popcorn, smart snack selections include pretzels, flavored rice cakes, and sunflower seeds. Honey-mustard pretzels tend to have more fat than regular varieties, so go easy on them. Sunflower seeds also have a lot of fat (most of it unsaturated), so they're not for everyday munching.

Canned Foods

Fruits and vegetables. Canned produce has at least one advantage over fresh: a longer shelf life. It also helps ensure that you're meeting the six- to seven-serving quota for fruits and veggies (one vitamin C, one folate, two phytochemicals, one carotenoid, one to two fiber) that's recommended in the *Prevention* Food Pyramid for Women.

Although some vitamins can be lost in the canning process, one University of Illinois analysis found that some canned fruits and vegetables, like pineapple and carrots, contain as much vitamin A and C as the fresh or frozen varieties. Because they're canned without their skins, however, they don't have quite as much fiber as their fresh and frozen counterparts. Look for products that are packed in water or light syrup, with little or no added sugar.

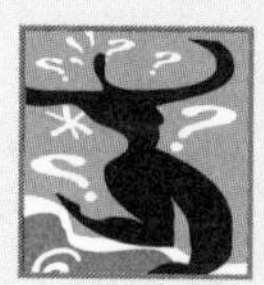

WOMEN ASK WHY

Why does a can of soup have 2½ servings instead of an even 2 or 3?

In terms of calories and nutrients, that extra ½ serving can make a big difference! But if you're cooking for yourself, it's a pain to freeze those fractional leftovers for later. Better to eat the extra than toss it down the garbage disposal, right? Probably, but the Food and Drug Administration (FDA) food labels are going to tell you what you're getting into, nutritionally speaking.

The FDA has created 140 product categories, each of which has a reference amount that roughly determines the serving size of the different foods in that category. For example, the reference amount for snack foods is 30 grams, a weight based on U.S. Department of Agriculture surveys of how much people actually eat. If you have a bag of pretzels and each pretzel weighs 11 grams, the serving size is going to be three pretzels (33 grams). It doesn't have to be exactly 30 grams, but it has to be close. The reference amount for soup turns out to be 1 cup. If you have 2½ cups in a can—or a concentrated soup that makes 2½ cups—you have 2½ servings, not 2 or 3. Splitting that 2½-cup can into 2 servings really gives you a serving size of 1¼ cups. And that extra ¼ cup is going to give you a quarter more fat,

Best choices: Among canned fruits, choose chunky applesauce, mandarin oranges, peaches, and pears. Healthy selections among canned vegetables include kale, asparagus, green beans, spinach, and yams.

Soups. Depending on what kind you choose, soup serves up an array of nutrient-dense vegetables in every spoonful. It's a simple, satisfying way to boost your consumption of these good-for-you foods. Choose nonfat or low-fat products, taking note of the serving size. Sometimes it's smaller than people think. Skip the cream soups.

Best choices: Black bean soup offers a good amount of iron—about two milligrams, or 12 percent of the DV—but very little fat and no cholesterol. Lentil soup, another low-fat selection, is also an impressive source of iron (three milligrams, or 14 percent of the DV) as well as folate (50 micrograms, or 12.5 percent of the DV).

Meats and Poultry

There are three grades, or qualities, of beef sold in most supermarkets. Prime cuts have the most fat, select cuts have the least, and choice cuts fall somewhere in between. You want to sodium, and everything else of what's listed on the label.

With a huge bag of pretzels, an extra ½ serving isn't as crucial. Instead of being spread over just 2 servings, the extra ½ serving would be spread over, say, 20 servings, making the difference in fat, sodium, and other nutrients negligible. That's why the FDA only requires food companies to round to the nearest ½ serving for up to 5 servings.

As far as soup goes, you're probably still wondering why Campbell's hasn't made their cans larger or smaller by a half-cup so the serving size is an even 2 or 3. Well, before the nutrition labeling laws went into effect—and before nutrition as a concept became so widespread—soup plants like Campbell's were set up to produce a different-size can. Campbell's has been producing 10½-ounce cans since the first can of condensed soup was made in 1897. Sure, they've come up with other sizes (26 ounces, 19 ounces, 15 ounces), but making a whole new can to line up perfectly with the FDA reference amount would mean that consumers would have to be willing to pay for the expense of building new plants. We'd probably be better off just dealing with that extra ½ serving.

Expert Consulted
Ellen Anderson, Ph.D.
Chemist at the Food and Drug Administration Office of Food Labeling
Washington, D.C.

look for cuts stamped select. The less marbling a piece of meat has, the leaner it is.

Choose chicken pieces labeled "extra-lean" or "lean." White meat is a healthier choice than dark, but dark meat has more iron and zinc, so you don't necessarily want to completely eliminate it from your diet. Do be very cautious with ground chicken, though. The high-fat skin may have been mixed in with the meat during processing. Check the label for fat content or ask the butcher to grind some plain chicken breasts for you.

When serving meat or poultry, remember to stick with a three-ounce portion. That's roughly the size of a deck of cards or about the size of the palm of your hand.

Best choices: Chicken breast and turkey breast have less than half the fat of most cuts of meat. Among meats, pork tenderloin is among the leanest cuts, as are select-grade bottom and top round.

Seafood

Almost any fish or shellfish you can think of has nutritional benefit. Some, like Atlantic herring, canned salmon, fresh tuna, and Atlantic mackerel, are rich in omega-3 fatty acids. Medical evidence indicates that omega-3's can reduce heart-unhealthy triglycerides, inhibit the growth of breast cancer cells, and even prevent gallstones. Some seafood does contain fat, but it's not enough to raise the level of cholesterol in your blood. Shellfish are a good example: They don't have a lot of saturated fat, which is the real culprit in raising blood cholesterol levels. Do steer clear of prepared seafood salads, though. They're bound to be loaded with fat.

Best choices: In addition to being a top-notch source of omega-3's, canned salmon (with bones) delivers roughly 20 percent of your recommended daily calcium intake in a three-ounce serving. Fresh salmon, while not as rich in omega-3's as the canned kind, contains a wealth of B vitamins. You get over 80 percent of the DV of B_{12}, along with lots of niacin and some riboflavin, thiamin, and B_6. Fresh tuna is also a stellar source of these B vitamins, supplying almost one-third of the DV of B_{12}. White and light-meat tuna, canned in water, are low-fat, high-protein staples that you shouldn't pass up.

Cereals

No matter what you choose in this aisle, you really can't lose. Even sugary cereals fulfill roughly one-quarter of your nutrient needs for an entire day. That's because cereals are fortified. Still, you should compare sugar contents and pick the product that has less. (For a ravenous sweet tooth, though, consider munching on cereal rather than candy. At least cereal has some nutritional value.)

You can't beat cereal as a fiber source, either. In fact, some products have as much as 13 grams of fiber per serving, nearly three-quarters of the minimum recommended daily intake.

Best choices: Top fiber sources in the cereal aisle include Fiber One from General Mills (14 grams per ½ cup) and Kellogg's All-Bran (almost 10 grams per ½ cup). Also check out the various brands of raisin bran and anything whole-grain.

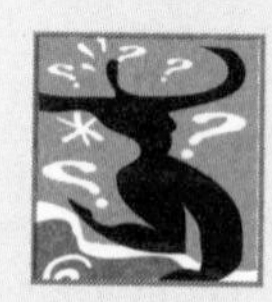

WOMEN ASK WHY

Why does all-fruit spread, which is supposed to be made from real fruit, have no vitamins or minerals listed on the label?

If you're looking for your daily dose of vitamin C in that little glass jar, you're going to be in a bit of a jam! Since the spread is made of fruit, you might expect to find *some* vitamins and minerals on the label. But unless the spread is fortified, you're not going to find much in a tablespoon (or two) of jam.

If your spread does have some vitamins and minerals in it, it could be that they're just not listed on the food label. Back in the 1940s and 1950s, nutritional labels often had long lists of vitamins and minerals because, at that time, the real health concern was vitamin and mineral deficiency. People were worried about scurvy, beriberi, and other deficiency diseases, and the government helped solve the problem by fortifying foods that everyone eats, such as grains and cereals.

In the last 10 years or so, however, we've been dealing with diseases of overnutrition. Now we're concerned about the effect of getting too much of something. The new food labels focus on what we need to know about now—particularly how much fat, saturated fat, cholesterol, and sodium we

Condiments

Oils. All oils are 100 percent fat. What differs is their proportions of monounsaturated, polyunsaturated, and saturated fats. You want an oil that is high in monounsaturates and low in saturates. Spray oils work well because they have built-in portion control. Rather than spending more money for the fancy packaging, you can make your own spray oil by pouring oil into a spray bottle.

Best choices: Canola oil has the best fat profile. Of its 14 grams of fat, 8 are monounsaturated, while only 1 is saturated. Olive oil has a high monounsaturated fat content, too, but it also has a strong flavor, so it's not usually recommended for baking.

Salad dressings. Dressings don't have a lot to offer nutritionally, but at least they get people to eat their veggies. Pay attention to serving size: The label usually says one to two tablespoons, but most folks use a lot more. You can add flavored vinegar to an oil-based dressing to reduce its fat content. If it's a non-oil-based dressing, just add water.

Best choices: Dressings with an oil-and-vinegar base have less sugar and additives than dressings that are creamy. If you're making your own, try red-wine, raspberry, or balsamic vinegar. Their robust flavors mean you can go easy on the should have in our diets. The only vitamins and minerals the labels must show are vitamin A, vitamin C, calcium, and iron. Cereals and other fortified foods will list others, but all other foods list them voluntarily.

In an all-fruit spread, which is probably made of mostly fruit and sugar and a little pectin, iron and calcium probably won't show up at all. Vitamin A isn't typical in fruits, but you probably won't find vitamin C, either, for a couple of reasons. First, vitamin C is the most fragile of all the vitamins—if you open up a carton of orange juice and leave it sitting out overnight, a lot of the vitamin C is going to disappear. Second, vitamin C is heat labile, meaning it will be driven off when heated. Making jams and jellies involves a heat step, so chances are most of the vitamin C is going to be lost.

Another reason why you won't find vitamins and minerals listed for something like fruit spread is that the serving size is so small. If you're talking a tablespoon, the amount of vitamin C is going to be negligible—if there's any at all. Sure, you could eat the whole jar, but knowing how fragile vitamin C is, you're better off reaching for a glass of OJ. Just make sure you keep it in the fridge.

Expert Consulted
Ellen Anderson, Ph.D.
Chemist at the Food and Drug Administration Office of Food Labeling
Washington, D.C.

oil—and they have very little sugar and fat. Light mayo has better flavor than the nonfat variety.

Frozen Foods

Believe it or not, frozen produce has a nutritional advantage over fresh. Because the fruits and veggies are in a deep freeze, they retain the nutrients that fresh varieties lose as they age and eventually spoil. Since you don't know how long fresh produce has been on display, you can't be sure that you're getting all of its nutrients. Try a variety of frozen fruits and veggies for a healthy mix of vitamins and minerals.

The rest of the frozen foods aisle is a mixed bag, nutrition-wise. There are some decent heat-and-serve foods, like pizzas and microwavable dinners. But you have to watch their calorie and fat content. In general, steer clear of anything that's breaded, because it has added fat. And try to limit your intake of frozen foods that contain more than five grams of fat per serving.

Ice cream is okay as an occasional treat. A one-cup serving has nearly 20 percent of the DV for calcium. Just be sure to pay attention to the serving size when you indulge. One cup of vanilla ice cream also has 270 calories and 14 grams of fat, making half of those calories come from fat.

Best choices: Among frozen vegetables, asparagus, broccoli, and spinach all deliver a diverse array of nutrients. Pick up some pierogies: They're low in fat, as long as you prepare them by boiling, microwaving, or pan-frying with spray oil. Soft pretzels make a good low-fat snack, too—but check out the serving size before buying.

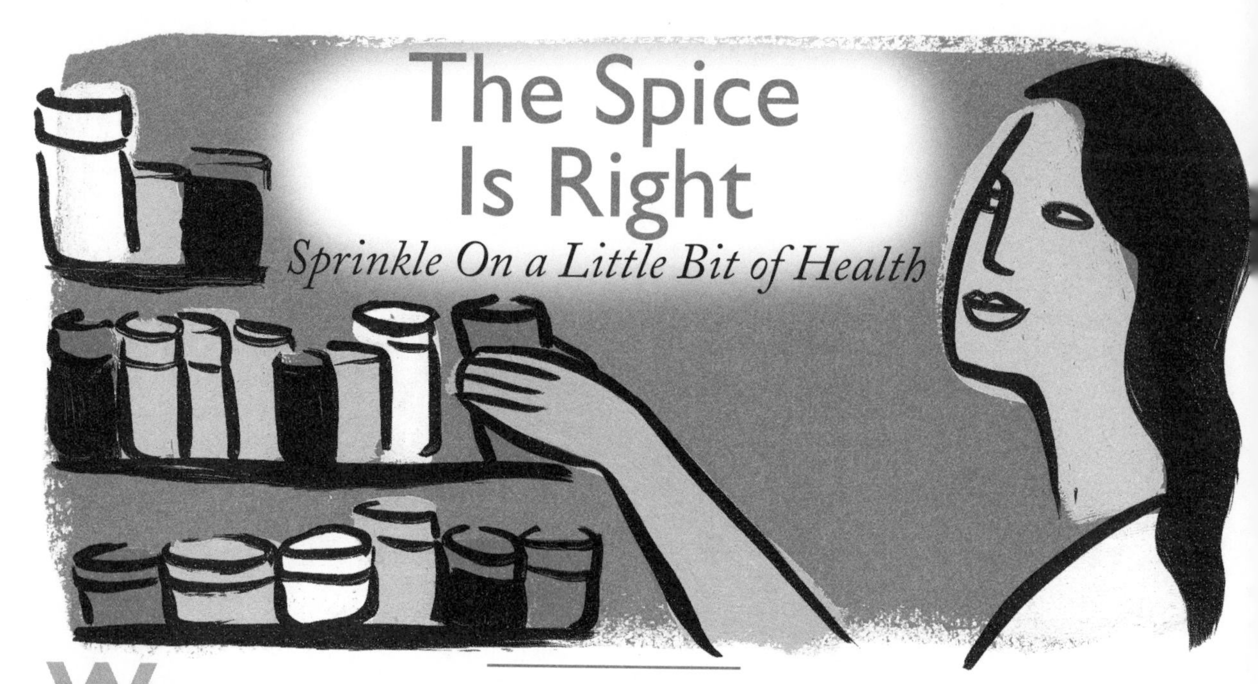

The Spice Is Right

Sprinkle On a Little Bit of Health

Women have been exploring the secrets of seasonings for thousands of years. Some of the earliest-known references to the use of herbs in cooking date back to the first century. Spices have an even longer tradition in the kitchen, referred to in writing on 4,800-year-old Egyptian papyri.

By one estimate, the use of various seasonings in this country has jumped by 50 percent over the past decade. These days, the average American consumes about three pounds of spices every year.

Why the surge? Our changing eating habits are at least partly responsible. While we once relied on fat and salt to give our foods taste, we now know that we need to cut back on this dastardly duo for the sake of good nutrition. Herbs and spices more than fill this flavor void, while also supplying barely any fat, sodium, or calories.

There's something else about herbs and spices that makes them an essential part of a health-promoting diet: Many of these pungent products have therapeutic properties. Studies have shown that they can do everything from easing cold symptoms to protecting against cancer. Of course, these "discoveries" come as no surprise to practitioners of Eastern medicine, who have been prescribing herbs and spices for centuries.

Must-Have Herbs and Spices

If you've ever browsed the herb-and-spice display in your grocery store, you've spotted dozens of different seasonings. Each imparts a very distinct flavor and aroma. Which ones you choose depends as much on the foods you're preparing as on the preferences of your palate. If you haven't used herbs and spices a whole lot, you'll need to experiment to figure out which ones best suit your cooking and your tastebuds.

The following selections make an ideal starter kit that should cover many of your cooking needs. Besides being quite versatile, these seasonings offer so many important health benefits that they're almost too good to pass up.

Basil. A common ingredient in tomato

sauces, this intensely flavored herb also works well in soups, salads, and vinaigrettes. There's good reason to make the most of basil in your cooking. Preliminary research suggests that the herb may help block the biochemical chain reaction that leads to the development of cancer.

Bay leaves. These woodsy-tasting green leaves are being studied as a potential treatment for Type II (non-insulin-dependent) diabetes. In Type II diabetes, the body doesn't produce enough of or becomes resistant to the hormone insulin, which it needs to help convert food into energy. But bay leaves can actually help regulate insulin levels. You can use the herb as a flavor enhancer in soups, stews, and marinades. Just remember to remove it from a dish before serving: The leaf is so sharp and stiff that it can damage the throat or digestive tract if swallowed.

Cloves. With their intense orangy scent and piquant flavor, cloves nicely complement autumn-ripe vegetables such as pumpkin and squash. Cloves also spice up rice dishes and baked goods. They contain a compound called eugenol, a powerful antioxidant, that can help keep your arteries clear of cholesterol.

Cumin. If you've ever eaten a Mexican, Middle Eastern, or Indian dish, you've probably tasted cumin. The spice is also used as an ingredient in chili powder. The seeds have an earthy taste. Evidence suggests that cumin may have the most potent cancer-fighting properties of all herbs and spices. Add it to salsa and hummus.

Garlic. Okay...so technically, garlic doesn't qualify as an herb or a spice. (It's actually a member of the onion family.) Nevertheless, the medicinal benefits of this "wonder bulb" definitely merit mention. Perhaps the most compelling research so far focuses on the link between garlic consumption and cancer risk. A study at Pennsylvania State University in University Park found that garlic inhibits formation of breast cancer cells. And researchers in Iowa concluded that eating garlic at least once a week cut women's risk of colon cancer by one-third, compared with women who never ate garlic.

Garlic is so versatile that you can incorporate it into all but the sweetest dishes. Worried about garlic breath? Roasting or boiling the bulb before use will make it milder and less pungent. Or try chewing parsley sprigs after eating garlic.

Ginger. Many Chinese and Indian dishes call for this spicy-sweet ingredient, which, like garlic, has therapeutic properties. Ginger is perhaps best known for its ability to relieve motion sickness. Now researchers in Denmark and India have uncovered evidence that ginger can also ease migraine pain and help lower cholesterol. Use it in stir-fries, cakes, and marinades and as a complement to meat dishes.

Paprika. Paprika can boost your pound-burning power by accelerating your metabolism while curbing your appetite. The spice is available in a range of "temperatures," from mild to hot. It also tends to give foods a reddish hue. Use paprika to liven up broiled fish, chicken, and roasted or mashed potatoes.

Parsley. Nibbling that delicate green sprig on your dinner plate just might do you a world of good. Parsley contains compounds that act as natural diuretics, which means the herb can help prevent premenstrual water retention and flush out bacteria that lead to urinary tract infections. Besides using fresh parsley as a garnish, mince it and sprinkle it on soups, pasta, grains, and potatoes.

Red pepper. As with paprika, eating red pepper may speed up your metabolism. Red pepper also makes a good home remedy for a cold: The heat it produces can unclog a stuffed-up nose and stimulate a more productive cough. A natural in spicy-hot dishes such as chili, red pepper can also add flair to soups, stews, sauces—even salad dressings.

Rosemary. Common in French and Italian

PERFECT BLENDS

The following herb-and-spice blends can add a palate-pleasing punch to various dishes. Combine them in a small stainless steel bowl, and store them in three-ounce containers for later use. Then simply add them during cooking or set the containers on the table in place of the saltshaker.

CAJUN SPICE

This fiery mix of seasonings can jazz up a Creole or Cajun meal with some Louisiana zip.

- 2 teaspoons paprika
- 2 teaspoons ground black pepper
- 1½ teaspoons garlic powder
- 1 teaspoon crushed red-pepper flakes
- 1 teaspoon dried thyme
- 1 teaspoon dried oregano
- 1 teaspoon onion powder
- ¼ teaspoon dry mustard

MAKES ABOUT 3 TABLESPOONS

ITALIAN HERB SEASONING

Here's a versatile blend to go with everything from soups and stews to potatoes and pizza.

- 1 tablespoon dried oregano
- 1 tablespoon dried basil
- 1 teaspoon dried thyme

MAKES 2⅓ TABLESPOONS

SAVORY ALL-PURPOSE BLEND

This simple mix lives up to its name: It goes with just about anything!

- 1 tablespoon dried basil
- 2 teaspoons celery seed
- 2 teaspoons dried savory
- 1 teaspoon dried thyme
- 1 teaspoon dried marjoram

MAKES 3 TABLESPOONS

cuisines, this aromatic herb complements the flavors of a variety of dishes, especially poultry and lamb. On the health front, evidence suggests that rosemary helps protect against cancer.

Turmeric. Turmeric is what gives prepared mustard its distinctive golden glow. Its mild flavor and yellow hue complement curries and rice dishes. This spice can contribute to your heart health, too, by lowering blood levels of triglycerides and by preventing cholesterol from sticking to your artery walls. Other studies have linked turmeric to a reduced risk of cancer and possibly to stronger immunity.

Seasoning Savvy

If you're psyched to start sprinkling these healing seasonings on your favorite foods, the following guidelines can help you make the most of these condiments.

Get fresh. Certain herbs are much better fresh than dried. Basil, dill, parsley, cilantro, and mint are among the most notable. Since fresh herbs are so perishable, keep them refrigerated. Your best bet is to pat the herb sprigs dry with a paper towel, stand them in a jar that's filled halfway with water, and loosely cover them with a plastic bag. They'll keep for a week.

Keep them in the dark. Spices and dried herbs that haven't been ground can retain their potency for six months to two years if stored properly. Ground spices lose their potency on the shelf more quickly—usually in six months or so. To keep them flavorful as long as possible, take all spices out of your wall-mounted or countertop spice rack and store them in a cool, dry, dark place. Heat, moisture, air, and light are dried seasonings' worst enemies.

When possible, buy spices and dried herbs in whole form rather than ground, then grind them as you need them. This will help these seasonings stay fresh and flavorful.

Take a whiff. Before using a spice or dried herb, take a pinch from the jar, lightly rub it between your fingers, and sniff it. If it doesn't have much of an aroma, it is probably past its prime.

Time it right. Add spices and dried herbs early in the cooking process, so the heat and moisture can coax them into releasing their flavors. But don't hold an open jar of seasoning right over a simmering pot. The rising steam can get trapped in the jar and cause the seasoning to become moldy.

Unlike their dried counterparts, fresh herbs give up their flavors quite readily. Wait until the cooking process is almost done before throwing them into the pot.

Proceed with caution. If you're modifying a recipe to use less salt, a good rule of thumb is to increase the quantities of any herbs and spices by 25 percent and decrease the salt by half or more. For unseasoned dishes, add a pinch at a time—constantly taste-testing as you go—until the taste suits your palate.

WOMEN ASK WHY

Is salt really so bad for me?

In itself, salt is just the innocent grainy white substance formed when some sodium hooks up with some chloride. But only the sodium raises concern.

Ironically, sodium is an essential nutrient. Our bodies need some sodium to regulate blood pressure, transmit nerve impulses, and maintain normal muscle activity. The problem is that we usually take in much more sodium than the job requires. We need only about 500 milligrams a day—the equivalent of a quarter-teaspoon. The average adult eats 4,000 to 7,000 milligrams a day.

Studies have linked excessive sodium intake to high blood pressure, which is associated with stroke and heart disease. You may, however, remember reading some reports to the contrary. That's because not everyone is sodium sensitive.

In sodium-sensitive people, too much salt creates an imbalance with the way water gets transported through the cells of our bodies. We have fluid outside our cells as well as fluid inside our cells. The fluid outside our cells is largely governed by sodium, while the fluid inside is governed by potassium. When sodium levels rise too high, it can throw this delicate balance out of whack, calling in a host of hormones that constrict blood vessels, making our blood pressure surge.

The thing is that there's no way to tell if you are salt sensitive or not. So to play it safe, most health professionals still recommend that you hold your sodium intake to 2,400 milligrams per day.

Don't think of cutting back on salt as a curse. People who reduce their salt intake usually find that they can actually taste other flavors better, so they enjoy food more, not less.

Expert Consulted
Barbara O. Schneeman, Ph.D.
Professor of nutrition
Dean of the College of Agriculture and Environmental Sciences
University of California
Davis

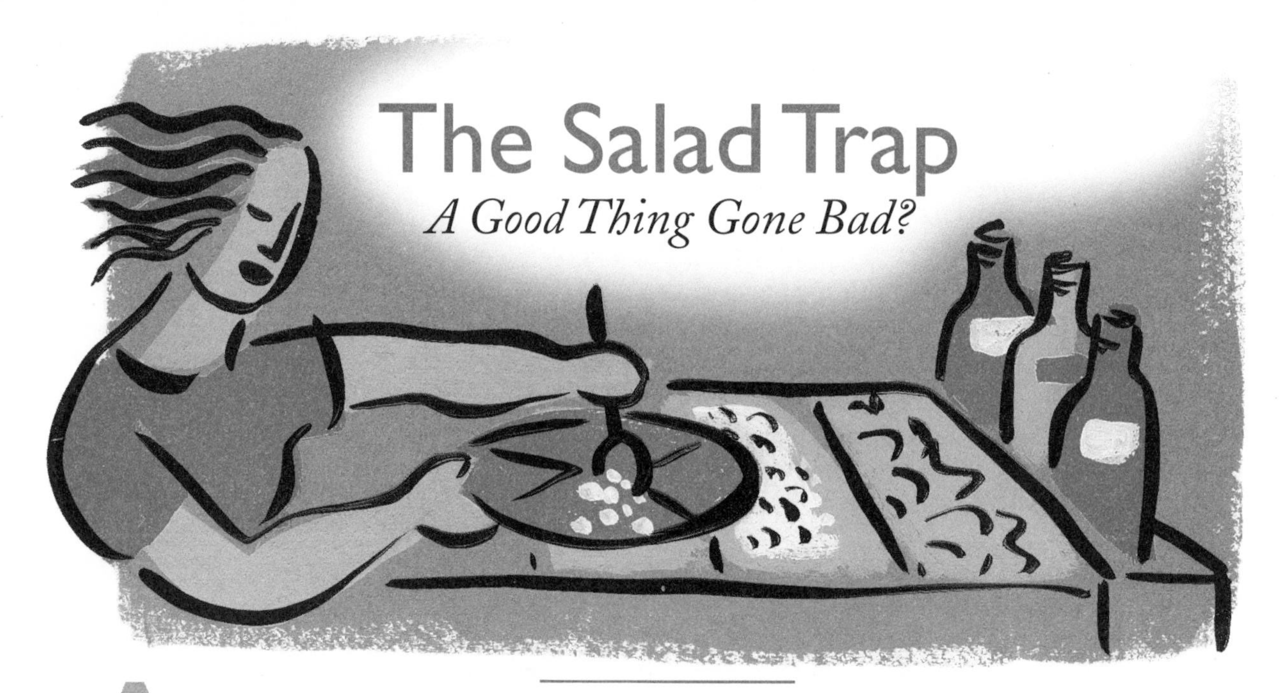

The Salad Trap

A Good Thing Gone Bad?

A salad may seem like a better choice than, say, a burger. But garnish your greens with the wrong choices, and you might just as well eat the ground round—and maybe even have some fries on the side.

To its credit, a salad is an easy way to boost your daily intake of vegetables and fruits. According to the *Prevention* Food Pyramid for Women on page 26, you should eat at least six servings of produce every day. One cup of raw, leafy vegetables counts as a serving, as does ½ cup of chopped raw vegetables, berries, or cut-up fruit. Based on these amounts, a typical main-dish salad could probably get you as much as halfway toward your six-a-day goal.

What's more, all those veggies and fruits often contain loads of nutrients that your body needs, such as vitamins A and C, folate, and fiber. And many are rich in phytochemicals, disease-fighting, health-promoting chemical compounds that scientists have just begun to isolate in foods.

Unfortunately, the natural goodness of these ingredients is routinely undermined by the fat we pour on top to make it all taste good. "Salad dressing is the biggest source of fat in a woman's diet," notes Jayne Hurley, R.D., senior nutritionist with the Center for Science in the Public Interest, a nonprofit consumer group in Washington, D.C., and a writer for *Nutrition Action Healthletter*. In fact, according to statistics from the National Cancer Institute and the U.S. Department of Agriculture Human Nutrition Information Service, salad dressing accounts for almost 10 percent of the average woman's fat intake—more than even margarine, cheese, or ground beef.

Then there are the other high-fat salad toppings: olives, croutons, cheeses, bacon bits, and chow mein noodles, to name just a few. Pair them with a ladle or two of creamy dressing, and that formerly nutritious salad can easily surpass the 1,000-calorie mark. By comparison, even a Burger King Double Whopper with Cheese has only 960 calories.

Good Grazing

The salad, of course, has a place in a healthy diet—if you know how to navigate the salad bar.

SIZING UP THE SALADS

"I'll have a salad."

Not so fast. A salad isn't always the healthiest choice on a restaurant menu. Depending on what's in it, it can have an even worse nutritional profile than that classic dietary demon, fast food.

We asked the folks at the Rodale Test Kitchen to evaluate the nutrient content of four popular main-dish salads: chef, grilled chicken Caesar, niçoise, and taco. They based their calculations on serving sizes of 2 to 3½ cups—typical of the humongous portions that many restaurants serve. The results, which are shown below, may surprise you.

CHEF SALAD

Menu description: A large bed of greens heaped with ham, salami, and chicken breast and garnished with eggs, tomatoes, cucumbers, carrots, Cheddar cheese, and Gruyère cheese. Served with ranch dressing.

Per 3-cup serving:
Calories: 743
Fat: 48 grams; 59 percent of calories
Cholesterol: 389 milligrams
Sodium: 1,340 milligrams

GRILLED CHICKEN CAESAR SALAD

Menu description: A classic Caesar salad topped with slices of grilled chicken breast. (Translated, "classic Caesar" consists of romaine lettuce, anchovies, garlic, Parmesan cheese, croutons, olive oil, and lemon juice.)

Per 3- to 3½-cup serving:
Calories: 941
Fat: 46 grams; 44 percent of calories
Cholesterol: 114 milligrams
Sodium: 2,342 milligrams

SALADE NIÇOISE

Menu description: Grilled marinated fresh tuna on a bed of mixed greens with green beans, onions, potatoes, tomatoes, eggs, anchovies, capers, and black olives. Served with French vinaigrette. (Don't let the word *vinaigrette* fool you—its base is olive oil.)

Per 2-cup serving:
Calories: 680
Fat: 48 grams; 64 percent of calories
Cholesterol: 236 milligrams
Sodium: 860 milligrams

TACO SALAD

Menu description: Mounds of lettuce topped with simmering ground beef, black beans, pinto beans, tomatoes, onions, Monterey Jack cheese, olives, salsa, and sour cream served in a tortilla shell.

Per 3-cup serving:
Calories: 886
Fat: 62 grams; 63 percent of calories
Cholesterol: 112 milligrams
Sodium: 539 milligrams

The following tips from nutrition experts can help you create salads that draw the line at fat and calories.

Turn over a new leaf. Iceberg lettuce is standard at most salad bars, but truth be told, it doesn't hold a candle to its darker green brethren in terms of nutrient content. Romaine lettuce, for example, has twice as much calcium and iron and eight times as much vitamin A and vitamin C as iceberg. As a good rule of thumb, the darker your leafy greens, the more nutritious they are. Other smart selections to look for include kale, spinach, watercress, and arugula.

Veg out. Fresh, raw vegetables add flavor and color to a salad, not to mention healthy doses of important vitamins and minerals. You can beef up your salad's nutritional profile with any combination of the following toppings.

- **BEETS:** One-half cup of these red gems supplies a whopping 68 micrograms of folate, a vitamin that moms-to-be need to protect their babies against birth defects. There's also evidence to suggest that folate may protect against cervical dysplasia, the development of abnormal cells in the cervix that is sometimes a precursor to cancer.
- **BROCCOLI FLORETS:** One-half cup provides 41 milligrams of disease-fighting vitamin C, or 68 percent of your Daily Value (DV).
- **CARROTS:** You won't find a better food source of vitamin A—½ cup has 17,159 IU, or over 300 percent of the DV. You get a good amount of fiber, too.
- **CAULIFLOWER:** Like its cruciferous cousin broccoli, cauliflower is rich in vitamin C—about 23 milligrams in ½ cup.
- **CELERY:** Except for small amounts of folate, vitamin C, fiber, and potassium, celery doesn't have a whole lot of nutritional value. But it does give your salad a lot of crunch for just a few calories and practically no fat.
- **CUCUMBERS:** Another "crunchable," cucumbers contribute small amounts of fiber, folate, potassium, and vitamin C to your salad.
- **MUSHROOMS:** Along with copper, mushrooms provide a B-vitamin boost of folate, niacin, and riboflavin.
- **PEPPERS:** Sweet red peppers are another stellar source of vitamin C, providing 87 milligrams per ½ cup chopped. Their green counterparts supply a not-too-shabby 66 milligrams. You can't beat either variety for vibrant color and satisfying crunch.
- **RED CABBAGE:** With more vitamin C than the pale green variety, red cabbage also supplies some vitamin B_6 and fiber.
- **TOMATOES:** There's no better source of lycopene, a relatively unknown "supernutrient" that scientists believe helps to protect against a number of different cancers as well as cervical dysplasia.

Be fruit-full. Many salad bars feature nutrient-rich fresh fruits, from melon wedges and pineapple spears to kiwifruit and berries. Enjoy them on the side—or add them to your greens to give your salad just a touch of natural sweetness.

Pick some protein. Scout the salad bar for legumes such as kidney beans, chickpeas, black beans, lentils, and split peas. They're low in fat and high in fiber and protein—perfect as a meat substitute in a healthy salad.

If you have a hankering for the real thing, choose turkey breast or chicken breast. They're not as low in fat as legumes (they get about 20 percent of their calories from fat), but they're not nearly as bad as most lunchmeats.

Sprinkle on the cheese. When sprinkled on your salad sparingly, cheese supplies a nice-size dose of bone-building calcium. It's best to choose low-fat or nonfat varieties, but you can't always tell what you're getting at a salad bar. Grated Parmesan is usually a safe bet. It's higher than most other cheeses in calcium, and one or two tablespoons can go a little farther than a shredded type.

Fake out fat. Anything can look healthy when it's surrounded by a sea of greens and veggies. But beware the usual salad bar fat traps: nuts and seeds, sliced olives, croutons, chow mein noodles, and bacon bits. Any of these can sabotage your salad by driving up its calorie and fat content.

Sample with restraint. Just because something is called a salad doesn't mean it's good for you. Take potato salad: Just ½ cup can add 179 calories and 10 grams of fat to your plate. In general, it's a good idea to avoid this and other mayonnaise-based, deli-style concoctions.

But if you do want to sample, wait until your second trip to the salad bar. Fill up on the healthy stuff first, so "just a taste" doesn't turn into an entire plateful.

BETTER LEFT UNDRESSED

Those ladles in the salad dressings at the salad bar can hold anywhere from ¾ to 2 ounces. That may not sound like much—until you consider how much fat and calories those ounces contain.

Here's how some popular full-fat dressings measure up in terms of fat content per 2-ounce serving (four tablespoons).

Dressing	Fat (g.)	Calories
Blue cheese	32	308
French	26	268
Italian	28	275
Russian	31	302
Thousand Island	22	234

Dressing Down

Your salad may not seem complete without your favorite dressing drizzled over the top. But before you grab the ladle and pour, consider this: If you overdo it, you can turn a perfectly healthful plate of greens and vegetables into unhealthy fare that gets as much as 70 percent of its calories from fat.

The obvious solution is to stick with a nonfat or low-fat salad dressing, but even that should be used with a light touch. You may want to try one of these options instead.

Give it a squeeze. Lemon or lime juice makes a nice substitute for traditional salad dressing, and it gives your salad a burst of vitamin C to boot. Simply squeeze a slice or two of the fruit right onto your salad for a light yet zesty taste.

Try something new. If you're an oil-and-vinegar fan, sample some of the more exotic vinegars that some salad bars offer these days, such as balsamic, champagne, raspberry, and white- or red-wine. Their robust flavors mean you can get by with a lot less oil—say, three parts vinegar to only one part oil.

Make your own. At home, you can combine a couple of salad bar staples to create a "dressing" with less fat and fewer calories than their premade counterparts. For example, spoon out some low-fat yogurt and add just enough reduced-calorie mayonnaise to thicken it, then add it to your salad. Or mix just a small amount of low-fat dressing with some low-fat cottage cheese and use that as your salad topping.

Think thin. Among regular, full-fat dressings, thin ones such as French and Italian tend to be better choices than thicker ones such as blue cheese and Thousand Island. This is true not because they have less fat but because they spread more easily, so you can use less.

Keep it on the side. Rather than ladling the dressing right over your salad, put it in a small container. Then lightly dip your fork into the container before spearing your salad. This method gives you better portion control.

Water—Liquid Gold

Drink to Your Health's Content

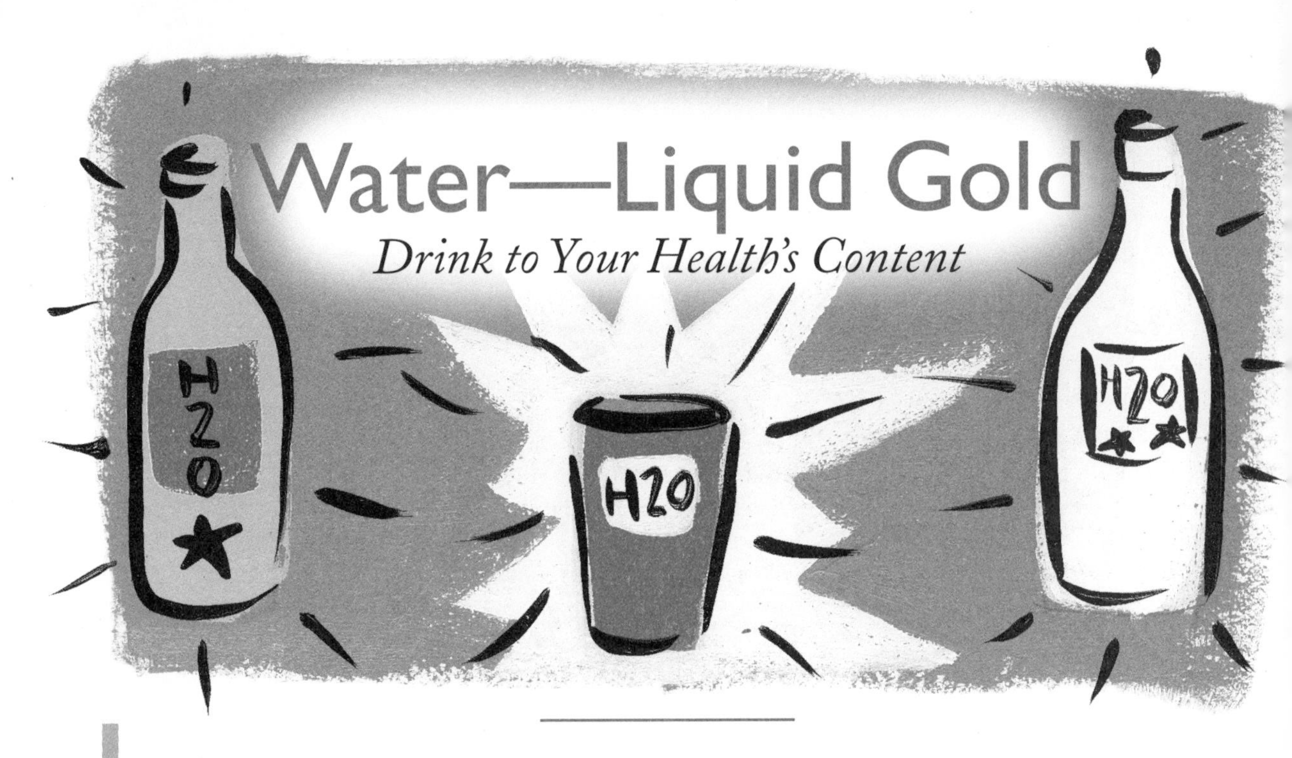

In the 1970s, we were singing in *"per-fect har-mo-ny"* to a catchy commercial jingle that wanted us to drink Coke. Years later, we became enchanted by a comely couple being romantic over their cups of Taster's Choice coffee. Then milk became the commercial drink of choice with its celebrity-mustached ad campaign.

It's about time for water to get its due. After all, water is the only fluid that you truly can't live without. Every cell in your body depends on it to function properly. In fact, your body processes about two to three quarts a day to transport nutrients to where they're needed, get rid of body wastes, regulate temperature, support chemical reactions, and perform other critical tasks.

That's why drinking water is so important. If you don't replenish your internal water supply, you can easily become dehydrated—which in turn prevents your body from performing as it should. This is more of a problem for women than for men, notes Felicia Busch, R.D., a nutritionist in St. Paul, Minnesota, and a fellow of the American Dietetic Association. Unlike men, women tend to have more body fat than muscle. And body fat doesn't hold water as well as muscle.

Benefits by the Glassful

Clearly, water plays a vital role in keeping all of your body's systems running smoothly. But this versatile nutrient can do a whole lot more for your good health. Here are some examples.

Water burns fat. Like every other chemical reaction in your body, fat-burning can occur only in the presence of water. And some scientists believe that running low on H_2O can actually cause your body to store fat.

Water satisfies your appetite. Water takes up a lot of room in your stomach, so you feel full and don't want to eat as much. And you won't find a better "diet drink" than water: It contains no calories or fat.

Water quashes cravings. Sometimes what you interpret as a hunger pang is really your body telling you that it's thirsty. Try sipping a glass of water before you raid the refrigerator—your urge to eat may subside within minutes.

Water combats the effects of stress. Stress can really do a number on your body. Staying hydrated keeps your body's systems in balance and counteracts stress "symptoms" such as perspiration, dry mouth, and heart palpitations.

Water fends off fatigue. If you feel like you're running on empty, maybe you need to fill up on fluids. Tiredness is a common—though often unrecognized—sign of dehydration.

Water boosts your brainpower. Dehydration can also leave you with a bad case of mental fuzzies. In fact, some researchers have suggested that too little water in your body can cause your brain to shrink ever so slightly, affecting your ability to think and concentrate.

Water turns back the clock. Instead of spending a small fortune on facial creams and lotions, generously sip Nature's own beauty fluid. Water helps fend off wrinkles and other signs of aging, leaving your skin smooth and supple.

Water keeps you moving. Your body uses water as a natural lubricant. It cushions your joints and helps them stay limber so you don't stiffen up like a statue.

Water douses urinary tract infections. In a survey of 16,000 women, 82 percent named water as the most effective home remedy for bladder infections, the most common type of urinary tract infection (UTI). Doctors agree that drinking plenty of fluids can help flush UTI-causing bacteria out of your system.

REAL-LIFE SCENARIO

Kick the Coffee and Cola Habit

Sara loves coffee and counts on it to keep her going all day long. She nurses her first cup while packing lunches for her husband and kids, then pours a big one to take with her on her morning commute. After two more refills at work, she switches to diet cola: one with lunch and another to get her through the afternoon. At 5:00, she fills her coffee cup one last time. At dinner, she has a big glass of water, but afterward she likes to relax with a glass or two of wine. Sara's daily fluid intake is high—after all, she has all those trips to the bathroom to prove it! But her doctor says she's not getting enough fluids. Can this be?

Absolutely! That's because everything Sara drinks—except that single glass of water at dinner—has either caffeine or alcohol in it, and both act as diuretics. Although coffee, cola, and wine all contain water, anything containing caffeine or alcohol forces water out of the body. If you only drank beverages with caffeine or alcohol, you could conceivably release more fluids than you take in!

Sara's best move would be to cut out some of those coffees and colas, but she obviously relies on the effect of their caffeine to get her through the day. Two cups of high-test in the morning are okay, but at work she might try gradually switching over to decaf by mixing a little with the regular stuff. Eventually, Sara may be able to drink decaf straight.

Sara's afternoon diet colas serve the same purpose as coffee—they keep her going. As with the coffee, she needs to gradually switch to decaffeinated soft drinks, and she should consider replacing some of that cola with a glass or two of juice.

As for Sara's dinnertime wine—a glass for good health is okay, but she should limit it to one glass. Alcohol has the same diuretic effect as caffeine. For every alcoholic beverage that she drinks, Sara needs to drink a comparable amount of water.

Expert Consulted
Neva Cochran, R.D.
Private nutrition consultant
American Dietetic Association spokesperson
Dallas

Water staves off colon cancer. Researchers at the Fred Hutchinson Cancer Research Center in Seattle have uncovered a possible link between water consumption and colon cancer. In a survey they conducted, women who drank more than five glasses of water a day had about half the risk of colon cancer of women who drank less than two glasses of water a day.

Getting Your Fill

To replenish the water your body uses up, you need to drink at least eight eight-ounce glasses of water a day. And we're talking water here—not Diet Coke, coffee, or other popular drinks. Many of the bottled beverages on the market contain sodium and caffeine, which are diuretics. You may not notice it, but they'll dehydrate, rather than hydrate, you.

"You do get water through certain foods, too, such as fruits and vegetables, which are about 90 percent water," says Judy E. Marshel, R.D., director of Health Resources in Great Neck, New York. "And your body chips in another ½ cup or so as a by-product of metabolism, your body's calorie-burning mechanism." But that's not enough. You should try to drink 64 ounces of water every day, recommends Marshel.

If downing 64 ounces of water daily seems hard to swallow, relax. With the following strategies recommended by nutrition experts, drinking water will become an enjoyable habit.

Drink up when you wake up. Start your day with a glass of water. It will help make up for the fluids you lost while you were sleeping.

Contain yourself. Here's an easy way to keep track of your daily water intake: Invest in a 32-ounce container that you can carry with you as you go about your daily business and can refill throughout the day.

Sip, don't gulp. Take just a little bit of water at a time. If you try to down all 64 ounces in one, two, or even three sittings, you'll get tired of it mighty quickly.

Beat thirst to the punch. Don't wait until you feel parched to start sipping. By the time your thirst mechanism kicks in, you're already well on your way to empty. In fact, you can lose as much as 2 percent of your body weight through perspiration or urination before you get the urge to drink something.

Consider the conditions. There are times when you may need to increase your water intake beyond the usual 64 ounces a day. For instance, to stay hydrated during a workout, you should drink a large glass of water 30 to 60 minutes beforehand, then take a few sips every 15 minutes or so while you exercise. Likewise, you should up your ounces of H_2O if you're sick, pregnant, or breastfeeding; if you spend a lot of time in a heated or air-conditioned environment; or if you're traveling by plane. (The recirculated air in the cabin of the plane can easily leave you dehydrated.)

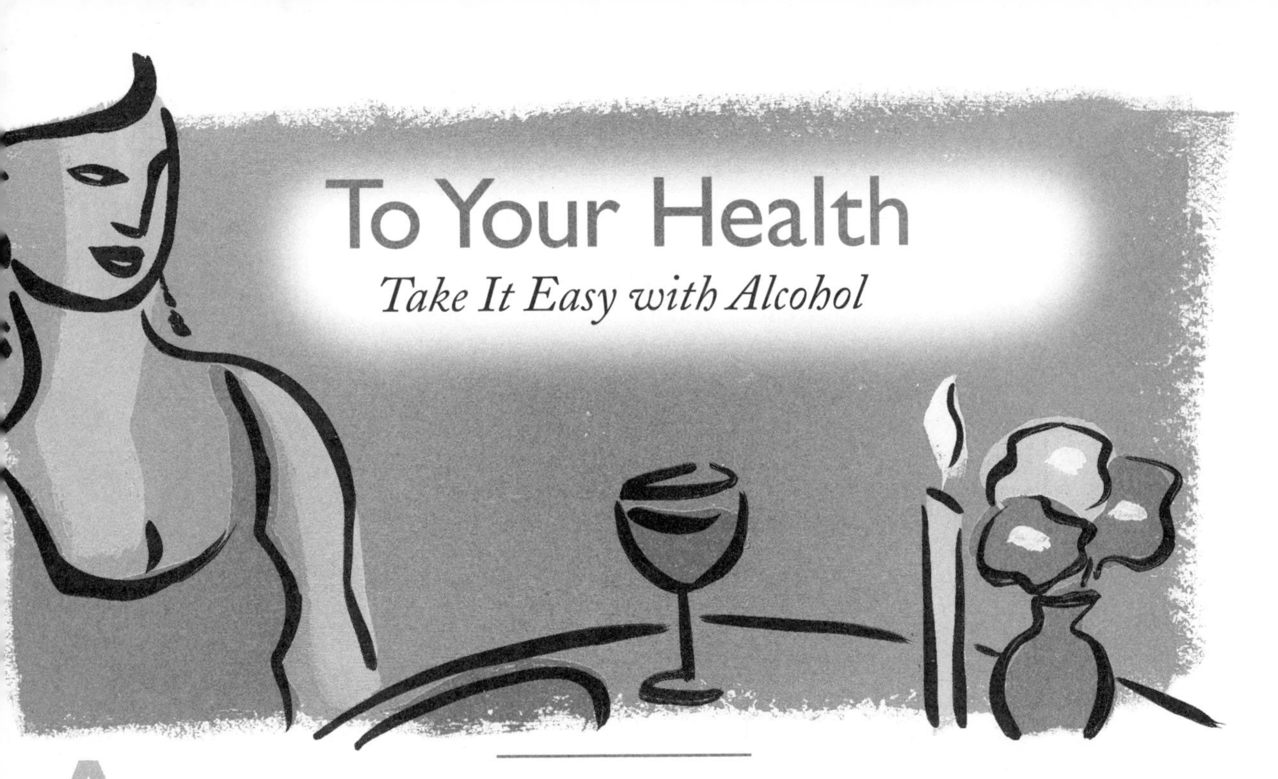

To Your Health

Take It Easy with Alcohol

Alcohol has sure come a long way, from social scourge in the Roaring Twenties to acclaimed elixir at the turn of the twenty-first century. Indeed, the news that alcohol can protect against heart disease may have you poised to drink a toast to your favorite spirits.

Not so fast, experts say. While alcoholic beverages may offer some health benefits, they also have some very real risks. "The fact remains that alcohol is a general toxin—in other words, it can travel anywhere in your body because there's nothing to stop it," says Anne Geller, M.D., chief of the Smithers Addiction Treatment and Training Center at St. Luke's–Roosevelt Hospital Center in New York City. "And anywhere it goes, it can potentially cause problems."

This is especially true for women, Dr. Geller explains, because we experience the negative effects of alcohol at much lower levels than men do. By one estimate, the harmful amount of alcohol for women is about 60 percent of the harmful amount of alcohol for men.

Now we're not suggesting that you take to the streets, a one-woman army marching for the return of Prohibition. We are saying that you need to consume booze wisely by weighing the pros and cons before you take your next sip.

The French Connection

Those revolutionary French. They're the ones who flambéed conventional nutrition wisdom a few years back, when researchers determined that folks who live in the land of rich cream sauces and decadent pastries are 2½ times less likely than we Americans to die from heart disease. This, despite the fact that they eat four times as much butter as we do.

The secret to their seemingly Teflon-coated cardiovascular systems? Researchers suspect it has something to do with the red wine that the French savor so much.

Red wine is loaded with natural compounds called flavonoids. Research suggests that these supernutrients may protect the heart in two ways. First, evidence indicates that flavonoids may prevent harmful low-density lipoprotein cholesterol from sticking to artery walls and

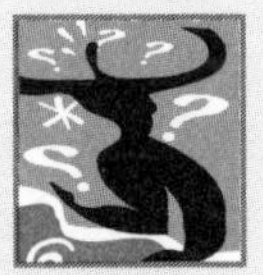

WOMEN ASK WHY

Why is it that women can't hold their liquor as well as men?

You'd think that the most obvious answer is the difference in size, which is true, but it's only part of the reason. More significant is the fact that men's bodies contain more of the natural "mixer"—water.

A woman's body weight is about 45 to 50 percent water, compared to 55 to 60 percent in men—mainly because guys have a higher proportion of lean muscle tissue, which holds almost three times as much water as fat tissue does. When you drink alcohol, it runs through your bloodstream and is eventually distributed to your tissues, where it is metabolized. It's the alcohol in your blood that gives you the buzz, and it's the amount of water that you have in your tissues that determines how quickly the alcohol moves to safe ground.

So if you try to stay one-on-one with the boys, chances are that you're going to get drunker faster.

The best solution is to forget trying to keep up with the Jacks and Daniels and drink sensibly. That means limiting yourself to one drink an hour and sipping plenty of water to help metabolize the alcohol.

Expert Consulted
Johanna Dwyer, R.D., D.Sc.
Professor of medicine and community health
Tufts University Schools of Medicine and Nutrition Science Policy
Director of Frances Stern Nutrition Center
New England Medical Center Hospital
Boston

clogging up the works. And second, flavonoids may stop blood platelets from clumping together and forming dangerous clots.

While red wine has the strongest protective effects, other alcoholic beverages can give your heart a boost, too. Though more research is needed, some studies have shown that any alcohol—whether it's white wine, beer, or a mixed drink—can raise your blood level of high-density lipoprotein cholesterol, the good kind that helps keep your arteries clean.

To Drink or Not to Drink

Once you get past all the heart-health headlines, however, alcohol begins to show a decidedly mean streak. Among the most provocative findings so far: A four-state study of 15,000 women revealed that moderate alcohol consumption—just one drink a day—increases breast cancer risk by 30 to 40 percent.

If you're trying to lose weight, alcohol won't do you any favors, either. For one thing, it contributes a lot of extra calories to your diet—105 in 5 ounces of wine and 150 in a 12-ounce beer. At a rate of just one drink a day, that's more than 700 unwanted calories per week. In just five weeks, you'd consume enough calories to gain one pound.

What's more, alcohol appears to inhibit your body's fat-burning mechanism and promote fat storage. And it pumps up your appetite: One study at the Mayo Clinic in Rochester, Minnesota, found that a person consumes about 350 extra calories when she has an alcoholic beverage with her meal.

Excessive alcohol consumption, defined as three or more drinks a day, presents its own set of health problems. For starters, heavy drinking wreaks havoc on your hormones, according to

Dr. Geller. You may experience irregular menstrual cycles and, eventually, premature menopause. "Your body composition changes, too," Dr. Geller says. "You gain fat and lose muscle." You become more vulnerable to osteoporosis as alcohol leaches calcium from your bones. Your odds of developing colorectal cancer also jump—perhaps by as much as 78 percent, according to Harvard University researchers.

Smart Sipping

Understandably, all these issues have left many experts reluctant to endorse alcohol consumption as a healthy habit. "The question is not 'Is alcohol safe?' but 'What amount of alcohol is safe?' " Dr. Geller says.

Of course, finding the answer will require a lot more research. In the meantime, if you don't drink, don't start. And if you do drink, keep these guidelines in mind.

Know your limit. Guidelines established by the National Institute of Alcohol and Alcohol Abuse suggest that women can safely consume one drink a day without experiencing any ill effects. (A drink, incidentally, is defined as 12 ounces of regular beer, 5 ounces of wine, or a cocktail made with 1½ ounces of 80-proof distilled spirits.)

Some experts advocate a more conservative limit—say, two or three drinks per week, tops. "A woman has to weigh her own benefits and risks," Dr. Geller says. "If you have a family history of breast cancer, then you'd be wise to restrict your alcohol consumption. On the other hand, if breast cancer doesn't run in your family but heart disease does, a drink a day won't hurt."

Wash it down. If you do have a drink, follow it with a glass or two of water, suggests Felicia Busch, R.D., a nutritionist in St. Paul, Minnesota, and a fellow of the American Dietetic Association. The reason: Alcohol is a diuretic, which means that it makes you urinate more frequently. Following up with an H_2O chaser helps replenish lost fluids and prevent dehydration.

Consider the source. Red wine doesn't hold a monopoly on heart-healthy flavonoids. They're plentiful in a variety of foods, including onions, apples, broccoli, tea—and, of course, grapes. So instead of imbibing to get your fill of flavonoids, choose one of these nonalcoholic alternatives instead.

Give baby a healthy start. If you're a mom-to-be, abstain from drinking for the duration of your pregnancy. Alcohol can cause fetal alcohol syndrome, the number one cause of mental retardation.

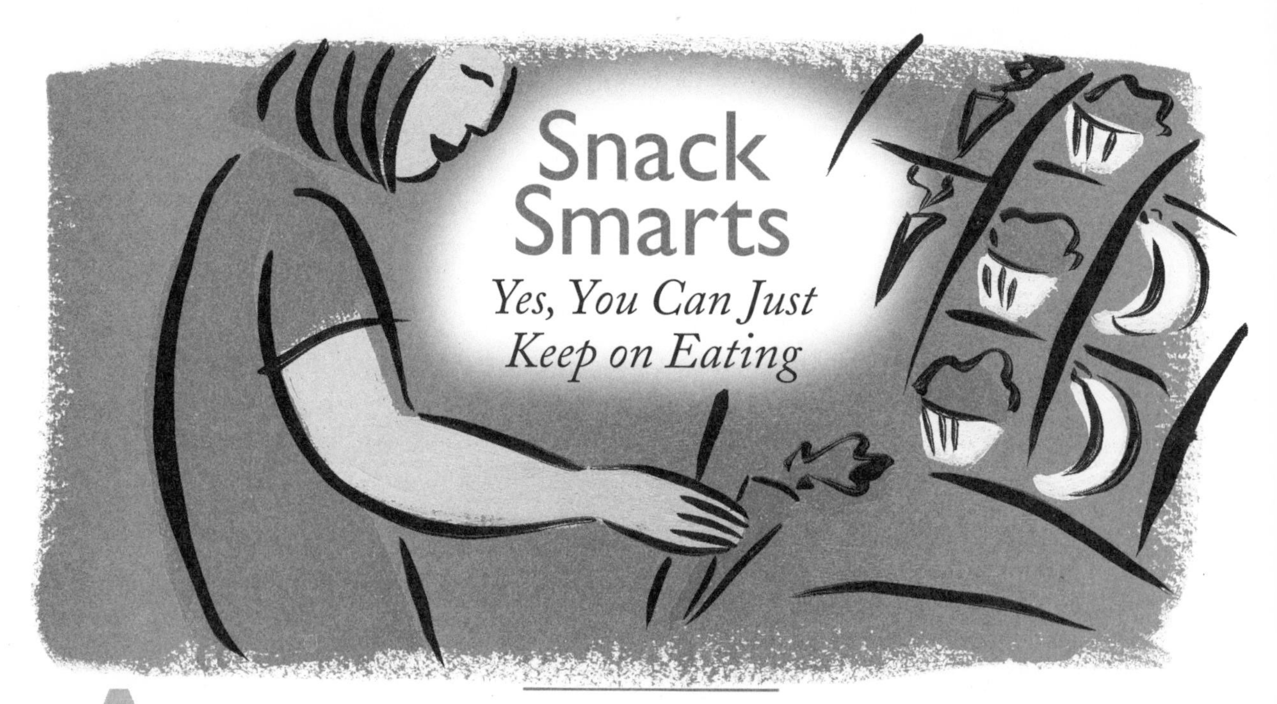

Snack Smarts

Yes, You Can Just Keep on Eating

According to the head-counters who track such things, at least three-quarters of us women eat one or more snacks every day. The rest of us may be missing out on the healthiest dietary habit this side of breakfast.

It seems that the experts have begun to rethink the long-accepted notion that snacking expands your waistline, spoils your appetite, rots your teeth, and commits various other nutritional offenses against your health. Many now believe that between-meal nibbling, combined with smaller versions of the traditional three squares, can keep your body functioning on a more even keel and reduce your risk of some big-ticket health problems.

"Your body needs food—its fuel—in moderate doses throughout the day so it always has nutrients available," says Pat Harper, R.D., a nutrition consultant in Pittsburgh. "I find that having four or five 'mini-meals' daily helps most people prevent cravings and ultimately achieve and maintain a healthy weight."

This new way of eating—or "grazing"—has put snacking in the nutritional mainstream. But you have to know how to do it right. "Try thinking of snacks as foods eaten between meals rather than as treats or rewards," suggests Barbara Whedon, R.D., a dietitian and nutrition counselor at Thomas Jefferson University Hospital in Philadelphia. "You should choose them just as you would plan a meal—with variety, balance, and moderation in mind."

Big Benefits from Grazing

Researchers have only recently begun investigating the possible health benefits of the small-meals-plus-snacks style of eating. But what they've uncovered so far is quite compelling. Here is just a sampling of what grazing can do for you.

Snacking sends pounds packing. Women who want to lose weight often skip breakfast as a way to lower their calorie intakes. Studies have shown that this practice does more harm than good. Not eating your morning meal actually makes you more likely to compensate for the missing calories—and then some—by overeating later in the day. On the other hand, eating small meals and snacks more frequently helps you to manage your appetite better, so you never get too hungry.

Grazing can also keep your metabolism, or calorie-burning mechanism, running high. Your body uses calories when you eat and digest food. By consuming smaller amounts of food more frequently, you can end up burning calories very efficiently. You'll be less likely to gain weight, even though it may seem like you're eating more than you did before.

Snacking fights fatigue. When more than four hours go by between meals, your body's energy supply—your blood sugar, or glucose—dips low enough to allow fatigue to set in. Well-timed snacks give your body a steady supply of fuel, so you're at your best physically and mentally throughout the day. Studies have shown that a snack between 2:00 and 4:00 in the afternoon can improve cognitive skills such as memory, arithmetic reasoning, reading speed, and attention span, notes Harper.

Snacking combats high cholesterol. Research comparing people who eat six or more mini-meals a day with people who eat the customary three squares has consistently shown lower cholesterol levels in the nibblers. In one study, consuming six mini-meals a day shaved cholesterol levels by 8 percent, which translates to a 16 percent reduction in heart attack risk. To put it another way, a 1 percent reduction in cholesterol

REAL-LIFE SCENARIO

The Compulsive Snacker

Kathryn loves to snack—ice cream, potato chips, and chocolate are her weaknesses. But she knows that they're high in fat and calories, so she only indulges in them once in a while. The problem is that Kathryn is such a snack-lover that she's eating all the time—popcorn, pretzels, cheese, peanut butter, low-fat cookies, bagels, yogurt—you name it. So by the time mealtime rolls around, she's not really all that hungry and either picks at or skips the meal altogether. Kathryn says she can handle the weight problem; she's been 10 to 20 pounds overweight all her life. But lately she's fatigued a lot and wonders if taking a multivitamin will solve the problem.

Although Kathryn is eating almost constantly, she rarely eats fruits and vegetables, which means that her diet is sorely lacking in important vitamins and minerals. While a daily multivitamin may help, she still won't get the full benefit of eating a balanced diet, including all the fiber and complex carbohydrates that her snack foods seem to be lacking. She's getting way too many calories and probably too much fat with very little nutritional return.

Kathryn can't be sure, though, that her poor diet is the cause of her fatigue. A nutritional shortage is only one of many possible causes of fatigue. She also needs to examine her lifestyle. The fact that she eats poorly is an indication of a lifestyle out of whack.

The first thing Kathryn needs to do is to get on a meal plan, beginning with breakfast. If she can't do it on her own, she should seek the aid of a nutritionist, who can help her evaluate everything from her lifestyle to her food habits to her physical activity. She'll probably also find that replacing her snack habit with a balanced diet will help her lose those extra pounds. Then maybe her fatigue will be a thing of the past.

Expert Consulted
Rebecca Reeves, R.D., Dr. P.H.
Chief dietitian
Baylor College of Medicine Nutrition Research Clinic
Houston

lowers the risk of heart attack at least 2 percent, according to evidence from several other studies.

Snacking fends off heart attacks. A small-meals-plus-snacks eating strategy can help reduce your risk of heart attack by keeping your heart's workload during digestion to a minimum. Whenever you eat, your heart has to pump extra blood to your stomach and intestines to aid the digestive process.

One study demonstrated that meal size can make a difference in terms of cardiovascular demand. When women ate a 240-calorie meal of cornflakes and skim milk, their hearts pumped an extra 84 quarts of blood over the next two hours. When they ate a 720-calorie meal with added sugar, bread, and honey, their hearts pumped an extra 258 quarts of blood—enough to fill your car's gas tank five times over. This might help explain why doctors see an increase in the number of heart attack patients within 24 hours after big holiday meals.

The 10 Healthiest Snacks

Looking for something to munch? We've ferreted out 10 noteworthy low-fat noshes recommended by the American Dietetic Association that will more than satisfy your tastebuds while sneaking in generous amounts of some very important nutrients. No, cookies, ice cream, and potato chips didn't make the grade. But we'll guarantee that once you get used to this new way of snacking, you won't even miss that high-fat, high-calorie fare.

Bagel. One two-ounce enriched bagel supplies two milligrams of iron—11 percent of the Daily Value (DV)—along with good doses of the B vitamins niacin, riboflavin, and thiamin. Instead of topping it with full-fat cream cheese, try cottage cheese or part-skim ricotta.

Banana. Widely recognized as a good source of potassium, bananas are also surprisingly rich in vitamin B_6. One four-ounce fruit contains about 0.7 milligram of B_6, or 35 percent of the DV.

Bran muffin. A tasty way to boost your fiber intake: One 1½-ounce muffin provides three grams of the nutrient. You also take in 1.8 milligrams of iron, which is about 10 percent of the DV.

Broccoli. You get over half a full day's supply of vitamin C—41 milligrams, or 68 percent of the DV—in ½ cup of chopped, raw broccoli. This nutrient-rich veggie offers some

Chews Wisely

Now before you get caught up in the grazing craze, just remember that "snack" does not mean a doughnut at midmorning, potato chips at midafternoon, and rocky road ice cream for a nightcap. Whatever you choose to nosh on, it should be reasonably good for you.

To get in the swing of smart snacking, give these tips a try.

Set up a schedule. To get the most benefit from grazing, plan to eat a little something every three to four hours over the course of a day, advises Elizabeth Somer, R.D., author of *Nutrition for Women* and *Food and Mood.* Perhaps the simplest way to do this is to divide each of your usual big meals into two smaller ones. Here's what a typical day's eating might look like.

- Breakfast: cereal, milk, and orange juice
- Morning snack: bagel or banana
- Lunch: turkey sandwich with romaine lettuce, tomato, and nonfat mayo or mustard
- Afternoon snack: pretzels or baked sweet potato
- Dinner: vegetable-bean soup and two small pumpernickel rolls
- Evening snack: baked apple crisp with low-fat yogurt

folate and a good amount of vitamin A, too. Eat it with low-fat dip.

Cantaloupe. Another stellar vitamin C source: One cup of cubed cantaloupe provides 68 milligrams of C, or more than 100 percent of the DV.

Carrot. Eat a single medium-size carrot, and you'll more than satisfy your vitamin A needs for an entire day. Just one contains 17,158 international units of A, which is close to 3½ times the DV.

Mexican-style beans. A ½-cup serving of this filling, flavorful fare provides an impressive 7 grams of fiber—about 26 percent of the DV. Just be sure that the brand you buy doesn't go overboard on sodium.

String cheese. This lower-fat variation on mozzarella cheese supplies 250 milligrams of calcium per 1½-ounce serving. That's about 25 percent of the DV.

Tuna. Three ounces of tuna, canned in water, is an excellent source for your daily requirement for vitamin B_{12}. You'll get 2 micrograms of the nutrient, or 32 percent of the DV. If you need to add mayonnaise to your tuna, just make sure it's low-fat.

Yogurt. Here's another top-notch source of bone-building calcium, with 415 milligrams—about 42 percent of the DV—in every one-cup serving. Be sure to choose nonfat or low-fat varieties.

Be careful not to just add snacks on top of your usual diet. That's a surefire way to gain weight.

Play to your tastebuds. "When we choose a snack, we often simply grab whatever is closest at hand," Whedon observes. "We don't think about what we're really hungry for. And that can lead to overeating because we're not satisfying our cravings."

In general, she says, a snack feeds a need for something chewy, crunchy, smooth, creamy, cold, sweet, salty, or some combination of these qualities. "If you want creamy and sweet, yogurt may be your perfect choice," she notes. "If you desire crunchy and cold, try slices of green pepper."

Feed your hunger, not your head. Stress, boredom, and frustration can all nudge you to nibble when you're not actually hungry. If you suspect that your urge to eat is emotion-driven, distract yourself by taking a walk or listening to music.

Think. It's much too easy to overdo portion size, cautions Margo Denke, M.D., associate professor of internal medicine at the Center for Human Nutrition at the University of Texas Southwestern Medical Center at Dallas. You need to pay attention to every bite, especially if you munch while watching television. Otherwise, you could end up taking in more calories than when you were eating three meals a day.

Stash a stash. Ensure nutritious snacking wherever you go by keeping a stash in your office, car, purse, and briefcase. Some foods that make wonderful travel companions are snack-size boxes of raisins and cereals, cans of low-sodium vegetable juice cocktail, and whole-wheat hard pretzels.

Learn to love leftovers. "Leftovers make great snacks, provided they aren't loaded with fat," says Harper. What you choose ultimately depends on what's in your refrigerator. But don't overlook leftover pasta, cold pizza made with low-fat cheese, half a tuna sandwich, or that three-bean salad you didn't have room for at lunch.

Don't retreat from treats. "Some snacks can be just for fun," says Dr. Denke. If you have a hankering for a cupcake or chips, dig in. Just be sure to compensate by choosing leaner foods for the rest of the day to keep your daily fat intake to about 25 percent of calories.

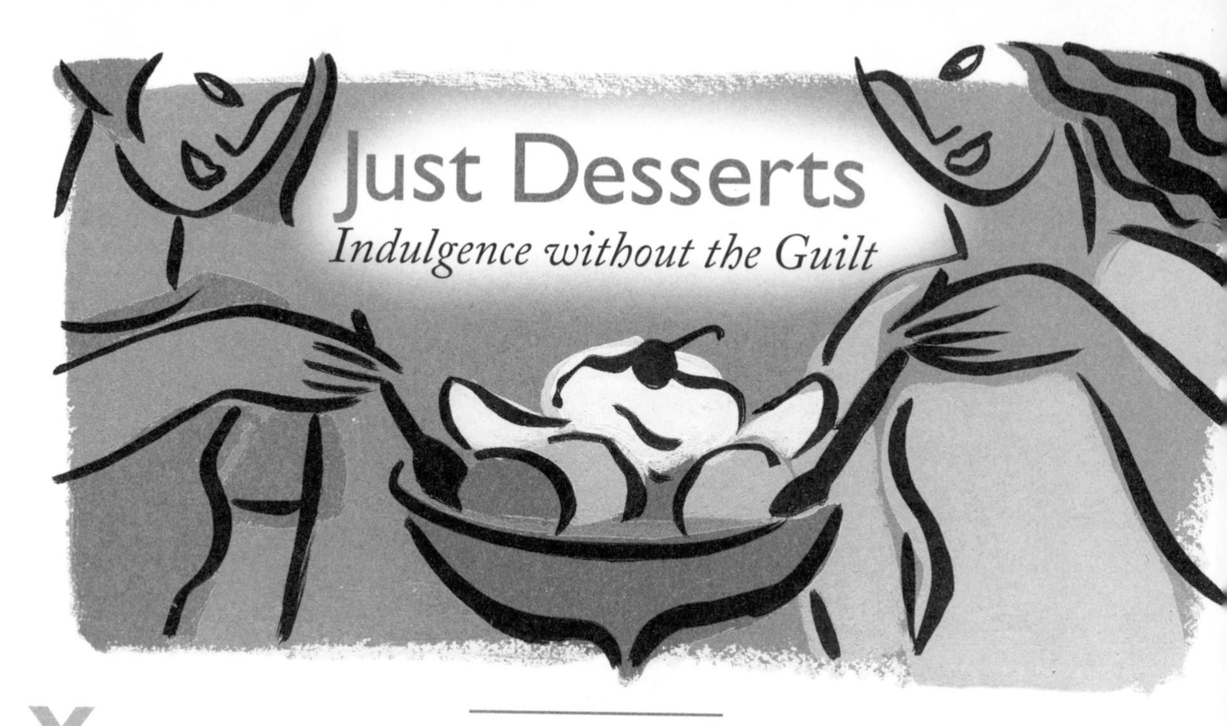

Your brain says, "Strawberries." Your tastebuds say, "Sure—if they're piled high in a piecrust and buried under a mound of whipped cream."

Your brain says, "Well, then, how about a banana?" Your tastebuds say, "Great—as long as it's hugging three scoops of ice cream, all smothered with syrup and coated with nuts."

And so the great dessert debate rages on, and your best intentions are smack in the middle of it. You want to make a healthful choice—and nutrition-wise, nothing beats fresh fruit as an after-dinner treat. But you can't ignore your tastebuds' contention that fruit alone is not dessert.

No, indeed, it's not. So go ahead. Indulge.

In fact, there are a couple of reasons why you should. First, when you deny yourself food that you really want, you may eventually end up stuffing yourself with much more of it once you finally cave in. And second, the sweetness of dessert may signal your brain that feeding time has officially ended. You feel satisfied, so you won't spend your evening browsing your kitchen for munchies.

Besides, if you're going to eat a sweet, it's best that you tack it on to a meal, says Nancy Clark, R.D., director of nutrition services at SportsMedicine Brookline in Brookline, Massachusetts, and author of *Nancy Clark's Sports Nutrition Guidebook*. That way, the fiber, protein, and tiny amount of fat in the other foods can slow the absorption of sugar into your bloodstream. Your blood sugar level holds steady, which in turn keeps your energy supply on a more even keel.

Happy Endings

While dessert has its place in a healthy diet, you do need to exercise some restraint. Cheesecake, hot fudge sundaes, and other high-fat goodies are not everyday fare. Go for the gooey once a week, at best. When you do feel the urge to splurge, here's how to do it right.

Make the most of every mouthful. Don't polish off your dessert so fast that you barely taste it. Instead, eat *sloooowly*, allowing every bite to linger on your tongue.

It takes a while for your brain to acknowledge the fact that you're having dessert. If you relax your pace, you will have eaten less by the time your brain gets the message and calls off your craving for a sweet.

Stay single. Another way to limit how much dessert you eat is to stick with individually wrapped goodies. "It's better to buy a box of Fudgsicles than a half-gallon of ice cream," says Georgia Kostas, R.D., director of nutrition at the Cooper Clinic in Dallas and author of *The Balancing Act Nutrition and Weight Guide*. "That gives you built-in portion control."

Check the label. Buyer beware: Some manufacturers are able to "reduce" the fat content of a packaged food by changing the serving size. Take Twinkies snacks as an example. For the regular variety, the number of fat grams is based on two cakes per serving. For the low-fat variety, it's based on only one cake per serving.

Spot the sneaky treats. Some desserts taste like they have much more fat than they actually do. Among them are angel food cake (0.1 gram of fat per serving), fig bars (1 gram), fortune cookies (0 gram), ladyfingers (2 grams), and rice pudding (4 grams). Any of these can satisfy your sweet tooth without guilt.

Grab your toothbrush. Once you've swallowed your last bite, brush your teeth right away. No, you're not trying to get rid of the evidence. Like eating the dessert itself, brushing sends your brain the message that you're finished eating—and that can switch off late-night cravings.

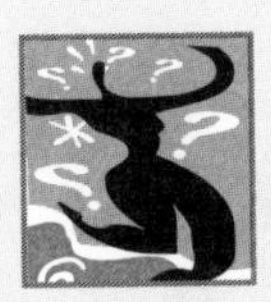

Women Ask Why

Since it has no fat and only 16 calories per teaspoon, why does sugar have such a bad reputation?

Sugar itself isn't necessarily bad; it's the fact that we overuse it that gives sugar such a bad name. In the United States, the per capita consumption of caloric sweeteners went up from 129 pounds to 153 pounds over the past decade. Most of this sugar isn't "table sugar" that we add ourselves; it's the refined sugar and corn sweeteners that are added to the sweets we love, including the many fat-free processed foods we buy today.

If you're among those who consume more than a spoonful or two a day, you're getting a lot of calories with little nutritional return. For example, one bottle of a popular brand of flavored iced tea contains over 10 teaspoons of sugar and 200 calories—about 1⁄10 of a typical woman's caloric intake—with zero nutrients. Further, you will most likely gain weight. The hidden sugar in soft drinks, sweets, and processed foods adds up quickly. Plus, excess refined sugar, like too much of any carbohydrate, is stored as fat.

So, sugar's bad reputation is really associated with quantity. If you use it sparingly, it's not going to cause you too much trouble; just a spoonful (or two) isn't going to sabotage your nutrition, your health, or your weight. Admittedly, it's tough to keep your sugar intake in check with all the good-tasting, empty-calorie foods and beverages around, but nutritionally speaking, it's worth it to read food labels and set some limits.

Expert Consulted
Barbara Whedon, R.D.
Nutrition counselor
Thomas Jefferson University Hospital
Philadelphia

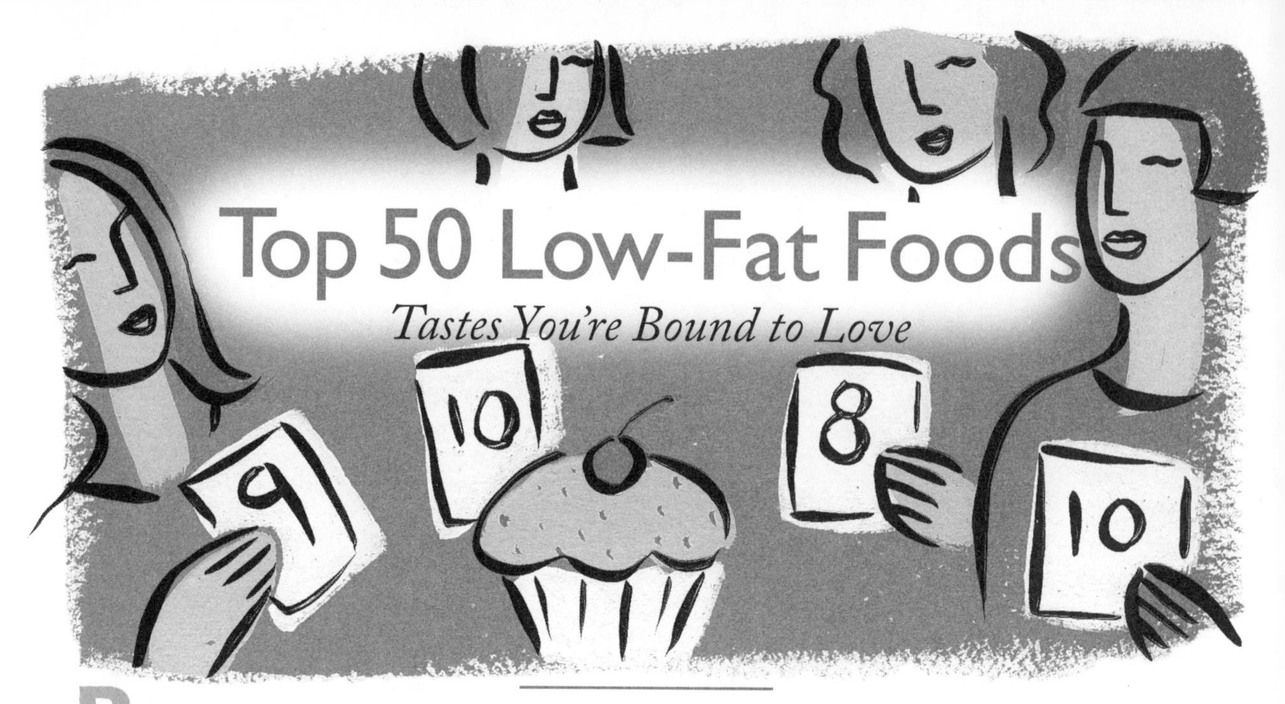

Top 50 Low-Fat Foods

Tastes You're Bound to Love

Beethoven or the Beatles. Pinstripes or polka dots. Ballet or baseball.

So much in life is a matter of taste—especially what you eat. Regardless of how wholesome a food is, if it doesn't please your palate, it will never make it past your bicuspids without throwing your tongue into turmoil.

But good taste and good nutrition don't have to be mutually exclusive. These days we have more eating options than ever, from the growing assortment of exotic fruits and vegetables in the supermarket produce aisle to the expanded selection of packaged nonfat and low-fat products. Thanks to modern technology, junk foods have become healthier, and health foods have undergone a flavor face-lift.

What all this means, of course, is that there are countless ways in which you can satisfy your hunger without one iota of guilt. Now all you have to do is choose.

Rating the Favorites

So when it comes to making choices from the vast new assortment of low-fat flavors, what appeals most deliciously to a woman's tastebuds?

To find out, we conducted an informal survey of 100 health-conscious women to get their vote on the most flavorful low-fat foods. Then, just to make sure these low-fat faves actually are low in fat and good for you, we ran the list by Toni Ferrang, R.D., owner of Food for Thought Nutrition Consulting in Burlingame, California.

Here, then, are the top 50 low-fat foods, rated by a random sampling of American women and arranged from A to Z.

1. Angel food cake. "Great!" Ferrang says. "Make it even better by topping it with cut-up fruit and some nonfat or low-fat yogurt."

2. Apples. Our survey-takers love apples for their crunch and portability. They're a good source of fiber, too, Ferrang notes.

3. Bagels. "The best low-fat food God ever made," one respondent raves. "Just keep in mind that a typical bagel-shop bagel has 200 to 350 calories," Ferrang says. "You'd be better off eating half of one with some fruit."

4. Baked potato chips. Based on our respondents' experiences, baked potato chips taste better than previous attempts at low-fat potato chips, and they aren't as greasy as regular chips. Even better, Ferrang adds, some brands have only one gram of fat per serving.

5. Baked potatoes. "To get the fiber, eat the skin," Ferrang says.

6. Bananas. "A banana is the easiest thing in the world to stick in your bag and carry to work or wherever," one woman observes.

7. Beans. These fiber-rich legumes win kudos for their versatility. "And they seem to give you substance without weight," noted one woman.

8. Berries. Blueberries, raspberries, and strawberries are all low-calorie and practically nonfat, and they're loaded with vitamins and minerals to boot, Ferrang says. One woman likes to eat fresh berries that are semifrozen—"kind of like Popsicle bites," she explains.

9. Brownies. The low-fat kind, of course. "If you combine a low-fat brownie with a piece of fruit, you have a good snack," says Ferrang.

10. Cantaloupe. This sweet-tasting fruit makes summertime low-fat eating a breeze. "It's loaded with beta-carotene," Ferrang notes.

11. Carrots. Many women like to keep carrots handy—washed, cut up, and ready to eat. "A great taste that takes the edge off my appetite," says one respondent.

12. Cereals. "I love cereals because they're really crunchy and I can get the sweetness I like," offers one woman. She thinks Cheerios leads the pack for flavor.

13. Chocolate syrup. For chocoholics, nothing beats chocolate syrup since it has plenty of flavor but no fat. Ferrang recommends mixing it in skim or low-fat (1 percent) milk for a healthy treat.

14. Corn on the cob. "A great choice," comments Ferrang. One woman recommends seasoning it with spices instead of the usual butter and salt.

15. Cottage cheese. Many women have ingenious ways of enjoying this old diet staple. One suggests adding herbs such as chives for a super-easy dip or spread. Another adds it to tomato soup for an interesting mix of flavors.

16. Couscous. "Serve this grain with veggies—lots of veggies—for a more nutritionally rounded meal," Ferrang suggests.

17. Crackers. You have to be very careful with crackers, Ferrang says. "You can easily eat the calorie equivalent of three or four slices of toast." Be sure to choose a nonfat or low-fat version, she adds.

18. Cupcakes. The low-fat varieties can cure a craving for sweets quite nicely, our survey-takers say. "But be aware that you're getting virtually no nutritional value for the calories you're consuming," Ferrang cautions.

19. Fig or fruit bars. Great to satisfy a sweet tooth.

20. Frozen yogurt. No food evokes as much passion as this one. Women rhapsodize about their favorite brands and flavors, from nonfat peach to low-fat Death by Chocolate. And all agree that it tastes even better than ice cream. Frozen yogurt isn't the same as "regular" yogurt, however, and doesn't supply the amount of calcium that its namesake does, Ferrang says.

21. Graham crackers. Just like "regular" crackers, you can overdo with graham crackers quite easily, Ferrang notes. Still, she says, they're better than cookies.

22. Grapefruit. "I love the tart, fresh flavor of a grapefruit—even though peeling one sometimes takes a while," one respondent writes. It's worth the time, Ferrang replies, since the fruit is so rich in vitamin C.

23. Grapes. They taste great frozen, noted several women.

24. Hot chocolate. "I make mine with skim milk," one respondent says. "It turns out really creamy, and it's a great chocolate fix." Choose a nonfat, sugar-free mix to save calories, Ferrang suggests.

25. Ice cream. Nonfat and low-fat varieties of ice cream hold their own against the real thing, women agree. Ferrang says to try topping it with fruit to make it more nutrient-dense—and to keep you from going for a second serving.

26. Italian ice. Sweet and refreshing—a perfect summertime treat, respondents say. But watch the sugar content, Ferrang advises.

27. Licorice. A number of women applaud the chewy texture of this low-fat sweet. But licorice also packs a hefty amount of sugar, Ferrang warns.

28. Mixed greens. Many supermarkets now carry ready-to-eat mixed greens that have already been washed and cut up. "They make preparing a salad so much more convenient," one respondent points out. Dress up your greens healthfully with lemon juice, balsamic vinegar, and a dash of soy sauce, Ferrang suggests.

29. Oatmeal. A classic comfort food for many women. "Stick with plain oatmeal that you can season yourself," Ferrang advises. "The flavored varieties (in the packets) have a lot of sugar."

30. Oranges. This citrus superstar supplies lots of vitamins and minerals—especially vitamin C—for hardly any calories or fat, according to Ferrang.

31. Pasta. Ferrang says your best bet is to downsize the portion of pasta and add lots of veggies.

32. Pears. One woman described them as "low-fat art."

33. Peppermint patties. "You get the satisfaction of eating chocolate

WHERE'S THE FAT?

From candy to chips, from ice cream to sour cream, many of our high-fat favorites have gone on a diet. You name it—if it has a reputation as being high-fat, chances are that some manufacturer has found a way to offer a low-fat version of its former self.

But where, we wonder, does the fat go? And, even more important, what do they put back to replace it?

How fat is taken out of a food really depends on the food itself. Often manufacturers use mechanical means. In the case of milk, for instance, the full-fat, straight-from-the-cow liquid is put in a centrifuge and separated. Voilà—skim milk. Other foods, like nuts, undergo a defatting process called leaching. The nuts are placed over a barrel and coated with an approved food additive. As the additive drains off, the fat travels along with it.

With manufactured foods, it's not a matter of removing fat. The products are simply made without it. This is where fat-replacers come into play.

There are three different types of fat-replacers: carbohydrate-based, fat-based, and protein-based. Each is made a little differently, and each functions a little differently in foods.

Following is a rundown of the fat-replacers currently being developed by manufacturers. Watch for these names: They may someday make an appearance on the labels of your favorite packaged pickin's—if they haven't already.

CARBOHYDRATE-BASED REPLACERS

Cellulose. Cellulose is actually an insoluble fiber that's found in all plants. It has been chemically altered so that it can hold moisture and form gels. Cellulose may be listed on labels as microcrystalline cellulose, methylcellulose, or hydroxymethylcellulose.

Gums. These go by an array of names, including gum acacia, guar gum, xanthan gum, gellan gum, alginate, and agar. All are soluble fibers, found primarily in plant products such as tree bark, seeds, and seaweed. (The exceptions are xanthan gum and gellan gum, which are produced by microbes.)

Like cellulose, gums hold moisture and form gels. They're often used to thicken foods.

Pectins. More soluble fiber! Pectins come from fruits such as citrus, apples, prunes, dates, and pears. They hold moisture and thicken foods.

Modified starches. Derived from corn, potatoes, and tapioca, modified starches have been chemically altered to give foods bulk without a lot of calories. Watch for names like polydextrose and maltodextrin.

Oatrim. As its name hints, Oatrim is made from oat flour. It's being used as a fat-replacer in baked goods, milk, and processed meats.

Z-trim. A relative newcomer, Z-trim has as its "active ingredient" the insoluble fiber found in grains such as oats, rice, and soybeans. (The Z, incidentally, means zero—as in zero calories.)

Fat-Based Replacers

Emulsifiers. Emulsifiers are fatty substances such as lecithin, monoglycerides, and diglycerides. Manufacturers use them in very small amounts to hold mixtures together.

Olestra. You may know olestra by its brand name, Olean. It's actually a combination of sugar and fatty acids. It has no calories, mainly because your body can't digest or absorb it. It just slides right through your system. Eaten in quantity, olestra may deplete your body of vitamin A and other fat-soluble vitamins.

Salatrim. Fatty acids usually contain nine calories per gram. But the fatty acids used to make Salatrim contain only about half that amount—five calories per gram. This fat-replacer is most often found in baked goods and chocolate.

Protein-Based Replacers

Whey proteins. Probably the best-known of the whey protein bunch is Simplesse. These fat-replacers are actually milk proteins that have been processed into microparticles so round and tiny that they convince your tastebuds that you're eating fat.

without overindulgence," says one woman. "And they come in minis, which is the perfect serving size. Mini patties are a good idea because, as with any candy, they're loaded with sugar," Ferrang says.

34. Peppers. Votes for this veggie ran the gamut from fresh bell peppers to spicy pickled peppers. It's the crunch factor that seems to win women over. And as Ferrang points out, peppers have lots of vitamin C, too.

35. Pickles. "I like to eat garlic dill pickles when I get home from work," one woman says. "They don't spoil my appetite for dinner, and they have just a few calories."

36. Popcorn. This snack gets great accolades. Most go for the air-popped kind, though some favor low-fat microwavable varieties. Popcorn is higher in fiber than most snacks, Ferrang adds. You can flavor it with spices or with nonfat butter spray.

37. Pretzels. For many women, pretzels defuse cravings by delivering a one-two punch of salt and crunch. Most have no fat, Ferrang adds, and you can get them without salt, which really is better for you.

38. Prunes. "Prunes satisfy my craving for sweets," one woman notes. "They're filling without being fattening, and they give me an energy boost, too."

39. Pudding. Chocolate pudding made with skim milk, to be exact. Ferrang suggests opting for the sugar-free mix to save on calories.

40. Raisins. Munch on these for healthy doses of fiber, iron, and vitamin C, Ferrang says. Your sweet tooth will get a quick fix, too.

41. Refried beans. The low-fat or nonfat kind, of course. "They're just as spicy and filling and satisfying as the lard-laden kind, but with none of the fat," one respondent points out.

42. Skim milk. A great way to get your calcium. If you shy away from skim, try it with a shot of chocolate syrup.

43. Sorbet. "I've successfully turned my deep need for ice cream into a sorbet fetish," one woman writes. Sorbet is a good alternative to full-fat ice cream, but keep an eye on those calories from sugar, Ferrang advises.

44. Strawberries. For a real treat, buy them in season and add them to low-fat cereal with skim milk.

45. Sweet potatoes. "I really like sweet potatoes because they're so sweet and yummy just plain—without adding all kinds of butter, salt, and other bad things," one woman writes. If you want, Ferrang says, you can add a little honey or orange juice for flavor.

46. Tomatoes. "In the summer, you can eat them just like an apple," says one woman. And they're packed with vitamin C, Ferrang says. Sprinkle tomato slices with fresh basil and pepper, then add a splash of olive oil or even a little feta cheese.

47. Tortilla chips with homemade salsa. "Wonderful, as long as the chips are baked," Ferrang says. "Add chopped peppers, onions, and mushrooms for extra flavor." The veggies provide bulk, too, so you'll feel full on fewer chips.

48. Watermelon. "It's refreshing and thirst-quenching—food and drink all in one," according to one respondent.

49. Whipped topping. Several survey-takers nominate whipped topping as the best medicine for an aching sweet tooth. If you must eat it, stick with the nonfat version, Ferrang advises.

50. Yogurt. Our survey-takers express strong brand loyalty here. But overall, it's the creamy texture of nonfat and low-fat yogurt that appeals to their tastebuds. You can add some fiber to this healthy treat by slicing some fruit on top, Ferrang suggests. Other favorite toppings include cinnamon, low-fat granola, and Grape-Nuts cereal.

Part Three

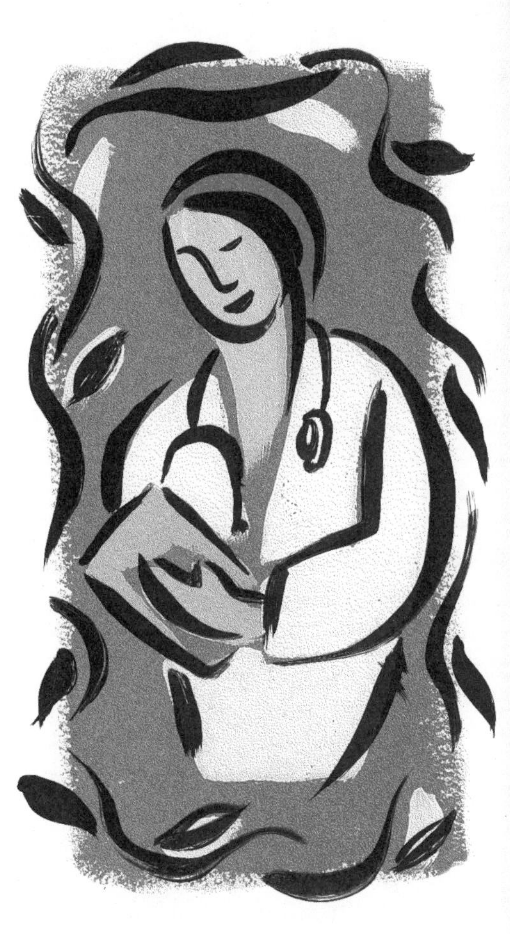

Eating for the Health of It

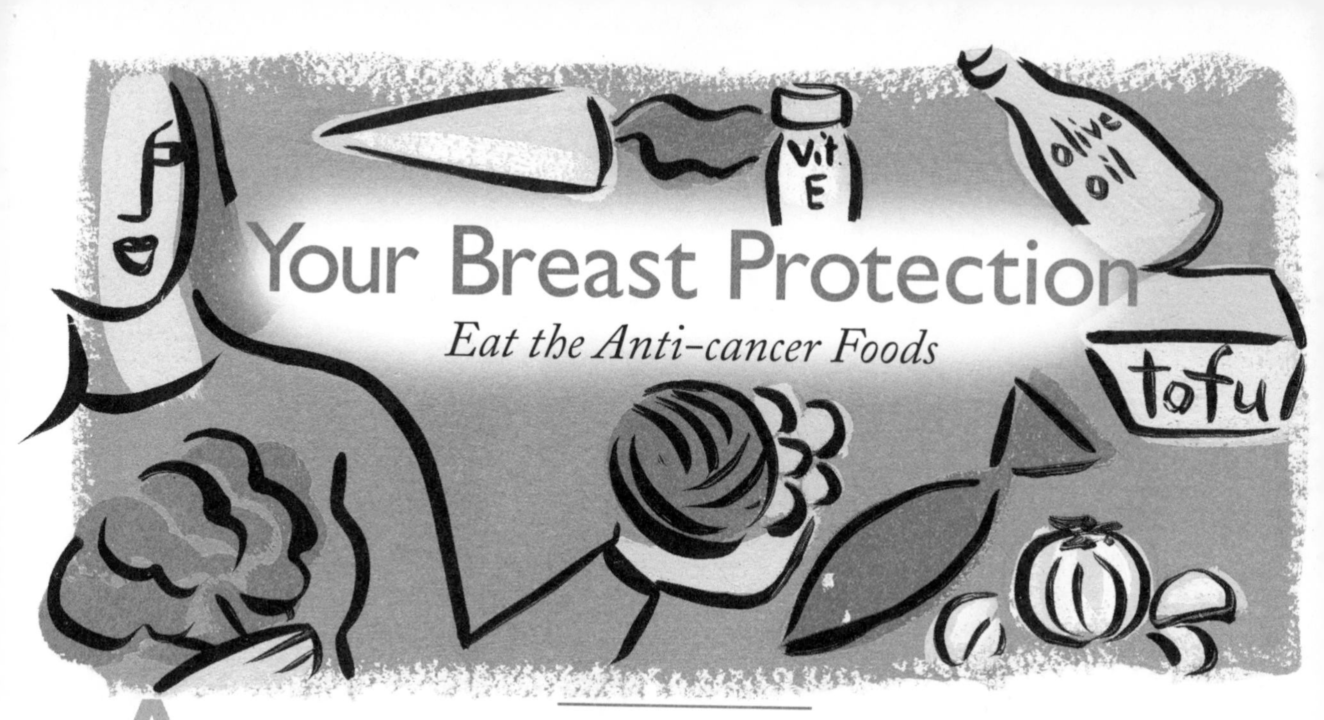

Your Breast Protection

Eat the Anti-cancer Foods

At age 30, your odds of developing breast cancer are 1 in 2,525. They climb to 1 in 93 by the time you're 45. And by the time you're 85, they stand at 1 in 9.

Thankfully, advances in both detection and treatment have dramatically improved the survival rate for the disease. But if given a choice between surviving breast cancer and preventing it, wouldn't you prefer the latter?

Granted, some risk factors you can't control, such as genetics and family history. But they account for a mere fraction of all breast cancer cases. Even if they do apply to you, that doesn't mean cancer is inevitable. But there is one risk factor you can do something about: your eating habits. According to nutritional epidemiologist Regina Ziegler, Ph.D., of the National Cancer Institute, the majority of breast cancer cases are due to something in our daily environment, with diet a likely player.

Weighing the Evidence

Scientists have yet to isolate the cause—or causes—of breast cancer. But they have firmly established a link between diet and the disease. Much of their work has centered on women in Asian countries such as China and Japan, where breast cancer rates are four to seven times lower than in the United States.

Interestingly, when Asian women come to live in this country, their breast cancer risk doubles in just 10 years, according to Dr. Ziegler. And as generations pass, the women's risk eventually catches up with that of the "native" population.

What causes their breast cancer rates to skyrocket? Dietary changes are at least partly to blame, Dr. Ziegler says. The women start eating a lot more meat—and, consequently, more fat—while cutting back on vegetables, grains, and soy, the healthy staples of Asian cuisine.

Dietary fat promotes breast cancer in two ways. First, a high-fat diet causes your body to produce more free radicals, renegade molecules that not only damage healthy cells but also increase damage to the cell's genetic material. The greater the amount of damage, the greater the odds of developing tumors.

Second, dietary fat easily converts to body fat. And body fat, in turn, churns out the hormone estrogen. Normally, estrogen acts as a reproductive regulator, maintaining the menstrual cycle and supporting fertility. But when too much of the hormone floats around your system, it can prompt breast cells to multiply, mutate, and form cancerous breast tumors.

Your Bosom Buddies

Within the medical community, not everyone agrees on the extent to which dietary fat influences the development of breast cancer. But even those who favor a "wait and see" approach to the issue generally regard a well-balanced, low-fat diet with plenty of fruits, vegetables, and whole grains as one of the best things you can do for your overall health. Many experts are convinced that eating this way can substantially reduce the amount of estrogen in your body—and with it your risk of developing breast cancer.

And guess what? If you follow the dietary guidelines presented in the *Prevention* Food Pyramid for Women (see page 26), you'll give yourself a big head start in the battle against breast cancer. You can make your eating habits even more breast-friendly by trying these tips from the experts.

Go easy on alcohol. In a major study on the alcohol–breast cancer link, researchers concluded that a woman who averages one drink a day over a lifetime could increase her breast cancer risk by 30 to 40 percent. Up the ante to two drinks a day,

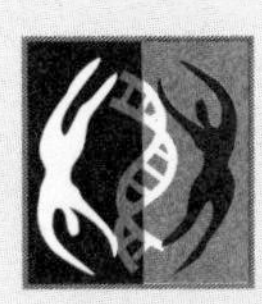

Woman to Woman

She Banished Caffeine—And Breast Pain with It

For four years, Dorothy Walker, a publishing consultant in Whitehall, Pennsylvania, tolerated excruciating breast pain—until she learned that her bad dietary habits could be the culprit. Not long after cutting out all caffeine, she returned to a practically pain-free life. Here's her story.

I remember dealing with breast pain for years—it was the same on-and-off aching feeling that many women experience during their menstrual cycles. It wasn't until age 33, however, that the pain became chronic and everyday activities turned unbearable: Any accidental brush against my breasts made me cringe. Even taking a shower and lying in bed were painful. I tried several over-the-counter pain relievers, but nothing worked.

It wasn't until my breasts became increasingly hard that my doctor thought he had an answer. He discovered some questionable growths, which turned out to be benign fibroid cysts, and removed two after a breast biopsy. The pain, however, continued.

Then I read a magazine article touting the pain-relieving benefits of avoiding caffeine. I immediately eliminated all caffeine from my diet—cold turkey. What I hadn't bargained for was the extreme withdrawal. I didn't realize it, but I was a caffeine addict. Each day I'd drink several pots of coffee plus lots of cola and iced tea. And I smoked constantly. Cutting these out brought on headaches and lightheadedness, followed by nausea and vomiting. I was bedridden for one week. The severe symptoms lasted a couple of months, but it took almost a year to ride out the remaining symptoms.

In retrospect, I realize that I should have gradually tapered off from my heavy caffeine intake. But the results, nonetheless, have made it all worthwhile. Many of the cysts have disappeared, and the ones that remain are much smaller. I have a spot on my left breast that is sometimes sore, but other than that, the pain is gone. The difference is incredible!

and her risk could grow by almost 70 percent.

Alcohol of any kind appears to increase the amount of estrogen circulating in the body. So if you do imbibe, try to limit yourself to just two or three drinks a week, advises JoAnn E. Manson, M.D., associate professor of medicine at Harvard Medical School and co-director of women's health at Brigham and Women's Hospital in Boston. (A drink is defined as 5 ounces of wine, 12 ounces of regular beer, or a mixed drink made with 1½ ounces of 80-proof distilled spirits.)

What about reports that a drink a day can protect you from heart attacks? "If you don't have risk factors for heart disease, then the benefit from alcohol consumption is small and in younger women is outweighed by the higher risk of breast cancer," says Dr. Manson.

Aim low. Some experts recommend that you get no more than 25 percent of your calories from fat. Other experts say that you would boost the benefit to your breasts by knocking the fat content down a few more notches—to, say, 20 percent of calories. As a bonus, at least one study has found that this lower fat intake can help to relieve painful breasts.

Favor fiber. Fiber should be part of every woman's anti–breast cancer arsenal, according to nutrition researcher Jean H. Hankin, R.D., Dr.P.H., of the etiology program of the Cancer Research Center of Hawaii and professor of public health at the University of Hawaii in Honolulu. Scientists believe that fiber may reduce breast cancer risk by binding with excess estrogen and ushering it out of the body before it has a chance to do harm. Fiber also appears to interfere with the absorption of dietary fat, which, as you'll recall, ultimately serves as a catalyst for estrogen production.

The National Cancer Institute recommends an intake of 20 to 30 grams of fiber a day. You can hit the mark by eating lots of whole grains, beans, fruits, and vegetables.

Crunch crucifers. Time and again, research has shown that women who eat lots of fruits and vegetables are much less likely to develop breast cancer than women who don't. Among the best cancer-fighters in the supermarket produce aisle are the crucifers—broccoli, brussels sprouts, cabbage, and cauliflower. These veggies contain a number of compounds, called phytochemicals, that put the squeeze on estrogen and prevent it from becoming destructive.

To preserve their phyto punch, eat crucifers raw. If you don't like them that way, then cook them until they're just tender. Canadian researchers have found that prolonged cooking can reduce the amount of at least one of the cancer-combating compounds in crucifers by as much as 50 percent.

Go fishin'. Fish such as Atlantic herring, canned pink salmon, and bluefin tuna are rich in omega-3 fatty acids. Laboratory evidence suggests that these fatty acids can stymie the growth of cancerous breast tissue.

Gobble garlic. Researchers at Memorial Sloan-Kettering Cancer Center in New York City have isolated four compounds in garlic that appear to stop breast cells from becoming cancerous in laboratory tests. These compounds also help to convert estrogen to a weaker form that isn't as likely to instigate breast cancer.

Savor soy foods. Soy is a staple in many Asian countries, and researchers believe that it's responsible for keeping the breast cancer rates among Asian women so low. It contains isoflavones, phytochemicals that mimic the hormone estrogen in the body but are 100,000 times weaker than the real thing. The isoflavones occupy places on breast cells called receptor sites, blocking estrogen from doing so.

The average Asian consumes 50 or more milligrams of soy isoflavones daily. But research suggests that if you eat just one serving of soy, that may be enough for you to experience some of its protective effects. Try adding cooked soybeans to chili, stir-frying tofu in place of meat for a variety of dishes, or drinking soy milk, which can be found in health food stores and some grocery stores. Keep in mind, however, that soy sauce and soybean oil don't contain isoflavones.

Favor flaxseed. Flaxseed contains compounds called lignan precursors. Scientists have just begun investigating how these phytochemicals work. Early studies show that lignan precursors change into a weak form of estrogen in the body and then act pretty much like isoflavones.

Try sprinkling two heaping tablespoons (about 25 grams) of ground flaxseed on cereal or in juice if you want to get the same amount that breast cancer researchers are studying at the University of Toronto. Check your favorite health food store or baking catalog to find flaxseed.

Opt for olive oil. In a study involving more than 2,000 Greek women, those who consumed olive oil at least once a day were 25 percent less likely to develop breast cancer than those who didn't. Scientists can't yet explain how the oil protects against cancer, but they believe it has something to do with antioxidants in the oil. (Antioxidants help to neutralize free radicals.)

Lean toward E. Vitamin E flexes its cancer-fighting muscle in several ways. First, it's an antioxidant, which means it helps mop up those damaging free radicals and prevents them from doing harm. Second, it keeps your immune system in good working order. And third, it appears to thwart the formation of cancer-causing compounds in your body.

Vitamin E can be difficult to get through foods. One of the best sources is wheat germ: A serving of 1⅔ tablespoons contains four international units of E. You'll also find the vitamin in vegetable oils, including olive oil. Just make sure that the oil you choose has mostly unsaturated fat.

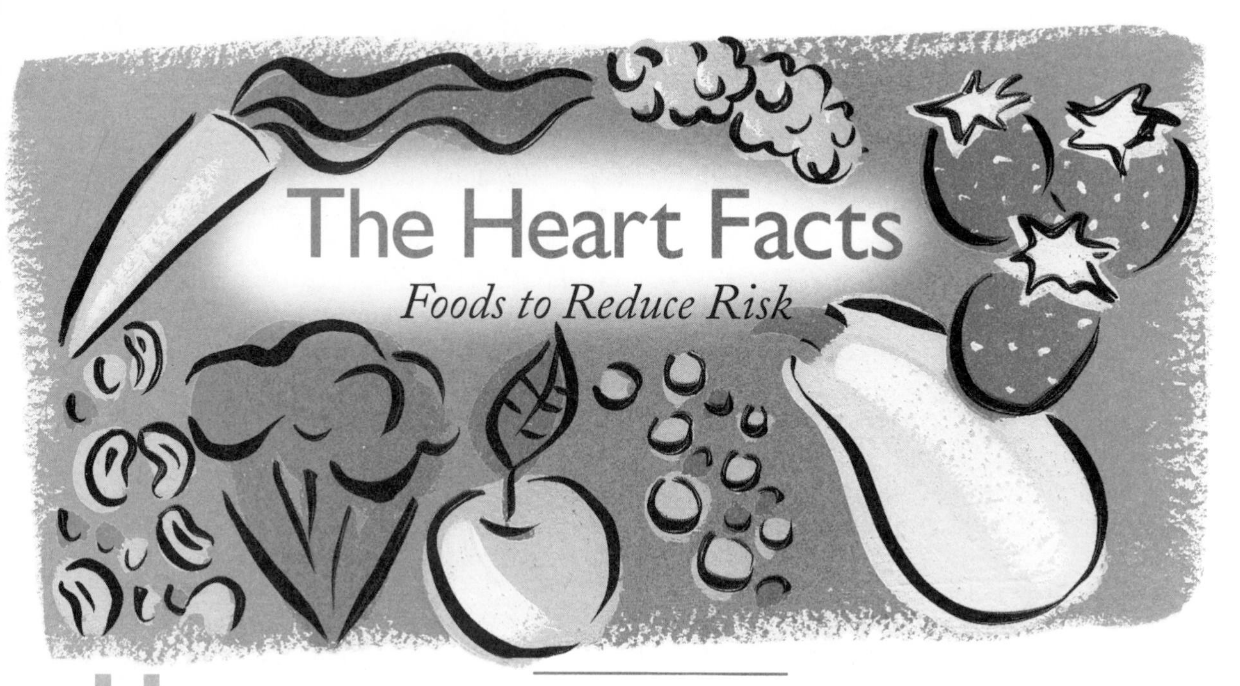

The Heart Facts

Foods to Reduce Risk

Heart disease has long had a reputation as a strictly male malady. True, it tends to affect men earlier in life—we women get about a 10-year grace period. But once we reach menopause, any female advantage quickly dissipates. In fact, 11 times as many women die from heart disease as from breast cancer, earning it the dubious distinction as the number one cause of death among adult women in the United States.

What happens at menopause that causes your heart disease risk to skyrocket? Doctors suspect it has something to do with the hormone estrogen. Estrogen circulating in your bloodstream helps keep your arteries clear by regulating cholesterol levels—increasing "good" high-density lipoprotein (HDL) cholesterol while lowering "bad" low-density lipoprotein (LDL) cholesterol. But as you pass through menopause, your body's production of estrogen dwindles—and with it goes some protection from heart disease.

Other health and lifestyle issues can pump up your risk of heart disease, too. Among them are family history (a parent diagnosed with heart disease before age 60), diabetes, high blood pressure, high cholesterol, overweight, physical inactivity, smoking, and high levels of stress—and not necessarily in that order. Any one is a serious risk in and of itself, and the overall risk only climbs as the risk factors add up.

None of these risk factors, however, is a guarantee that you're going to develop heart disease in your lifetime. In fact, every one can be offset to some degree simply by eating right.

How to Avoid a Broken Heart

What qualifies as "eating right"? Doctors say it's a combination of cutting your fat intake and filling up on fruits, vegetables, and fiber-rich grains and beans. *Hmmm*...just what the *Prevention* Food Pyramid for Women on page 26 recommends. Let's take a closer look at each of these heart-healthy nutrition strategies.

Skimp on fat. Most doctors recommend that you limit your fat intake to about 25 percent of calories—much less than the 34 percent of calories that the average American consumes. And most of that fat should be unsaturated, suggests

Alice Lichtenstein, D.Sc., associate professor and research scientist at the Jean Mayer USDA Human Nutrition Research Center on Aging at Tufts University in Boston. The reason is that both monounsaturated fat (found in olive and canola oils and most nuts) and polyunsaturated fat (found in corn, safflower, and sunflower oils) actually support heart health by reducing LDL cholesterol while leaving HDL cholesterol unchanged. That's important because your body needs HDL to flush out LDL.

On the other hand, saturated fat, found mainly in animal foods, increases heart disease risk. The link between the two is so strong that the American Heart Association recommends getting no more (and preferably less) than 10 percent of your calories from saturated fat.

Feast on fiber. Fiber—especially the soluble kind found in grains, beans, and fruits—binds with cholesterol in the body and helps remove it along with the waste, explains Diane Grabowski-Nepa, R.D., a nutritional counselor at the Pritikin Longevity Center in Malibu, California. Researchers cannot yet explain how fiber works its cholesterol-clobbering magic. One popular theory is that it binds with bile acids in the intestines and escorts these cholesterol-laden compounds from your body. Your body then has to recruit more cholesterol to make more bile acids, reducing your blood cholesterol level in the process.

How much fiber does it take to

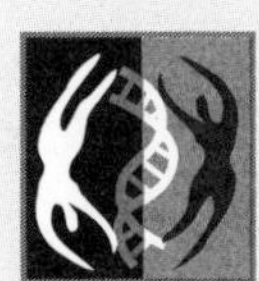

WOMAN TO WOMAN

She Fought Heart Disease with a Knife and Fork

For years, Donna Young, an Austintown, Ohio, salesclerk, misread the signs of her ailing heart. Fortunately, surgery opened her eyes—and her arteries—to give her a second chance at life. Here's how she fought back with food.

I can recall it vividly: I checked into the hospital just a woman complaining about back pain and came out a statistic.

At the age of 46, I finally learned what years of back pain had been trying to tell me. I had elevated cholesterol—and a suffering heart. Before long, I was undergoing coronary bypass surgery. It was in that hospital gown that I vowed to take an active role in nurturing myself back to health. I began reading all the medical literature I could get my hands on. I worked with the hospital's cardiac rehabilitation services and saw some success. But I still needed some direction after I moved to a new town.

I was relieved to find a local hospital's Slim Down clinic. Intrigued by its refreshing mind/body approach, I signed up. It was exactly what I needed. Along with the handfuls of self-help literature, presentations were sponsored weekly—for example, a cardiac rehabilitation therapist spoke on appropriate exercise, a doctor taught stress-management techniques, and a chef shared low-fat cooking tips and recipes.

My most prized lesson to date? Altering recipes. Now when I see a recipe, I immediately rework it into a healthier version, which is doubly important since my husband has diabetes. I've found that there's a substitute for every unhealthy ingredient. Whether it's applesauce instead of oil for buckwheat pancakes or egg substitute for omelets, my diet is the healthiest it's ever been.

At my most recent checkup, all my arteries were clear and my cholesterol had dropped from 280 to below 200. Being 15 pounds lighter is yet another bonus, but I don't need to see a skinny person in the mirror to feel good about myself. It simply feels good to know that I'm treating my body right.

safeguard your health? Between 20 and 30 grams a day, according to the National Cancer Institute.

Add some antioxidants. Vitamins C and E and beta-carotene are antioxidants. As their name suggests, the antioxidants protect against oxidation, a naturally occurring process in which renegade oxygen molecules called free radicals damage healthy cells and contribute to the artery-clogging process.

Just how protective are these nutrients? When researchers at Harvard University compared the diets of more than 87,000 nurses, they found that the nurses who ate the most antioxidant-rich foods were 46 percent less likely to develop heart disease than the nurses who ate the least.

At the very least, experts say, you should make sure that you're getting the Daily Values (DVs) of vitamins C and E—60 milligrams and 30 international units (IU), respectively. No DV has been established for beta-carotene—but you need a daily intake of about 5,000 IU to match the DV of vitamin A. (Your body converts beta-carotene to vitamin A.)

A Plateful of Prevention

To help you get in the swing of heart-smart eating, we've come up with a list of 20 foods that meet all three of the criteria outlined above. Most have less than one gram of fat, the two exceptions being chickpeas and wheat germ (which, incidentally, are still considered low-fat). Each one is high in fiber. All supply healthy doses of one or more of the antioxidants. And as a bonus, not one of these foods has even a smidgen of dietary cholesterol.

Apples. One medium-size fruit (about five ounces) has three grams of fiber, eight milligrams of vitamin C, and 0.6 IU of vitamin E.

Apricots. You get 111 milligrams of vitamin C—almost two times the DV—in three fresh apricots. They also provide two grams of fiber and one IU of beta-carotene.

Blackberries. One cup of berries contains 30 milligrams of vitamin C, along with seven grams of fiber and 0.1 IU of vitamin E.

Black currants. One cup of black currants meets the DV of vitamin C more than three times over, supplying 203 milligrams of the nutrient. You also get four grams of fiber and 0.7 IU of vitamin E.

Broccoli. One-half cup of cooked chopped broccoli offers almost a whole day's worth of vitamin C: 58 milligrams. The same-size serving also contains two grams of fiber and 0.3 IU of beta-carotene.

Brussels sprouts. You get 3 grams of fiber, 48 grams of vitamin C, and 0.2 IU of beta-carotene in ½ cup of boiled brussels sprouts.

Butternut squash. One-half cup of baked cubed butternut squash provides 16 IU of beta-carotene. It also provides a good amount of fiber (three grams) and a generous amount of vitamin C (15 milligrams).

Cantaloupe. Chow down on cantaloupe, and you can cover your vitamin C needs for an entire day. A one-cup serving of cubed fruit supplies 68 milligrams of vitamin C as well as one gram of fiber and 16 IU of beta-carotene.

Carrots. One of the best vitamin A sources around: One 2½-ounce carrot has 6,745 IU of the nutrient—all you need for an entire day. You also get a nice amount of fiber (two grams) and even a little bit of vitamin C (seven milligrams).

Chickpeas. You get a whopping seven grams of fiber in ½ cup of chickpeas—noteworthy even for a member of the fiber-rich legume clan. The same size serving also offers a small burst of vitamin C (five milligrams).

Grapefruit. Both pink and red varieties provide 50 milligrams of vitamin C as well as 0.7 gram of fiber.

Green peas. You can bump up your fiber intake a notch or two with these legumes. A ½-cup serving of boiled green peas offers a modest two grams of fiber, along with 11 milligrams of vitamin C.

Papaya. Yet another superb source of vitamin C: Half of a papaya supplies 94 milligrams of C—roughly 1½ times the DV. It also has a respectable three grams of fiber.

Passion fruit. It seems fitting that a food named "passion fruit" can do so much for your heart! A serving of five medium-size fruits (about 3½ ounces total) provides decent amounts of fiber (two grams), vitamin C (30 milligrams), and beta-carotene (0.2 IU).

Raspberries. One cup of berries gives you a hefty six grams of fiber as well as 31 milligrams of vitamin C.

Spinach. For beta-carotene, spinach is one of your best bets. A half-cup serving of boiled spinach provides 25 IU of beta-carotene as well as two grams of fiber and nine milligrams of vitamin C.

Strawberries. These bountiful berries offer 85 milligrams of vitamin C and four grams of fiber in every one-cup serving.

Sweet potatoes. Sweet potatoes pack a beta-carotene punch, with one baked four-ounce spud supplying 83 IU of the nutrient. As a bonus, it can boost your intake of fiber (three grams) and vitamin C (28 milligrams).

Sweet red peppers. One-half cup of chopped red peppers has only 0.8 gram of fiber and one IU of beta-carotene. But you get more than a day's supply of vitamin C—95 milligrams.

Wheat germ. One-quarter cup of toasted wheat germ contains three IU of vitamin E, making the grain one of the best food sources of E. You get a good four grams of fiber, too.

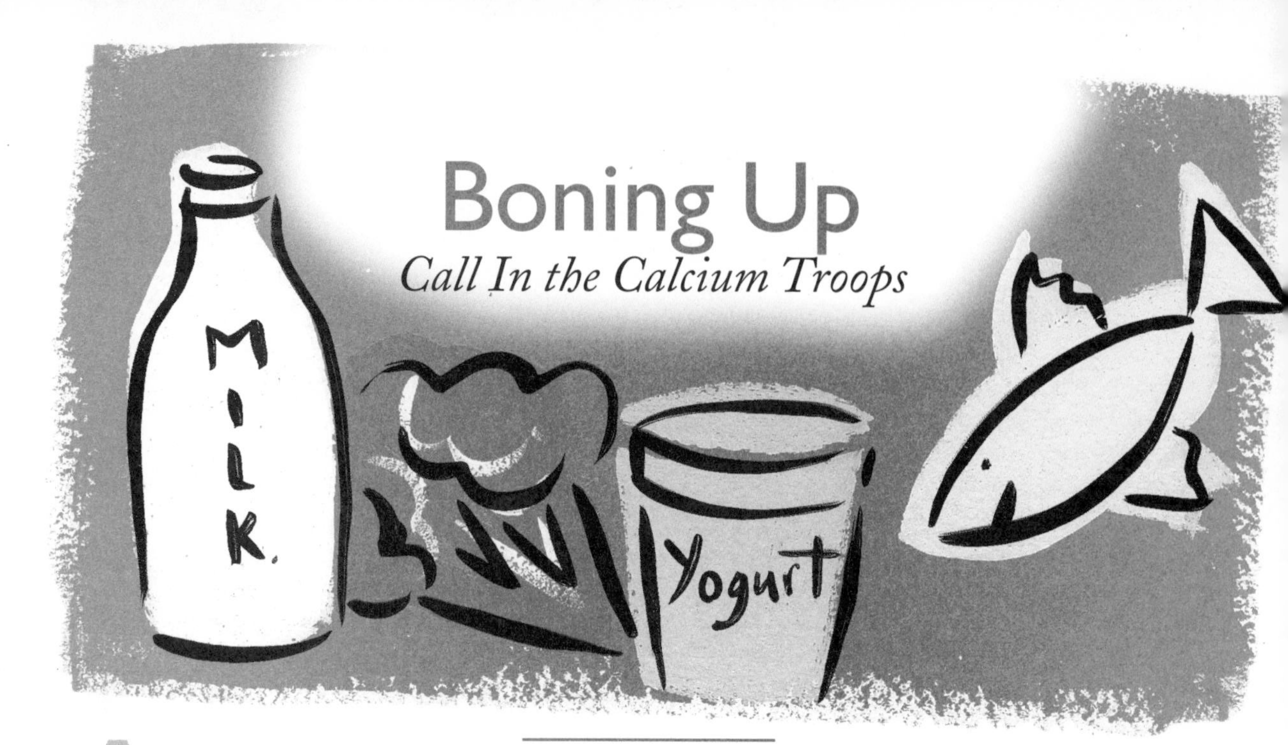

Boning Up

Call In the Calcium Troops

A woman bumps into her kitchen table and shatters her hip. Seem far-fetched? Well, about 240,000 women a year can tell you otherwise. They probably never would have believed such a minor incident could cause such a catastrophic injury—until it happened to them.

They're just a relative handful of the more than 22.4 *million* American women who face the threats of osteoporosis, a disease that weakens the bones and leaves them vulnerable to breaking. It's responsible for an estimated 1.5 million fractures every year—mostly of the hip, wrist, and spine.

While osteoporosis affects both sexes, it seems to target women with particular ferocity. By one estimate, as many as one in two of us is going to experience an osteoporosis-related fracture, compared with one in five men.

But there is a bright spot among all these bleak statistics. You see, osteoporosis doesn't happen overnight. It takes a lifetime to develop. So if you act now, you can help protect your skeleton from this insidious disease.

The best prescription for your bone health? Engage in weight-bearing exercise (such as walking, running, or aerobics), give up smoking (if you do), and—perhaps most important—eat lots of bone-friendly foods. In fact, one estimate suggests that the right diet alone could prevent as many as half of all osteoporosis-related fractures.

Growing, Growing...Gone

To understand how osteoporosis works, you should first know a little bit about the bone-building process itself. Throughout your life, your body constantly removes old bone tissue and replaces it with fresh stuff. The gains surpass the losses until sometime in your thirties, when you reach what is called your peak bone mass. Then your body institutes its own version of downsizing: It continues to get rid of old bone tissue, but it doesn't bother to fill all the vacancies. Demand exceeds supply, and you end up losing about 1 percent of your bone mass every year.

This rate of bone loss is considered normal. Everyone experiences it—women as well as men. But in osteoporosis, some additional factor kicks bone loss into overdrive. For women, that additional factor is usually menopause.

Up until menopause, your body has an abundant supply of the hormone estrogen. Estrogen helps to keep your skeleton healthy and strong. So when estrogen production declines at menopause, bone density does, too. In the five to seven years following menopause, you can lose 2 to 3 percent of your bone mass a year—or up to about 20 percent.

While it's true that you can't replace lost bone, you can do a lot to preserve the bone you have. You can start by reinforcing your diet with calcium, your best ally in the battle against bone loss.

DO YOU FIT THIS M.O.?

The National Osteoporosis Foundation has put together the following osteoporosis risk assessment for women. Keep in mind that a "yes" response to any question doesn't mean that osteoporosis is inevitable. You just have to take some extra precautions to protect your bone density.

1. Do you have a small, thin frame?
2. Are you Caucasian or Asian?
3. Do you have a family history of osteoporosis?
4. Have you been through menopause?
5. Have you had an early or a surgically induced menopause?
6. Have you been taking thyroid medication or high doses of cortisone-like drugs for asthma, arthritis, or cancer?
7. Is your diet low in calcium?
8. Are you physically inactive?
9. Do you smoke cigarettes or drink alcohol in excess?

In This Corner: Calcium

To show you just how important calcium is, in 1994 the National Institutes of Health convened a special panel to set optimum intake guidelines for women and men of all ages. Here's a quick recap of the panel's recommendations for women.

- Ages 25 to 50: 1,000 milligrams
- Ages 51 to 65 (postmenopausal) and taking hormone replacement therapy: 1,000 milligrams
- Ages 51 to 65 (postmenopausal) and not taking hormone replacement therapy: 1,500 milligrams
- Age 66 plus: 1,500 milligrams
- Pregnant or nursing: 1,200 to 1,500 milligrams

Unfortunately, most American women aren't hitting the 1,000-milligram mark—not by a long shot. The average intake is a paltry 450 milligrams a day. Why do we consistently come up short? Part of the problem, suggests Susan Broy, M.D., director of the Osteoporosis Center at the Advocate Medical Group in Chicago, is that we've forsaken some of the best food sources of calcium—namely, dairy products such as milk and cheese—because of their high fat content. It may very well be that in trying to protect our hearts and our waistlines from fat's follies, we're putting our bones at risk.

Befriend the Bone-Builders

By no means are we suggesting that you feast on high-fat fare for your bones' sake. Experts say that there are plenty of healthy ways that you can meet your daily calcium quota through diet.

The following nutrition strategies can keep your bone bank in the black—and save your skeleton for a lifetime.

Rediscover dairy. Have you paid a visit to

your supermarket's dairy case lately? If not, you should. You'll find an almost mind-boggling array of nonfat and low-fat dairy products, including milk, cheese, and yogurt. And just because the fat is gone doesn't mean the calcium is, Dr. Broy notes. For example, an eight-ounce glass of skim milk contains 300 milligrams of calcium. Drink 3½ glasses a day, and you'll get all of the mineral you need.

Graze on greens. They don't supply as much calcium as dairy products do, but dark green, leafy vegetables can definitely move you a few rungs up the ladder to your recommended daily intake. Among the calcium standouts in this produce group are kale, with 47 milligrams per ½ cup, and broccoli, with 36 milligrams per ½ cup.

Grow fond of fish. Certain fish have edible bones that are loaded with calcium. For example, three ounces of canned pink salmon has 181 milligrams of the mineral, while one ounce of canned Atlantic sardines has 92 milligrams. Canned fish does have a lot of sodium, though, so look for brands labeled "low-salt" and, in the case of sardines, rinse them well before eating.

Seek out surprise sources. Many manufacturers now add calcium to certain packaged foods. Calcium-fortified orange juice, for instance, supplies just as much of the mineral as skim milk: 300 milligrams in an eight-ounce glass.

Nosh at night. As mentioned earlier, your body is constantly dumping old bone tissue. But at least one study has shown that the process actually speeds up while you sleep, peaking at about 3:00 in the morning. Having a calcium-rich nightcap—maybe a glass of skim milk or some nonfat yogurt—may keep your blood level of the mineral more stable during the overnight hours.

Don't forget D. Calcium can't do its job without vitamin D to escort it across intestinal walls and into your bone cells. Your body can manufacture its own D with a little help from Old Sol. But if you live in a northern climate or don't spend 5 to 15 minutes in direct sunlight without sunscreen every day, you'll want to make sure that you're getting enough of the nutrient from food sources instead. Both milk and breakfast cereals are fortified with vitamin D. Aim for the Daily Value (DV) of 400 IU.

Watch your tempeh. Tempeh, tofu, and other soy foods contain estrogen-like compounds called isoflavones. Scientists at the University of Illinois found that women who consumed 90 milligrams of isoflavones a day experienced a 2 percent increase in their bone densities.

You can reach 90 milligrams—the amount used in the study—by eating one cup of roasted soy nuts (60 milligrams) and drinking one cup of soy milk (30 milligrams).

By the way, not all soy foods contain isoflavones. You won't find them in soy sauce or soybean oil, for example.

Beware the Bone-Robbers

Just as some foods can safeguard your skeletal strength, others seem to steal it away. To rid your diet of the leading bone-offenders, heed this advice from the experts.

Stop the a-salt. A high-sodium diet delivers a double whammy to your skeleton. Salt not only interferes with calcium absorption but also increases the amount of the mineral that's excreted from your body.

You don't necessarily have to give up salt entirely, says Edith Howard Hogan, R.D., a dietitian in Washington, D.C., and a spokesperson for the American Dietetic Association. But a little moderation is in order. Ideally, experts say, you should get no more than the DV of 2,400 milligrams of salt a day—the equivalent of about one teaspoon.

Quaff coffee with caution. Some studies suggest that drinking a lot of coffee—or any caffeine-laden beverage, for that matter—may raise your risk of a hip fracture. Based on what they know so far, experts believe that you can have up to two cups of java a day without any ill effects.

And rather than drinking your coffee black, try adding a little milk, suggests Jeri W. Nieves, Ph.D., a nutritional epidemiologist at Columbia University in New York City and director of the bone mineral measurement laboratory at Helen Hayes Hospital in West Haverstraw, New York. Milk prevents caffeine from stealing calcium from your bones.

Give cola the cold shoulder. It's not only the caffeine in cola that can be hard on your bones. Preliminary research suggests that phosphorus—a mineral found in cola as well as in many processed foods—contributes to higher rates of bone fracture.

Some scientists believe that phosphorus actually steps up calcium excretion. But others, including Mona S. Calvo, Ph.D., a member of the clinical research and review staff of the Office of Special Nutritionals at the Food and Drug Administration in Washington, D.C., suspect the real problem is that we're trading in milk for cola and running up a calcium deficit as a result. The combination of too much phosphorus and too little calcium leads to osteoporosis, she says.

Clearly, more research is necessary to flesh out the phosphorus-osteoporosis link. For now, experts recommend limiting your cola consumption to one 12-ounce serving per day.

Put a lid on alcohol. Research has shown that people who drink more than two glasses of wine or four ounces of hard liquor a day have less bone mass than teetotalers of the same age and sex. Why? Well, alcohol not only has a direct toxic effect on bone cells, it also seems to take the place of calcium-rich foods in the diet.

The bottom line is that if you must imbibe, do so in moderation—no more than two or three drinks a week. (A drink is defined as 5 ounces of wine, 12 ounces of beer, or a mixed drink made with 1½ ounces of liquor.)

Woman to Woman

Brittle Bones Are Her Family Heritage

Sandra Cheung, R.D., a homemaker and health educator from Wilmington, Delaware, saw a frightening genetic trend in the women in her family: osteoporosis. Her sister died of consequences of the disease at age 40. Not only has it spurred her to take drastic measures to protect her own bones but she now also volunteers at every opportunity to teach young girls the importance of bone health through good nutrition. Here's her story.

Osteoporosis has devastated my family. My mother has been left fragile from this disease, and my sister was diagnosed with osteoporosis at the early age of 37.

As a result, most of my adult life I have been very disciplined about my diet, and I am happy to say that tests show my bone density is normal. I eat lots of low-fat dairy products, including yogurt, as well as tofu. And I supplement my diet with plenty of calcium. I also try to avoid coffee and soda because they contain substances that make bones more susceptible to fractures. Too many women of all ages drink them without being aware of future potential consequences.

This is one of the reasons why I'm concerned about teen health. My job now is to teach teens the importance of bone-strengthening exercise and calcium-rich foods, especially milk. I educate them on risk factors that cause bone damage. I think it's important that children learn at an early age how to nourish their bodies with good foods and build up those bones.

Clobber Cholesterol

What the Numbers Are Telling You

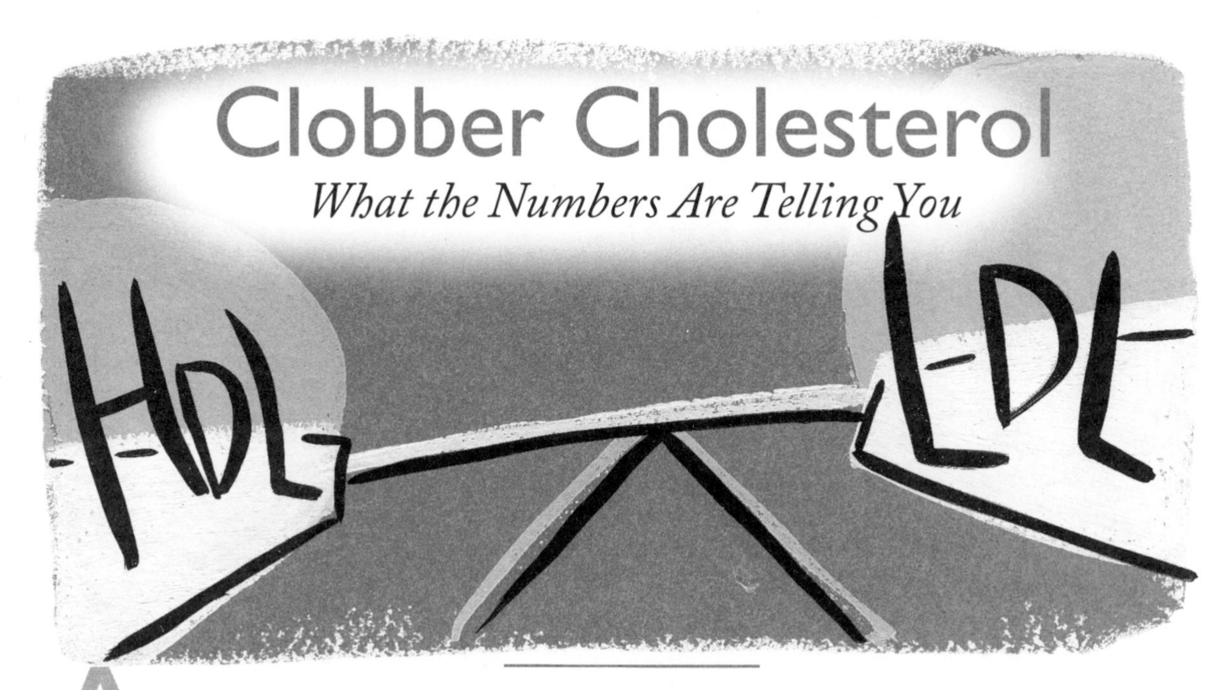

A generation ago, the word *cholesterol* would have had about as much meaning to the general population as *floppy disk* or *fax*.

These days, of course, most of us can recite our cholesterol readings as though they were our birth dates. We've taken heed of all the reports citing cholesterol as a leading risk factor for heart disease, the number one cause of death among American women.

Those reports don't paint a flattering image of cholesterol—nor, for that matter, an entirely accurate one. To begin with, you can get the impression that cholesterol is all bad, when in reality, your body *needs* it to manufacture cell membranes, sex hormones, bile acids, and vitamin D. Your liver produces about 2,000 milligrams of the waxy, fatlike substance every day just for these routine tasks. You literally couldn't live without it.

The problems arise when there's too much cholesterol floating around your bloodstream. While genetics, lack of exercise, and smoking can all contribute to high cholesterol, a high-fat diet is usually to blame, says Debra R. Judelson, M.D., a cardiologist in Beverly Hills and chair of the Cardiovascular Disease in Women Committee of the American Medical Women's Association.

But even then, not all cholesterol is bad. While one type, known as low-density lipoprotein (LDL) cholesterol, does most of the damage, another cholesterol, known as high-density lipoprotein (HDL), actually works to your health's advantage. And scientists now know that it's the ratio of the two rather than the total of the two that helps to determine your state of health.

That's great news for women because, as it turns out, we have different—and healthier—cholesterol ratios than men.

The Female Advantage

LDL is the cholesterol with the bad reputation because it likes to congregate on the walls of your arteries. Eventually, the buildup can become so severe that it slows and can eventually shut down blood flow to the heart and brain, explains Penny Kris-Etherton, R.D., Ph.D., professor of nutrition at Pennsylvania State

WHAT THE NUMBERS MEAN

The next time your doctor orders a cholesterol test, insist on two things: a total cholesterol reading and a breakdown of the total into high-density lipoprotein (HDL) and low-density lipoprotein (LDL) and triglycerides. Some doctors don't like to do separate HDL, LDL, and triglyceride testing because it's costlier and more time-consuming. Finally, when the results come in, don't settle for a verdict like "your cholesterol is fine"; ask for the numbers.

Incidentally, many doctors no longer go by your scores alone. Instead, they rely on the ratio of total cholesterol to HDL cholesterol as a more accurate predictor of heart disease risk. You can figure out your own ratio: Simply divide your total cholesterol reading by your HDL reading. According to the American Heart Association, if the answer is 3.5 or less, your cholesterol profile is in great shape.

According to experts, the following numbers will help you determine exactly where you stand.

	Total Cholesterol (mg./dl.)	HDL (mg./dl.)	LDL (mg./dl.)	Triglycerides (mg./dl.)
Desirable	Below 200	Above 55 (60 or higher is protective)	Below 130 (100 or lower if you have heart disease)	Below 200
Borderline	200–239		130–159	200–399
Undesirable	240 or higher	Below 35	160 or higher	400 or higher

University in University Park. HDL, on the other hand, plays good cop by rounding up loitering LDL and running it out of your body.

Ideally, then, a healthy total cholesterol reading consists of a low level of LDL and a high level of HDL. This is where women have a huge advantage. On average, our HDL readings are 10 to 12 points higher than men's.

Why the difference? Scientists suspect it may have something to do with the female hormone estrogen. Estrogen seems to boost your HDL level while at the same time holding down your LDL level. This may explain why a woman's risk of heart disease rises so sharply at menopause, just as the body slows its production of estrogen.

So what does all this mean for you? First and foremost, make sure any cholesterol screening that you have done breaks out your LDL, HDL, and triglyceride readings. (Triglycerides are a type of blood fat that, like cholesterol, appears to increase a person's risk for heart disease.) An HDL level of 55 to 60 is considered healthy for a woman—and the higher, the better, says Margo Denke, M.D., associate professor of internal medicine at the Center for Human Nutrition at the University of Texas Southwestern Medical Center at Dallas, a member of the American Heart Association's Nutrition Committee, and a member of the National Institutes of Health panel of experts on HDL and heart disease. But for LDL, you want to aim low: 130 or under. Levels of triglycerides and total cholesterol below 200 are considered ideal.

Conquering Cholesterol

The problem with cholesterol is that too few of us have ideal counts. If we did, heart disease would be way down. Research shows that for every 1 percent reduction in total cholesterol, the risk of heart attack drops 2 percent. For the most part, lowering your cholesterol is a simple matter of eating more of some foods and less of others.

Toss the yolks. Egg yolks and organ meats have no place in a low-cholesterol lifestyle. With 212 milligrams of cholesterol in a single large egg, it's just not worth it when you consider that we should be getting no more than 300 milligrams a day. Along with egg yolks, kidney and liver are the most notorious offenders.

Cut the fat. Some researchers believe that fat—especially saturated fat—may have more of an effect on your cholesterol level than dietary cholesterol itself. Like dietary cholesterol, saturated fat increases the amount of LDL circulating in your bloodstream, according to Mary Felando, R.D., a cardiovascular nutrition specialist in Los Angeles.

Conveniently, the foods that contain the most dietary cholesterol also contain the most saturated fat. Be especially wary of foods from animal sources, such as red meat and full-fat dairy products, especially butter.

Go for oil over butter. While saturated fat raises your cholesterol level, unsaturated fats have the opposite effect. Monounsaturated fat—the kind found in abundance in olive, canola, and peanut oils—lowers unhealthy LDL while preserving healthy HDL. Polyunsaturated fat lowers LDL, too, but at the expense of HDL. Still, experts agree, it's a better bet than saturated fat. You'll find polyunsaturated fat in corn, sunflower, and soybean oils.

Other food sources of unsaturated fats include whole grains, vegetables, avocados, olives, and legumes.

Give hydrogenation the heave-ho. Manufacturers use hydrogenation to harden vegetable oils into stick margarine and solid vegetable shortening. The process produces substances known as trans-fatty acids, which appear to not only raise LDL cholesterol but also lower HDL cholesterol. In fact, the Harvard University Nurses' Health Study, an ongoing study of 115,000 women, has reported that even modest daily consumption of trans-fatty acids can dramatically increase a woman's risk of heart disease.

If you prefer margarine over butter, stick with the tub or liquid variety. Also, go easy on fast foods and prepared baked goods—about 75 percent of the trans-fatty acids in the typical American diet come from sources such as these.

Have fish tonight. Fish such as salmon and tuna are rich in omega-3 fatty acids, a type of fat that appears to boost beneficial HDL cholesterol. To get the most benefit from omega-3's, try to eat a three- to four-ounce serving of fish twice a week, suggests Joanne Curran-Celentano, R.D., Ph.D., associate professor of nutritional sciences at the University of New Hampshire in Durham.

Fill up on fiber-rich foods. Soluble fiber—the kind found in beans, fruits, and grains such as oats, barley, and rye—dissolves in water to form a gel-like material that prevents cholesterol from being absorbed into your bloodstream, says Rosemary Newman, R.D., Ph.D., professor of foods and nutrition at Montana State University in Bozeman, who has studied fiber and its relationship to cholesterol since the early 1980s. And when cholesterol isn't absorbed, it gets excreted from your body instead.

There's another kind of fiber, too—insoluble fiber, found in vegetables, cereals, and grains such as wheat. It increases bulk and speeds the movement of waste products—including cholesterol—through the intestines, Dr. Newman explains.

The American Heart Association recommends a daily fiber intake of 25 grams, which is in the range of what other health organizations recommend. About 25 percent of that amount, or roughly 6 grams, should be in the form of soluble fiber. "And it's a good idea to eat most of your fiber with the fattiest meal of the day, so it does its job most effectively," Dr. Newman says.

Make pectin your pal. Fruits such as apples, grapefruit, oranges, and bananas contain a special kind of soluble fiber called pectin. Like other soluble fiber, pectin blocks the absorption of cholesterol into the bloodstream. But it also seems to affect the enzymes in the liver that produce cholesterol. The more pectin that you eat, the smaller the amount of cholesterol made in your liver.

Serve up soy. Tofu and other soy foods contain phytoestrogens, compounds that help transport LDL cholesterol from the bloodstream to the liver, where it's broken down and excreted. Based on what research has shown so far, experts suggest aiming for two or three servings of soy foods a day to reap the cholesterol-clobbering benefits of phytoestrogens. One-half cup of tofu counts as a serving, as does one cup of soy milk.

Savor the "stinking rose." Garlic contains a compound called allicin that apparently has the ability to alter the way your body uses cholesterol. An analysis of the findings of five studies found that eating ½ to 1 clove of garlic a day can lower blood cholesterol an average of 9 percent. If you decide to give garlic a try, remember to mince or crush it before eating it. That releases more cholesterol-combating allicin.

Drink to your health—maybe. Scientists don't yet know why, but alcohol can bolster beneficial HDL cholesterol—sometimes as much as moderate exercise can. Of course, this news is tempered by the finding that even moderate alcohol consumption can increase your odds of developing breast cancer.

Research is under way to identify the portion of wine that's beneficial to cholesterol to try to come up with a nonalcoholic substitute. Until then, Dr. Judelson advises that if you do choose to imbibe, keep it moderate: no more than two or three drinks a week.

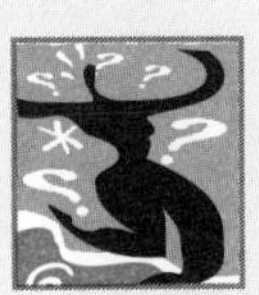

Women Ask Why

Why does my total cholesterol keep going up as I age?

Women have a natural prescription for keeping bad low-density lipoprotein (LDL) cholesterol levels low: the female hormone estrogen.

Estrogen protects us by acting as an antioxidant and fighting cholesterol buildup in our arteries. The problem is that when we go through menopause, our bodies produce less and less estrogen, making it easier for LDL to stick around and increase our risk for heart disease. (Protection against heart disease is one reason to consider estrogen replacement therapy; the other is the protection that estrogen gives your bones.)

No matter what your age, however, if you notice your cholesterol rising, the first thing you need to change is your diet. Cholesterol is only found in animal foods, so you should cut back on high-fat meats and choose low-fat dairy products. If you're overweight, limit calories. And you should increase your exercise as well. After diet changes, exercise has been found most effective in raising your good high-density lipoprotein (HDL) cholesterol. Smoking cessation also can raise HDL. So if you smoke, quit.

Expert Consulted
Barbara Levine, R.D., Ph.D.
Director of the nutrition information center
Cornell University Medical College
New York City

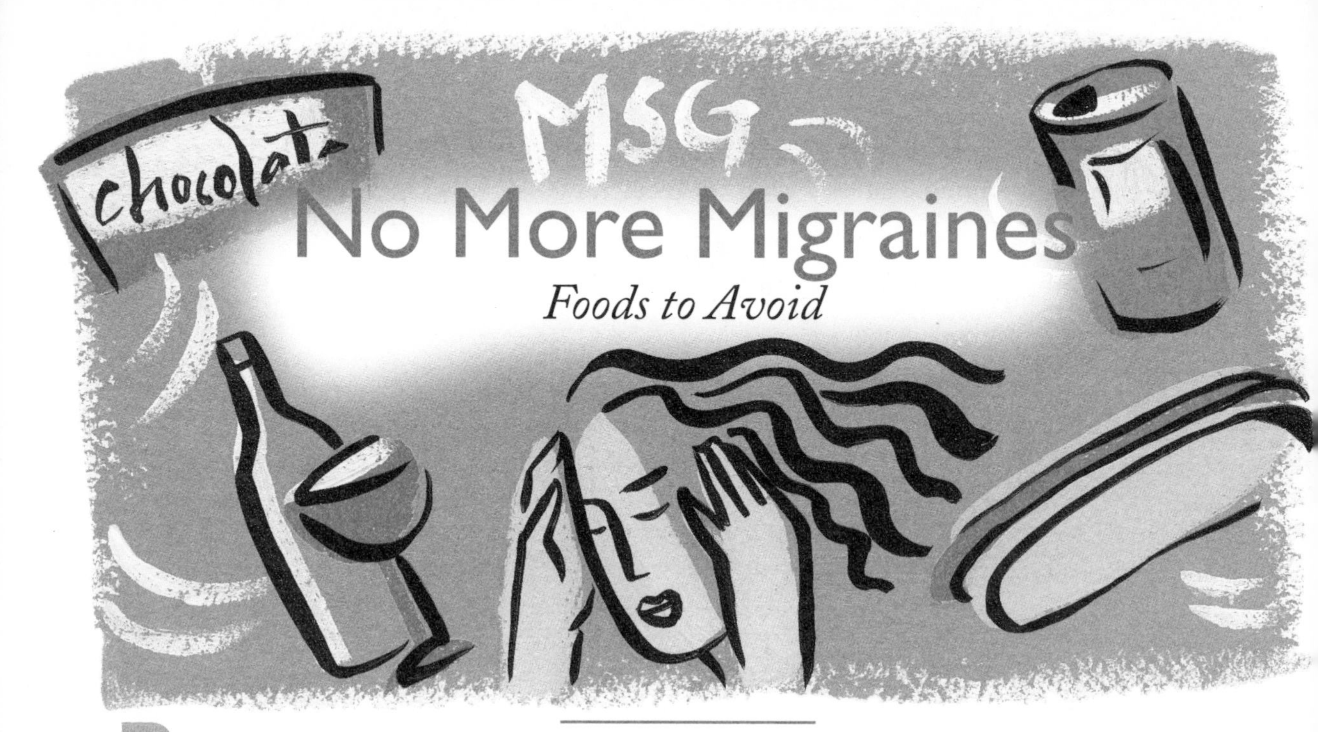

No More Migraines

Foods to Avoid

Referring to a migraine as a headache is like referring to a tornado as a breeze. Yes, a headache hurts, even throbs. But a migraine bludgeons, crushes, tortures, incapacitates. If you've never had one—lucky you—imagine having your skull squeezed in a vise while someone pounds on it with a sledgehammer, and you get the idea.

About 18 percent of women experience migraine, a condition characterized by rapid changes in the blood vessels of the face, head, and neck. The word *migraine* comes from the Greek *hemikrania*—literally, "half cranium." It alludes to the fact that migraine typically affects only one side of the head. But it doesn't stop there.

Migraine pain can envelop your entire body, treating you to a smorgasbord of symptoms that includes nausea, vomiting, dizziness, tremors, and sensitivity to light and sound. The misery can endure anywhere from a few hours to more than a day.

Scientists are still trying to figure out the chain of events that takes place in the brain leading up to a full-blown migraine. They do know that any of a number of factors can get the ball rolling, including stress, poor sleeping habits, even a change in altitude or the weather. But one of the most common triggers of migraine pain is food.

Foes in the Fridge

According to one estimate, one in every five migraine episodes can be traced to something you ate. Dozens of foods contain natural or added substances that can alter your brain chemistry in such a way that blood vessels on the outside of your skull undergo chemical changes that irritate sensitive nerve endings, explains Russell W. Walker, M.D., chief of the Head Pain Program at the Barrow Neurological Institute in Phoenix.

Women seem especially vulnerable to such food triggers. Perhaps that's why we are three times as likely to suffer from migraines as men.

Many doctors attribute this heightened susceptibility to the hormonal fluctuations that occur every month as part of the menstrual cycle. In fact, roughly 50 percent of migraine-prone women report that they most often experience attacks around the time of their periods.

You may be able to head off migraine pain, according to Dr. Walker, simply by avoiding foods that contain any of the following substances.

Aspartame. This artificial sweetener, which goes by the brand name NutraSweet, has caused its share of controversy. While researchers have not yet proven that it provokes migraines, people report experiencing more attacks when they eat foods and drink beverages that have aspartame as an ingredient.

Monosodium glutamate. Often used as a flavor enhancer in Chinese cuisine, MSG is also a common ingredient in lunchmeats, canned and dried soups, and frozen dinners.

Nitrites. Food manufacturers use nitrites to preserve the color of cured meats, such as hot dogs, bacon, ham, and salami.

Vasoactive amines. Perhaps the best-known member of this class of food triggers is tyramine, an amino acid found mainly in strong aged cheeses, pickled herring, chicken livers, and the pods of lima beans and snow peas. Other vasoactive amines include phenylethylamine (in chocolate) and synephrine (in citrus fruits and juices), says Merle Diamond, M.D., associate director of the Diamond Headache Clinic in Chicago.

Another common migraine provocateur: alcohol. "In fact, it tops the list of foods that affect the most people with migraine," says Dr. Diamond. "It is a vasodilator, meaning that it expands blood vessels, which can trigger migraine."

Making Headway against the Pain

If you are migraine-prone, you can control the frequency and severity of your attacks by identifying and eliminating the foods that cause you problems. The best way to accomplish that is to keep a migraine diary, according to Dr. Diamond.

Each time you experience a migraine, record the date, time, and severity of the episode, along with any foods you have eaten. Also make note of any details that you think may be relevant—perhaps you're stressed, or you're having your period, or you're taking medication. Then watch for a pattern to develop.

Once you've ferreted out the potential offenders, drop them from your diet and see if you notice a difference in how often migraine occurs and in how much it hurts. "You can prevent migraine at least 40 percent of the time just by making dietary changes," Dr. Diamond notes.

Just as some foods instigate migraine pain, other foods may actually help to prevent it. Here's what researchers know so far.

Count on carbohydrates. Eating more carbohydrate-rich foods can help boost levels of the brain chemical serotonin, which is responsible for transmitting messages from one nerve cell to another. A dip in your serotonin level can set the stage for migraine.

"There's no doubt that following a diet high in complex carbohydrates and low in fat can be very helpful for some people who experience migraines, although we don't know exactly why," Dr. Diamond says. So you may want to try stocking your diet with whole grains, beans, and fresh vegetables, all of which supply complex carbohydrates.

Note: If you have hypoglycemia, or low blood

sugar, eating lots of complex carbohydrates may make your migraine attacks worse instead of better. In fact, you may be better off cutting back on complex carbs.

Bank on B_6. Like complex carbohydrates, vitamin B_6 helps to increase the levels of serotonin in the brain. So make sure that you're getting at least the Daily Value (DV) of B_6 for women, which is 2 milligrams. One medium baked potato supplies 0.7 milligram of the nutrient, or 35 percent of the DV.

Mind your minerals. There's evidence to suggest that getting enough calcium, iron, and magnesium in your diet can also help to protect you against migraine attacks. Here are some of the latest findings about these minerals.

- ***Calcium.*** In one study, women who consumed 200 milligrams of calcium a day—just 20 percent of your recommended daily intake of 1,000 milligrams—experienced fewer migraine episodes than women who consumed less than that amount. Top food sources of the mineral include skim milk (302 milligrams per eight-ounce glass) and nonfat yogurt (452 milligrams per cup).
- ***Iron.*** If you run low on iron, your red blood cells can't transport oxygen the way they should. In response, your blood vessels dilate to allow more blood to flow through—and that may lead to migraine. You should be getting at least the DV of iron, which is 18 milligrams. Lean meats are your top choice, since they contain the type of iron that's highly absorbable. Three ounces of broiled top round steak, for example, supplies 2.5 milligrams of the mineral. An equal portion of roasted white turkey meat contains 1.2 milligrams.
- ***Magnesium.*** Research has shown that migraine-prone people often don't have enough magnesium in their brain cells. Correcting the shortfall may help protect against migraine pain. This "remedy" has proven especially effective for women who experience migraine during their periods. To meet the DV of 400 milligrams, check out the cereal aisle. Some brands supply more than 100 milligrams of magnesium per one-ounce serving.

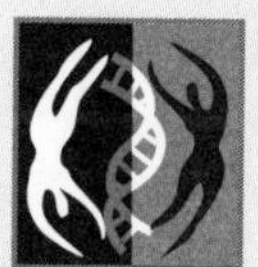

WOMAN TO WOMAN

Taking Out the Triggers, Taking Back Her Life

Jennifer Barber, a young woman from Alpharetta, Georgia, felt as though migraines were taking over her life. With lifestyle changes, she brought them under control. This is her story.

I had my first migraine at age 10. By the time I was a student in college, I was getting them every other day. They were persistent—the longest lasted for 20 days. Four or five times a month, migraines would severely interrupt my daily schedule. When I'm having one, I'm a leave-me-alone-to-lie-down-in-a-dark-room-and-be-quiet kind of person.

Then, one summer, I got fed up with my migraine attacks. I subscribed to a migraine newsgroup, accessed through the Internet. I discovered that by changing my lifestyle, I might be able to make the pain go away. I also went to a neurologist.

The neurologist prescribed some powerful medication. When the migraines abated a bit, I had more energy to think about my headaches and identify my major migraine triggers. By paying attention to what I was eating, I discovered that many of my migraines were caused by eating some very common foods.

I stopped eating processed meats, which contain nitrites.

That wasn't a big deal for me—I'm not a lunchmeat-eater. I do have the occasional hot dog craving, but if I eat one, it's an instant migraine.

I've also cut back on aged cheeses, like Cheddar, and I always avoid MSG. That's a challenge, because many packaged foods, even canned soups, contain it. The hard part is that labels don't always say "MSG." They refer to it by its full name: monosodium glutamate. So grocery shopping can be challenging.

I tried cutting back on caffeine and chocolate, which trigger migraines in some people, but I didn't notice a big difference. I was in college at the time, and I couldn't make it without Diet Coke.

Since I'm hypoglycemic, my blood sugar levels plummet if I don't eat regularly—which I know will lead to an immediate migraine. So I try to eat reasonable amounts of protein and complex carbohydrates, which keep my blood sugar steady.

I have seen some pretty weird tips on the migraine newsgroup. I'm willing to try anything, though. There are very few things that I wouldn't give up to get rid of the pain of migraines.

The changes I've made have helped—it has been amazing. I get one migraine a week now as opposed to four, and they're not usually as bad as before. I may not be able to uncover the cause of my migraines, but I sure can eliminate the triggers.

Quaff coffee. A jolt of java may help pull the plug on migraine pain since caffeine temporarily constricts dilated blood vessels, points out Dr. Diamond. But be careful not to overdo: Too much caffeine can actually trigger a migraine attack. She recommends that you limit yourself to two five-ounce cups of coffee a day, which amounts to about 200 milligrams of caffeine.

Size up soy. Based on very preliminary research, a team of scientists at Yale University School of Medicine has theorized that soy foods may help head off one particular type of migraine. Soy contains compounds called isoflavones, which the researchers found can short-circuit migraine associated with a rare disorder called hereditary hemorrhagic telangiectasia. The results of their study need to be confirmed on a much larger scale. But given all the other wonderful things that soy can do for your good health, you have nothing to lose—and everything to gain—by giving it a try.

Treat your pain gingerly. From Odense University in Denmark come preliminary reports that the spice ginger may counteract prostaglandins, substances that cause blood vessels to become inflamed and therefore produce migraine pain. It's too soon to say what the therapeutic amount of ginger may be. But if you want to give it a try, make yourself a cup of ginger tea by steeping a teaspoon of the grated root in a cup of boiling water for at least five minutes, suggests Dr. Walker. Sip the tea whenever you feel migraine coming on, she says.

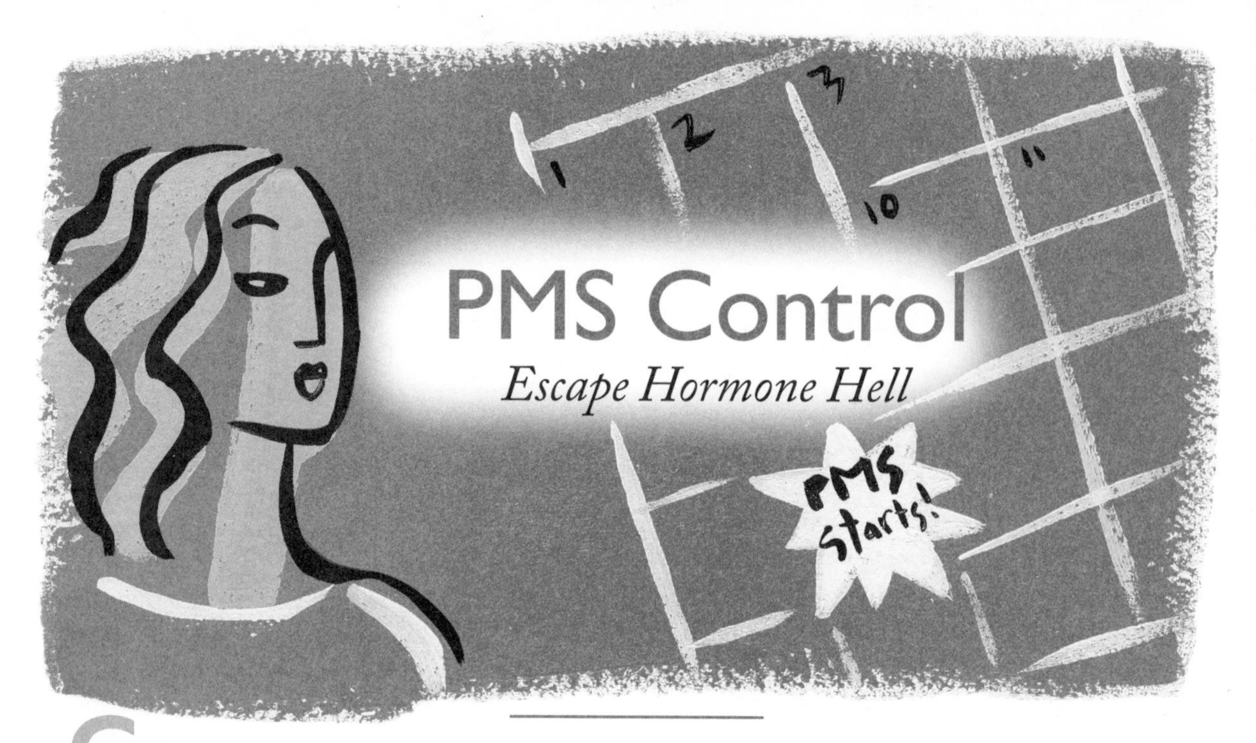

PMS Control

Escape Hormone Hell

Comedians build their stand-up routines around it. T-shirts, bumper stickers, and coffee mugs poke fun at it. Heck, even those little sticky notes feature snide one-liners about it.

But for those of us who actually have premenstrual syndrome...well, this monthly misery doesn't exactly evoke belly laughs.

Premenstrual syndrome—you may know it as PMS—is really an umbrella term for a whole suitcase of symptoms that drop in like an unwelcome houseguest a week to 10 days before your period. In fact, more than 150 specific physical and emotional maladies have ties to PMS.

Thankfully, no one—at least no one on record—experiences them all. Some of us may get only one or two, while others may get as many as a dozen. Among the most common complaints are irritability, depression, insomnia, bloating, headaches, edginess, constipation, fatigue, and breast tenderness—not to mention seemingly insatiable cravings for sugar, fat, and other dietary bad guys.

Scientists can't yet explain why PMS knocks some women for a loop while leaving others virtually unscathed. Nor do they understand why PMS bestows about 15 percent of women with premenstrual pleasantries such as increased sex drive and enhanced creativity. One thing is almost certain: If PMS makes you miserable, you'll do just about anything for relief.

No More PMS, Period

What you eat—and when you eat—has a lot to do with how you feel in the week or two leading up to menstruation. Some foods can ease your premenstrual symptoms, while others can make them worse. If your period is punctuated by PMS distress, heed this nutrition advice from the experts.

Think small. Instead of your standard three squares, try eating smaller meals more often throughout the day. "Anecdotal evidence suggests that you're more irritable about four hours after your last meal," explains Jean Endicott, Ph.D., professor of clinical psychology in the department of psychiatry at Columbia University College of Physicians and Surgeons and director of the premenstrual evaluation unit at Columbia-Presbyterian Medical Center, both in New York City. "So we suggest women don't go more than three to four hours without eating something."

Quiet cravings with complex carbs. "On top of all the other symptoms they're experiencing, a lot of women also have intense food cravings with PMS—especially for sweet foods, like chocolate," says Elizabeth Somer, R.D., author of *Nutrition for Women* and *Food and Mood.* "Sugar consumption can go up to 20 teaspoons a day for some women!"

You're better off sticking with foods rich in complex carbohydrates, Somer says. Complex carbohydrates have two advantages. First, they maximize your serotonin level. Second, they help to stabilize your blood sugar, which appears to take a premenstrual dip in women with PMS. Whole-grain cereals, beans, and fruits and vegetables are excellent sources of complex carbohydrates. Other choices include pasta, rice, and bagels.

Phase out saturated fat. Saturated fat—the kind found in meats, whole-fat dairy products, and many processed foods—elevates estrogen levels. And estrogen intensifies virtually all premenstrual symptoms.

Because dietary fat affects so many aspects of a woman's health, some experts advise that all women—whether or not they have PMS—limit their fat intakes to 25 percent of calories, with 8 percent or less of those calories as saturated fat and the rest as unsaturated fats.

Phase in the friendly fat. Researchers are now looking into whether another type of fat—omega-3 fatty acids, found in certain fish as well as in flaxseed and canola oils—may play a role in premenstrual symptoms. Preliminary evidence suggests that when we have too few omega-3's and too much linoleic acid (an unsaturated fat) in our systems, the imbalance leads to an overproduction of a certain type of prostaglandin. This hormonelike compound, in turn, can cause painful menstrual cramps.

Because we get so much linoleic acid in our diets from vegetable oils such as corn and safflower, some nutritionists suggest eating more omega-3–rich fish such as salmon and mackerel. You can also try using a little canola oil in your cooking and replacing other vegetable oils in salad dressings with flaxseed oil.

Count on calcium. In a study conducted at the USDA Human Nutrition Research Center in Grand Forks, North Dakota, researchers put two groups of women on either a high-calcium diet (1,336 milligrams a day) or a low-calcium diet (587 milligrams a day). Among the women consuming the most calcium, 70 percent reported fewer backaches and less cramping, 80 percent reported less bloating, and 90 percent reported being less irritable or depressed.

According to government guidelines, women between the ages of 25 and 50 should aim for at least 1,000 milligrams of calcium a day. An eight-ounce glass of skim milk has about 300 milligrams of the mineral, so 3½ glasses will put you over the top. If your stomach or your tastebuds don't tolerate milk well, you can opt for nondairy calcium sources like collard greens, dandelion greens, and canned salmon with bones.

Mine more minerals. In two separate studies, researchers found that women in the throes of PMS invariably come up short on the minerals magnesium and zinc. The researchers suspect that something—they don't yet know what—causes blood levels of these minerals to drop prior to menstruation. The nutrient shortfall, they theorize, affects the brain's chemical makeup. And that, in turn, triggers premenstrual symptoms.

More research is needed to determine the exact nature of the relationship between both

SMART SALTY FOOD SUBSTITUTES

If you're like most women, you can predict the impending arrival of your period by the fact that your once-comfortable jeans suddenly feel two sizes too small.

Bloating is a common premenstrual symptom—a sign that your body is hoarding water in preparation for the possibility of pregnancy. This filled-up feeling can last anywhere from a day or two to a week before your period. If you're routinely plagued with this waterlogged feeling, what you eat may be contributing to the problem, says Mary Lake Polan, M.D., professor and chairman of the department of gynecology and obstetrics at Stanford University School of Medicine.

The solution is simple: Drastically cut back on water-retaining salt. Here's a list of the high-sodium foods common to women's diets and some substitutions that you can make.

Instead of...	Choose...
Canned fish, meats, or pork and beans and processed lean meats	Cooked dried beans, fresh fish, fresh turkey or chicken, or tofu
Canned soup	Low-sodium canned soup
Canned vegetables	Fresh or frozen vegetables
Cheddar or Parmesan cheese	Monterey Jack, mozzarella, or ricotta cheese
Commercially prepared biscuits, muffins, or rolls	Whole-grain bread
Instant hot cereal	Cooked oatmeal
Olives, pickles, potato chips	Fresh fruit
Salted popcorn	Unsalted popcorn

minerals and PMS. In the meantime, it can't hurt to eat more foods rich in magnesium and zinc. For magnesium, choose leafy greens, beans, and whole grains. For zinc, your best bets are oysters and ready-to-eat cereals.

Bank on B_6. Vitamin B_6 appears to boost production of the feel-good neurotransmitter serotonin. When researchers in England gave women with PMS 50 milligrams of B_6 every day for three months, the women said they felt less depressed, irritable, and tired.

To reap the therapeutic benefits of B_6, you'd have to take 25 times the Daily Value of the nutrient, which is 2 milligrams. But experts say you can consume up to 100 milligrams of B_6 a day without any ill effects. Some of the best food sources include bananas, chicken breast, and baked potatoes.

Enjoy soy. Soy foods such as tofu and tempeh contain phytoestrogens, compounds that are essentially weak versions of human estrogen. For reasons that scientists can't yet explain, phytoestrogens actually reduce the amount of estrogen in your body, which in turn helps to relieve premenstrual symptoms. In Asian countries, where soy foods are a dietary staple, comparatively few women experience PMS.

Skip the salt. A high salt intake makes you retain more water, according to Peggy Gerlock, R.D., a spokesperson for the Washington Dietetic Association in Seattle. If you have a problem with premenstrual bloating, Gerlock suggests that you consume no more than 2,000 milligrams of sodium a day—that's about one teaspoon of salt—in the week or two leading up to your period. Try seasoning your foods with herbs rather than salt. And check the sodium content of packaged foods by reading their labels.

Can the caffeine. The caffeine in coffee, tea, cola, and chocolate appears to worsen premenstrual symptoms, especially breast tenderness. In a study at Duke University in Durham, North Carolina, researchers had 113 women with premenstrual breast discomfort limit their coffee consumption to two cups a day or less.

After six months, 61 percent of the women reported that their breasts felt better.

Cutting back on caffeine doesn't help everyone. But if you have premenstrual breast pain, you may want to give it a try. Just be sure to do it gradually. If you eliminate caffeine abruptly, you're likely to get bad headaches, Dr. Endicott says. So rather than going cold turkey with coffee, for example, you may want to slowly switch to decaf. Start with a mix of three-quarters regular coffee and one-quarter decaf, then graduate to half and half, then continue until you're completely on decaf.

Think before you sip. You may think that alcohol can douse your premenstrual tension and help you feel less anxious and irritable. In reality, alcohol is a depressant, which means it can deepen a dour mood. It also makes you more prone to angry outbursts and other impulsive, emotional reactions, Dr. Endicott says.

Your best bet—for a variety of health reasons—is to abstain from alcohol. But if you drink, do so in moderation: no more than one or two alcoholic beverages a week, advises Mary Lake Polan, M.D., professor and chairman of the department of gynecology and obstetrics at Stanford University School of Medicine.

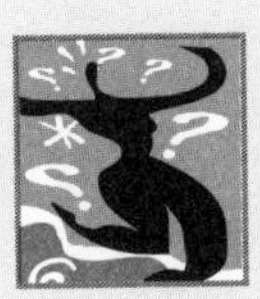

Women Ask Why

Why didn't I hear about PMS when I was growing up?

It wasn't until the 1950s that British doctor Katharina Dalton coined the phrase *premenstrual syndrome*. The term *PMS* didn't catch on until the 1960s, when the birth control pill was introduced, liberating women from previous sexual restraints. Before the 1960s, any mention of menstruation was taboo for the media. But following the sexual revolution, PMS and menstruation were openly discussed at colleges and universities, on television programs, and in newspapers.

The 1960s brought more than just talk. The decade also brought change. Instead of viewing the symptoms women experienced before their periods as a reason to deny them employment or even as a reason to excuse girls from gym class, the medical establishment and women themselves began looking for ways to ease and reduce the symptoms.

Is PMS more widespread today than in previous decades and centuries? In her book, *PMS: The Essential Guide to Treatment Options*, Dr. Dalton notes that women today have fewer children. Because they are pregnant less often, they have more periods and may more frequently seek a doctor's care to relieve their PMS symptoms. Also, women are under more stress than in previous times and tend to restrict their diets more often, both conditions that intensify PMS.

Expert Consulted
Maryanne Horowitz, Ph.D.
Professor of history
Title IX officer
Occidental College
Los Angeles

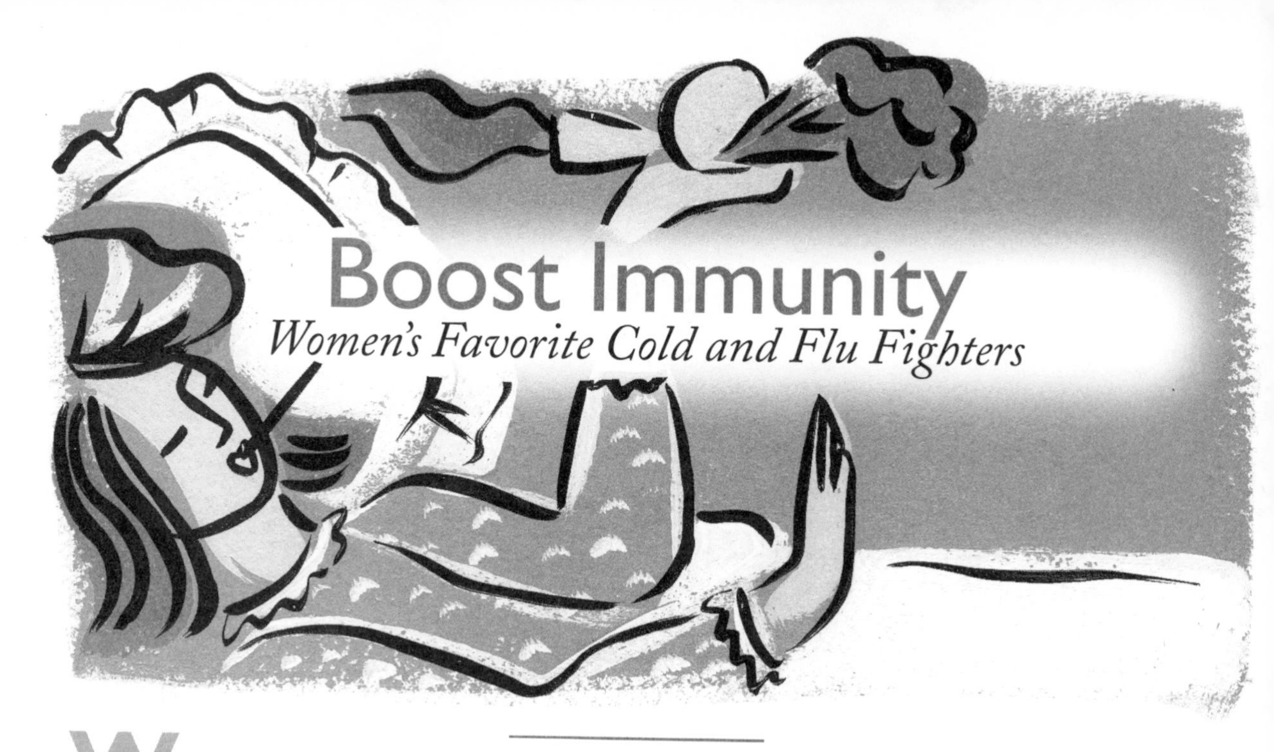

Boost Immunity

Women's Favorite Cold and Flu Fighters

"Wear your galoshes when it rains."

"Don't go out in the cold with damp hair."

"Stay out of drafts."

"Eat your vegetables."

Women do a pretty good job of passing along advice they heard as children for fending off colds and flu. Of course, doctors now tell us that wet feet, damp hair, and drafts don't make us sick—germs do.

Now more than ever, however, eating your vegetables (and fruit, while you're at it) seems to hold up as a valid strategy for boosting immunity. What's more, we should follow this advice ourselves—something we don't always do.

"When we don't eat well, the first thing that will be compromised is our immune system," says Susanna Cunningham-Rundles, Ph.D., associate professor of immunology at New York Hospital–Cornell Medical Center in New York City. "Because women experience additional stresses each month with menstruation and often in association with pregnancy and child care, women have a particular need to pay attention to getting the right nutrients to boost their immune systems. We are likely to be the ones caring for children, who are more readily exposed to viruses, exposing ourselves to germs, too."

The Defensive Lineup

Your immune system has special defense mechanisms that are constantly at work, protecting your body from bacterial infections or viral invasions that can cause colds and flu. Your skin and mucous membranes, and the secretions these membranes produce, constitute your first line of defense against foreign substances.

If a virus manages to slip past your outer barrier, it's met by the next level of defense, which works via immune cells in your bloodstream. Specifically, blood has two specialized types of white cells, or lymphocytes, called B cells and T cells.

B cells manufacture antibodies. T cells are the first to attack viruses and bacteria when they enter your body. They also manufacture interleukins, which carry signals through the immune system. Other immune cells, natural killer cells, kill infected cells and make interferon to protect healthy cells from infection.

The immune system is extremely selective, launching responses geared toward eliminating a specific invader. Your immune system also has an incredible memory. After your initial exposure to an infection, if this same infection ever returns, your immune system will recognize it immediately and issue a counterattack. In other words, you build immunity to infections encountered in the past.

Vitamins to the Rescue

Plant foods contain substances called antioxidants. These are disease-fighting compounds that keep our immune systems strong by protecting cells from harm. Of the many antioxidants found in nature, vitamins C and E and beta-carotene are the most powerful. And getting enough of these compounds in your diet is easy if you know what foods to eat, says Lillie Grossman, R.D., Dr.P.H., professor of nutrition at California State University, Northridge. Here's what experts recommend.

Consume citrus for C. Vitamin C strengthens white blood cells, which are critical for fending off infection. It also lowers levels of histamine, a chemical released by the immune cells that can trigger runny noses.

The Daily Value (DV) for vitamin C is 60 milligrams. Many researchers agree that 200 milligrams may be the optimal amount that your body needs every day to protect against disease. Some of the best sources of vitamin C are citrus fruits; an orange, for example, has 70 milligrams. Other fruits and vegetables such as kiwi, cantaloupe, and broccoli are also good choices.

Nibble seeds, nuts, and wheat germ. Vitamin E has been found to increase levels of interferon and interleukin, two of the chemicals produced by the immune system to fight off infection. In a study at Tufts University in Boston, researchers found that people taking 800 international units (IU) of vitamin E each day were able to increase their levels of interleukin.

Experts generally recommend 400 IU of vitamin E a day—well above the DV of 30 IU. Unfortunately, vitamin E is found mainly in nuts, seeds, and vegetable oils, which are also high in fat. But you don't have to eat nuts and seeds by the handful to reap their benefits. Just sprinkle a few almonds or sunflower seeds onto your salads to give them an extra antioxidant crunch. Wheat germ also supplies generous amounts of vitamin E, but without the fat and calories. Try adding it to cereal, baked goods, and casseroles.

Scout out beta-carotene. Beta-carotene stimulates the immune system's natural killer cells. Researchers at the University of Arizona in Tucson found that people getting 30 milligrams (about 50,000 IU) of beta-carotene a day produced more natural killer cells and immune-boosting lymphocytes than those getting less beta-carotene.

Beta-carotene is a plant pigment, so look for deep green, yellow, and orange fruits and vegetables when you're in the produce aisle. Dark, leafy vegetables like spinach, broccoli, turnips, and collard greens and bright orange and yellow vegetables like sweet potatoes and carrots are all excellent sources of beta-carotene. In fact, eating one carrot a day will provide 12 milligrams (20,000 IU) of beta-carotene, just under the recommended amount of 15 to 20 milligrams (25,000 to 33,000 IU) each day.

Munch Foods with Minerals

Vitamins aren't the only nutrients that help hold the line against infection. In various ways, minerals like zinc, copper, iron, magnesium, and

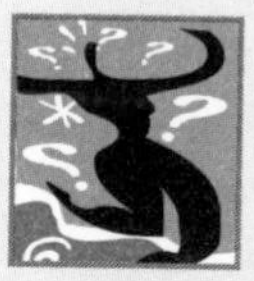

WOMEN ASK WHY

Why should I feed a cold and starve a fever?

Maybe there is something to this old wives' tale. When you come down with a fever, your immune system kicks into defense mode. It produces proteins called cytokines to protect your body from harmful invaders. Unfortunately, these proteins also affect your metabolic rate. It slows down and makes you feel like you don't want to eat, which isn't necessarily a bad thing. Not eating gives your digestive system a rest and allows your body's resources to be used to fight the invading infection.

On the other hand, feeding a cold can be very therapeutic because it helps to stimulate circulation. Further, by eating, you provide your immune cells with the vitamins and minerals they need to fight the cold. But you need to be careful about the foods you eat. This isn't the time to take in fatty, salty foods, because they are more difficult to digest. Fortunately, when they have a cold, many people crave soups and other hot foods. This is very beneficial since a steaming bowl of soup opens airways and keeps mucus flowing. Chicken soup is a well-known home remedy for a cold because it usually contains garlic and vegetables, well-known immunity boosters.

Whether you have a fever or a cold, however, it's important to drink plenty of fluids. Even if you aren't hungry, keep drinking juices such as orange juice and grapefruit juice, which are high in vitamin C, a potent immunity protector. Most important, listen to your body. If it says you're hungry, eat. If you can't bear the thought of food, don't push it. Just remember to keep flushing your system with liquids.

Expert Consulted
Susanna Cunningham-Rundles, Ph.D.
Associate professor of immunology
New York Hospital–Cornell Medical Center
New York City

selenium play a role in boosting immunity—and they're widely distributed in fresh foods. In fact, the less you rely on processed foods, the less apt you are to need mineral supplements to shore up immunity, says Dr. Grossman.

For mineral-smart eating, follow these guidelines recommended by Dr. Grossman.

Make seafood your zinc link. A deficiency in zinc can slow down your immune system's response to foreign invaders, and it can cause a decline in the production of T cells. Studies have shown that people deficient in zinc are more prone to infection and immunity weakness.

Among food sources of zinc, oysters are tops. Six medium-size steamed oysters supply 76 milligrams—about five times the DV of 15 milligrams. Lean meats are also good sources, as are wheat germ, green beans, and legumes such as pinto beans and black-eyed peas.

Do some ironing. Iron helps carry oxygen to cells, including your immune cells. In addition, your body produces fewer antibodies when it doesn't have enough iron, and as a result your immune defense becomes slowed and less destructive. During menstruation, iron reserves drop, so women need to be particularly aware that they are getting the DV of 18 milligrams of iron. Besides beans, good sources of iron include lean meats and steamed oysters and clams. Tofu and fortified cereals such as Cream of Wheat also supply an abundance of iron.

Serve up selenium-rich foods. Like vitamins C, E, and beta-carotene, selenium is an antioxidant. Needed in very small amounts, this trace mineral activates your body's infection-fighting cells and prevents oxidative damage to cells. The DV for selenium is 70 micrograms—the amount in half a tuna sandwich. Whole grains, fish, and shellfish provide the most selenium.

Mind your magnesium. This mineral helps your body manufacture infection-fighting white blood cells. The DV for magnesium is 400 milligrams. Magnesium is found primarily in whole grains, nuts, seeds, and a few of our finned friends such as mackerel.

Slip in some copper. As mineral deficiencies go, copper deficits are rare, since you need only two milligrams each day. Nevertheless, a deficiency of this essential trace mineral can lead to a low white blood cell count and, consequently, poor resistance to infections. Veal and organ meats such as liver are good sources of copper, but they are also high in cholesterol. Your best bet is to eat steamed oysters (without the butter bath), which have three milligrams of copper for a serving of six oysters.

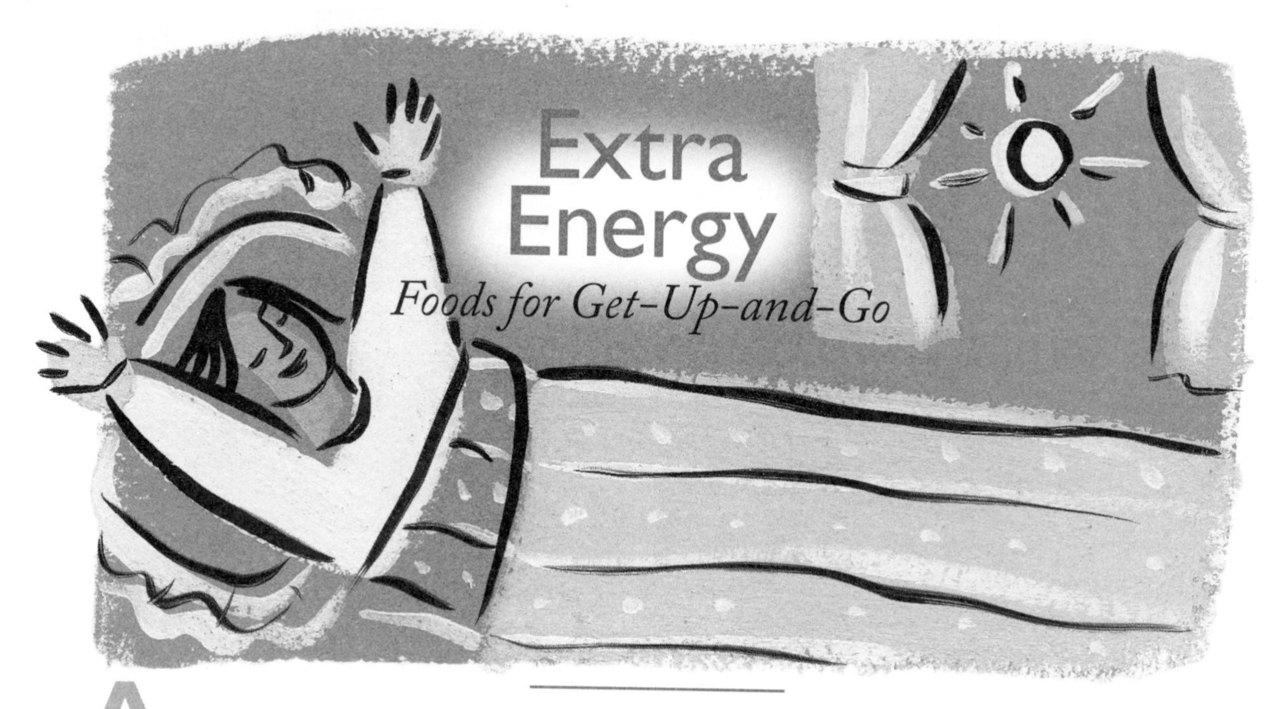

At age 5, you stubbornly refused to take an afternoon nap. At 10, you routinely pleaded with your parents to let you stay up for "just five more minutes." At 20, you lived for weekends, when you and your buddies would head out for a night on the town and not return home until the wee hours of the morning.

Well, all those years of brushing off Mr. Sandman have come back to haunt you bigtime. These days you don't defy sleep. You crave it. Some days you feel sluggish and worn out just hours after rolling out of bed. You rely on caffeine to get you going in the morning. You know Afternoon Slump all too well. By nightfall, you don't need to have someone nag you to go to bed. You go willingly.

It may be small consolation, but you are not alone in your quest for zest. About one-quarter of all Americans—more women than men—go through their days feeling fatigued. And 2 to 3 percent have fatigue so severe that it's almost disabling.

No matter what is responsible for your malaise, poor eating habits can magnify the problem. Quite simply, when you don't feed your body properly, it doesn't have the nutrients it needs to perform at its peak.

The Food Factor

To understand how food influences your energy level, you need to know a little bit about what's going on inside your noggin—even as you're reading this sentence. The nerve cells in your brain communicate with each other with the help of substances called neurotransmitters. These chemical messengers can drastically affect energy levels and how you feel at any given moment. "We're talking about a whole symphony of brain chemicals that ebb and flow throughout the day," says Elizabeth Somer, R.D., author of *Nutrition for Women* and *Food and Mood*.

To produce these neurotransmitters, your brain needs certain nutrients from foods. What you eat, in other words, influences which neurotransmitters are firing away in your brain.

Dopamine and norepinephrine, for example, are two neurotransmitters associated with physical and mental vigor. Studies have shown that when people have high levels of dopamine and norepinephrine, they feel more energetic. Your brain manufactures these neurotransmitters with a helping hand from tyrosine, an amino acid found in high-protein foods such as fish, chicken, and low-fat yogurt.

Serotonin, on the other hand, makes you feel relaxed and snoozy, which is great at bedtime, but not at two o'clock in the afternoon. To produce serotonin, your brain needs the amino acid tryptophan. And tryptophan is abundant in high-carbohydrate foods such as potatoes, pasta, and rice. In fact, just three to four tablespoons of rice can jump-start serotonin production.

Ideally, Somer says, you should choose foods that complement your energy peaks and valleys. For example, if you routinely crash in the afternoon, bypass the high-carbohydrate lunch for one that's rich in protein—perhaps a tuna sandwich, skim milk, and fruit. "Then, when you need to wind down at the end of the day, go for the spaghetti dinner," she suggests.

MAXIMUM-ENERGY MENU

To keep going strong all day long, you need a high-octane meal plan—like this one, designed by Elizabeth Somer, R.D., author of *Nutrition for Women* and *Food and Mood*. It fulfills all the requirements of eating for energy, combining protein- and carbohydrate-rich foods in six small meals spread throughout the day. This meal plan also delivers a healthy dose of fatigue-fighting iron while trimming stamina-sapping sugar, fat, and caffeine.

Breakfast: Toasted bagel topped with one tablespoon of peanut butter; banana; eight ounces of skim milk

Midmorning snack: Bran muffin topped with two tablespoons of apple butter; eight ounces of skim milk

Lunch: Three ounces of extra-lean roast beef on a whole-wheat roll with tomato, lettuce, and mustard; one cup of raw cauliflower florets, sliced carrots, and broccoli; piece of fruit

Midafternoon snack: Six ounces of vanilla low-fat yogurt sprinkled with ⅓ cup of low-fat granola and two tablespoons of dried cranberries, raisins, chopped dates, or other dried fruit

Dinner: Four to six ounces of broiled salmon with dill and lemon; baked potato topped with fat-free sour cream; 1 cup of steamed broccoli; 1 cup of tossed salad with two tablespoons of low-fat dressing; ½ cup of fresh blueberries or one-quarter of a honeydew melon

Evening snack: Frozen whole-wheat waffle topped with half of a banana and one tablespoon of maple syrup

You can also keep your energy on a more even keel by eating low-fat mini-meals instead of the standard three squares. When you don't eat for three to four hours at a shot, your blood sugar level drops slightly, explains Franca Alphin, R.D., nutrition director at the Duke University Diet and Fitness Center in Durham, North Carolina. Eating four or five small meals throughout the day stabilizes your blood sugar, which helps to fend off fatigue.

Edible Energizers

There's more to the energy equation than just protein and carbohydrates. Scientists have identified other key nutrients that keep your internal batteries charged. The following tips can help ensure that you're fueling your body properly, so you feel pumped up instead of pooped out.

Insist on iron. Fatigue is a classic symptom of iron-deficiency anemia. But even minor depletions of your body's iron stores can leave you feeling tired.

Unfortunately, about 40 percent of premenopausal women routinely run low on iron. The shortfall can be attributed in part to uniquely female events such as menstruation and childbirth. But in many cases, we simply don't get enough of the mineral in our diets.

The Daily Value (DV) for iron is 18 milligrams, an amount that you can easily obtain from foods. Among the best sources are lean meat, beans, tofu, and Cream of Wheat cereal.

Don't miss magnesium. Magnesium is a pivotal player in the energy production process. Your body needs the mineral to convert the food that you eat into fuel. To meet the DV of 400 milligrams, ply your diet with beans, tofu, wheat germ, nuts, and seeds.

Zero in on zinc. Like magnesium, zinc supports energy production. The mineral helps your pancreas to manufacture the hormone insulin, which in turn boosts delivery of blood sugar—your body's basic fuel—to cells.

Aim for the DV of 15 milligrams a day. Steamed oysters are an outstanding zinc source, as are wheat germ and lean beef.

B your best. A shortage of B vitamins can leave your body struggling to convert food into usable energy. If you're taking birth control pills, you need to pay special attention to your B vitamin intake. The Pill is known to deplete both B_6 and folate, which can set the stage for fatigue.

The DVs for vitamin B_6 and folate are two milligrams and 400 micrograms, respectively. You'll find B_6 in abundant supply in bananas, cabbage, cauliflower, and wheat germ. For folate, choose beans, carrots, pumpkin, and dark green, leafy vegetables such as spinach.

Real-Life Scenario

Her Lunch Habit Is Making Her Sleepy

Jenny can't understand why she feels so tired all the time. She gets plenty of sleep—in bed by 10:00 P.M., up by 7:00 A.M.—and she never skips breakfast (her usual: a cinnamon-raisin bagel with low-fat cream cheese and a cup of coffee). But by 10:00 A.M., she's dragging. She relies on coffee to get her through the morning, then tries to switch gears with a lunch of pasta salad and whole-grain bread. She feels good for a while, but by 2:00 P.M., she's nodding off at her desk. She hates these peaks and valleys. What can she do to keep her energy on a more even keel?

Half the problem is when and how often she's eating. Jenny's bagel breakfast is a great way to start the day, but if she's up at the crack of dawn, it's no wonder that her body dips into glucose debt by midmorning, driving her to drink mug after mug of caffeine to stay awake. Instead of drinking all that coffee, which provides zero nutrients, Jenny may want to either munch on a late-morning snack or move lunch up an hour.

The other half of Jenny's problem is *what* she's eating—particularly for lunch. What she experiences at two o'clock in the afternoon is not uncommon. While most people tend to feel a post-lunch slump, certain things can make it worse. One is eating a high-carbohydrate meal that's not balanced by pro-

Stay hydrated. You know what happens to your houseplants when you don't water them: They droop. Likewise, allowing yourself to run dry can sap your stamina and leave you feeling sluggish. Try to drink at least eight eight-ounce glasses of water a day.

Don't Let Them Fuel You

Many of the foods we normally turn to for a quick pick-me-up actually end up letting us down instead. To ID these energy impostors, heed this advice from the experts.

tein, and that's what Jenny does by having pasta and bread.

When you have a high-carb meal with little protein, your body starts producing insulin. That insulin causes most of the large amino acids in the bloodstream to be transported to your muscles. An exception is the amino acid tryptophan, the raw material for serotonin. With the competing amino acids cleared out of the bloodstream, more tryptophan can get carried into the brain. The more tryptophan the brain receives, the more serotonin is produced. Since serotonin is a chemical that's involved in a number of functions, including what is called the sleep onset mechanism, it makes you feel sleepy. That's why a pure carbohydrate lunch can trigger drowsiness a couple of hours later.

Consequently, in Jenny's case, a good night's sleep does very little to prevent her afternoon urge to nap. The best way to lift herself out of that midafternoon valley is to simply add some protein at lunchtime. To best keep insulin levels on an even keel all day, Jenny may even want to add a couple of small afternoon snacks—that way she'll be sure to last until dinner.

Expert Consulted
Bonnie Spring, Ph.D.
Professor of psychology
Finch University of Health Sciences/Chicago Medical School
North Chicago, Illinois

Go sour on sugar. Yes, sugar does give you a fast energy fix—but you end up paying for it. As the sugar floods your bloodstream, your pancreas responds by pumping out more insulin, which sweeps the sugar out of your bloodstream and into cells. As a result, your blood sugar level dips, so you feel pooped and may even get an overwhelming urge for a nap.

Nutritionists recommend limiting daily sugar intake to just 10 percent of calories. That means that if you eat 2,000 calories a day, only 200 of those calories should come from sugar. That's about the amount in a small slice of apple pie.

Forgo fat. Trying to get a kick-start from a fatty meal is like trying to start a campfire with a wet newspaper. Your body doesn't want to burn fat, Somer says. It wants to store it. What's more, it has to work hard to digest fatty foods. The process actually slows blood circulation, which impairs the delivery of oxygen to cells. That's when fatigue sets in.

For a variety of health reasons, many experts recommend that you limit your daily fat intake to 25 percent of calories.

Give joe the cold shoulder. A cup of coffee can get you started in the morning. But drink too much—or too late in the day—and you may find that your get-up-and-go has gotten up and gone. Not only does the caffeine in coffee disrupt your sleep, it also depletes B vitamins and disrupts the absorption of iron—nutrients your body needs to produce energy.

Limit your caffeine consumption to 300 milligrams a day, which is the amount in two eight-ounce cups of coffee, recommends Somer. Or slowly switch to a decaf brew, says Wahida Karmally, R.D, director of nutrition at the Irving Center for Clinical Research at Columbia University in New York City.

Rethink your drink. Don't let those frolicking, fun-loving folks in the beer ads fool you. Alcohol is a sedative, and even though it may give you a little buzz at first, it ultimately drops you like a lead balloon. And if you're already tired, you can end up feeling really beat.

Many experts believe that you're better off, health-wise, if you don't drink at all. But if you do drink, keep it moderate—two or three alcoholic beverages a week, at most.

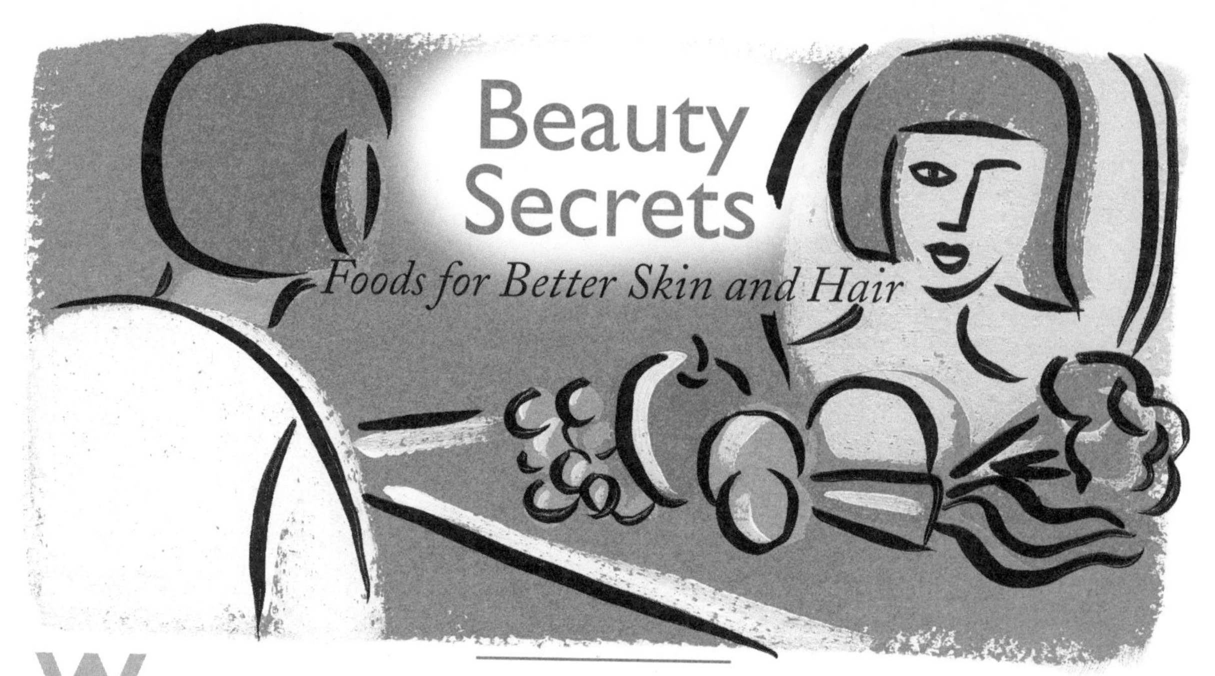

Wander into one of those bath-and-beauty boutiques at the mall, and you'll find shampoos made from kiwifruit, creams made from cucumbers, soaps made from almonds, and lotions made from mangoes. You might get the impression that you're standing before an upscale salad bar rather than a cosmetics counter.

Despite the elaborate packaging, these products press into service hair- and skin-care treatments that have been around for centuries. Even today, women in many parts of the world rely on Ma Nature to keep them looking their best. But you don't have to wear your food to reap its beauty benefits. There's compelling evidence that eating the right stuff—nutritious edibles such as cauliflower, fish, berries, and yogurt—can reward you with healthy hair, glowing skin, elegant nails, and more. It can also help protect against common conditions ranging from acne to wrinkles.

So instead of spending a small fortune on a veritable buffet of potions, why not achieve beauty naturally, from the inside out? The following food strategies can keep you in the pink, from the hair on your head to the nails on your toes.

Acne: Zits Aren't for Kids

You never thought you'd have to deal with one again. Yet here you are, poking and prodding the flaming red pimple that has sprouted on your chin. Sure, you wouldn't mind reliving your youth, but this is a bit too much.

As many adult women know all too well, acne doesn't automatically disappear with your teenage years. It can persist well into your thirties. In fact, some women experience their first breakouts as adults. Others develop rosacea, a condition characterized by pustules and enlarged blood vessels on the nose, cheeks, and forehead.

For blemish-free skin, heed this advice from the experts.

Sail away from seafood. Foods rich in iodine, including clams, crabs, and other shellfish, can cause some people to break out. So if you're acne-prone, leave these off your plate and see if you notice any improvement in the frequency or severity of your breakouts.

Cut out other culprits, too. Scientists have yet to prove that candy, chocolate, or greasy food causes acne. Yet many people swear that they get pimples when they eat too much of this stuff. If that's the case, experts say, then by all means avoid the offending edibles. "These aren't the most healthy foods anyway, so you're better off without them," says D'Anne Kleinsmith, M.D., a dermatologist affiliated with William Beaumont Hospital in West Bloomfield, Michigan.

Zap zits with zinc. The mineral zinc appears to deflate breakouts, perhaps because of its anti-inflammatory properties. Not everyone in the medical community is convinced that zinc works, but since women tend to run low on the mineral anyway, it can't hurt to get a little extra in your diet. Good food sources include wheat germ and nonfat or low-fat yogurt.

Age Spots: Calling Cards from Old Sol

Don't let their name fool you. Age spots can show up on your skin at any time, although they do become more common as you get older. These frecklelike brown splotches are your skin's attempt to protect itself from overexposure to the sun by producing too much melanin, or skin pigment. They're usually harmless, although you should see your doctor if you notice any change in their size, color, or texture.

To keep your skin spotless, give the following tips a try.

Lean toward E. "Vitamin E is an anti-inflammatory agent, and it reduces sun damage to your skin," says Karen E. Burke, M.D., Ph.D., a dermatologic surgeon and dermatologist in private practice in New York City. To get more of the vitamin in your diet, choose foods such as wheat germ, mangoes, and safflower, corn, and soybean oils.

Seek out selenium. "Selenium can also minimize sun damage to your skin," Dr. Burke says. "But because the selenium content of the soil varies across the country, not everyone is getting a protective amount of the mineral." Excellent food sources include tuna and baked tortilla chips.

Limit limes. Certain fruits and vegetables—especially limes, celery, parsnips, and carrots—contain psoralens, chemicals that can increase your sensitivity to the sun. Not everyone experiences a reaction after eating these foods. But if you do, even handling them can make you more susceptible to burning. That's why experts recommend washing your hands before venturing out. And be careful about drinking lime-garnished beverages when you're out in the sun.

Cold Sores: Beat Them to the Punch

Call them cold sores or fever blisters. Either way, they hurt like the dickens—and they don't look very nice, either.

Cold sores don't automatically follow a cold: You must first be exposed to a virus called herpes simplex type 1. (Type 2 causes genital herpes.) Once you have the virus, it stays with you for life. Most of the time, it keeps a low profile. But sometimes an aggravating factor—perhaps stress, illness, the onset of menstruation, or even a dental procedure—can trigger an outbreak.

The sores themselves usually occur around the mouth, although they've been known to show up inside the nose, on the fingers, and even on the eyelids. They start out as blisters, then break down into scabby lesions. It can take a week to 10 days for an entire episode to run its course.

Fortunately, cold sores tend to announce their impending arrival with a tingling sensation at the site of the eruption. That's your cue to take action. Here's what you can do.

Load up on lysine. An amino acid, lysine suppresses the growth of the herpes simplex virus, thus reducing the number of outbreaks. You can increase your lysine intake by consuming plenty of nonfat and low-fat dairy products and fruits such as apples and pears.

Avoid arginine. The herpes simplex virus needs arginine, another amino acid, in order to replicate. In some people, very small amounts of arginine can trigger outbreaks. So if you're prone to cold sores, try cutting back on the arginine-rich foods in your diet, including foods made from sesame seeds, peanuts, and soybeans. Then see if you notice any difference in the frequency or severity of your outbreaks.

FOOD AND BEAUTY: MYTHS AND MAGIC

When it comes to food and beauty, myths abound. Can you separate fact from fiction? Answer each of these questions true or false, then check out the answers that follow.

1. T F Chocolate causes blemishes.
2. T F Fried foods cause acne.
3. T F Drinking lots of water makes your skin healthier.
4. T F Eating gelatin makes your nails longer and stronger.
5. T F Eating lots of protein makes your hair stronger.

Answers

1. Maybe this is true, and maybe it isn't. One of every three people prone to acne may make matters worse by indulging in chocolate. "It's the richness of the chocolate that stimulates the production of excess oil, leading to more acne," explains Marianne O'Donoghue, M.D., associate professor of dermatology at Rush-Presbyterian-St. Luke's Medical Center in Chicago. Her advice: Eat chocolate in moderation.

2. Again, the answer is maybe. Fried foods have lots of fat, and for some people, fat may shift the oil-producing glands in their skin into overdrive. Choose foods that are baked

Fingernail Problems: A Sign That Something's Amiss

Have you taken a good, hard look at your fingernails lately? If not, perhaps you should. You see, your nails are built-in barometers of your body's nutrition status. When they become brittle or misshapen, it usually means that you're getting too little—or too much—of a particular nutrient.

Experts recommend the following strategies for healthy, sharp-looking nails.

Get a boost from biotin. A member of the B-vitamin family, biotin helps to build strong nails. In fact, researchers in Switzerland found that 2,500 micrograms of biotin a day could increase nail thickness by 25 percent.

The dose of biotin used in the Swiss study is more than eight times the Daily Value (DV), which is 300 micrograms. You can boost your intake of the vitamin by consuming soybean flour, cauliflower, lentils, and skim or low-fat (1 percent) milk.

Iron out the problem. If your nails appear spoon-shaped, you may have iron-deficiency anemia. You should see your doctor for a proper diagnosis. But in the meantime, try to get more iron-rich foods in your diet. Good sources include lean meat, Cream of Wheat cereal, baked potatoes, soybeans, and tofu.

Shed pounds slowly. Crash dieting can take a toll on your fingernails, leaving them riddled with horizontal ridges. If you want to lose rather than fried, suggests Dr. O'Donoghue. "I don't forbid my patients anything, though," she adds. "I just ask them not to be junk food junkies."

3. True. Drinking lots of water can reduce dryness and give your skin a healthy appearance, Dr. O'Donoghue says. Water also helps your body to shed old skin cells and replace them with new ones. So drink up. Nutritionists recommend at least eight eight-ounce glasses of water a day—and more, if you're able.

4. True, but not because there's anything special about gelatin. Gelatin is a source of protein, but any kind of protein helps your body grow. Any other protein-rich food would have the same effect, provided you're taking in enough calories to maintain your weight. Good dietary sources of protein include meat, fish, poultry, dairy products, and beans, Dr. O'Donoghue says.

5. False. A normal diet with adequate calories should keep most people's hair in fine shape, Dr. O'Donoghue says. Someone with an eating disorder such as anorexia nervosa would probably have weak, brittle hair because she's not getting enough calories. For the average person, though, nondietary factors like harsh brushing, lack of conditioning, and exposing color-treated hair to the sun may make hair more susceptible to breaking and damage.

weight, experts advise, don't eat so little that you lose more than two pounds a week.

Skin Cancer: Fry Now, Pay Later

Despite all the warnings about the sun's damaging ultraviolet rays, many women still cling to the notion that a bronzed body is the epitome of health and beauty. They don't seem to realize that every minute spent in pursuit of the perfect tan increases their risk of skin cancer. In fact, white women ages 65 and older have a 50-50 chance of developing this form of cancer. It's the most common in the United States, accounting for 40 percent of all diagnosed cancer cases.

Obviously, the best thing you can do for your skin's sake is to limit the amount of time you spend in the sun. When you do venture out, be sure to wear a sunscreen with a sun protection factor (SPF) of 15 or higher. Beyond that, you can try the following dietary strategies for a little extra insurance against skin cancer.

Get your fill of fish. There's some evidence that omega-3 fatty acids, found in fish such as mackerel and salmon, can help prevent skin cancer. Researchers at Baylor College of Medicine in Houston found that people who consume large amounts of omega-3's every day have less chance of developing the kind of cell damage associated with skin cancer during exposure to ultraviolet light, compared with people who don't consume large amounts of omega-3's.

Take time for tea. Laboratory research suggests that drinking green tea can reduce skin cancer risk. Scientists suspect that the tea's anticancer effects come from compounds called polyphenols. Like beta-carotene and vitamins C and E, polyphenols are antioxidants, which means that they protect cells from damage caused by radiation and other toxins. You can buy green tea in supermarkets and health food stores.

Eat lean. When a group of volunteers with histories of skin cancer followed a low-fat diet, they had fewer cancerous growths over a two-year period than a similar group that consumed twice as much fat. Scientists suspect that certain components in fat may cause skin cells to mutate in harmful ways. For this and other health reasons, many experts recommend limiting your daily fat intake to no more than 25 percent of calories.

Thinning Hair: Not for Men Only

We cut it, curl it, comb it, spray it, scrunch it, spray it some more. But never, ever do we *lose* our hair...right?

Well, it's true that we women don't go bald the way men do. But at least 25 percent of us have a problem with thinning hair, Dr. Kleinsmith says. Usually it's only temporary—the possible result of crash dieting, stress, or hormonal changes. If it persists, you should see your doctor.

The right diet can help keep your tresses in tiptop shape. Here's what the experts recommend.

Eye your iron intake. Iron-deficiency anemia can result in hair loss. To make sure that you're meeting the DV of 18 milligrams, pile your plate with iron-rich foods, suggests Mary Frances Picciano, Ph.D., professor of nutrition at Pennsylvania State University in University Park. Lean meat is perhaps the best source of the mineral. Other choices include Cream of Wheat cereal, baked potatoes, soybeans, and tofu.

Sup sensibly. Radical weight-loss programs can deprive your body of the nutrients it needs to function properly, and that can lead to thinning hair. If you want to lose weight, do it slowly and steadily—no more than two pounds a week. And hold your daily fat consumption to no more than 25 percent of calories.

Varicose Veins: Not Inevitable

Imagine pushing a car uphill with its brakes on, and you get a pretty good idea of what your blood is up against as it makes the journey from your legs to your heart. It has to fight gravity all the way. Valves, the gatelike structures in your veins, keep blood moving in the right direction. But sometimes a valve fails to shut properly—the result of too much sitting or standing. When that happens, blood pools in your leg, causing the vein to bulge toward the surface of your skin. That's what you know as a varicose vein.

What you eat—and what you *don't* eat—can influence whether or not you develop varicose veins in the first place. You can reduce your risk by heeding this advice from the experts.

Fight back with fiber. When you strain hard to move your bowels, you create pressure in your abdomen. That causes blood to back up into your legs, and this, over time, weakens vein walls.

To prevent constipation, include plenty of fiber-rich foods in your meals. Some top-notch sources are beans, whole grains, fruits, and vegetables. Some particularly high fiber foods to look for include chickpeas and dried pears.

Pick some berries. Deep-colored berries such as cherries, blueberries, and blackberries contain chemical compounds called bioflavonoids. Scientists believe that bioflavonoids make tiny capillaries less likely to distend or break down, preventing the appearance of so-called spider veins on the surface of the skin. Other good sources of bioflavonoids include grape juice and the white membranes of citrus fruits.

Go easy with the saltshaker. A too-high salt intake can cause your legs to swell. And that puts a lot of pressure on your veins if they are already damaged.

Wrinkles: Foods That Fight Father Time

Here's something to think about: Were it not for the sun, our skin would stay relatively wrinkle-free until we reach our seventies. Instead, most of us start noticing smile lines and crow's-feet years earlier, thanks to a process known as photoaging. In fact, at least 80 percent of the changes we see in our skin as we get older are the result of excessive sun exposure.

By adulthood, some damage has already been

done. But that doesn't mean you should sit around and wait for the wrinkles to appear. On the contrary, there's plenty you can do to delay their appearance. For starters, limit the time you spend in the sun—and when you are outside, protect your skin with sunscreen of at least SPF 15. Then round out your wrinkle-reducing plan with these nutrition strategies.

Up the ante. At least one study of animals has shown that exposure to ultraviolet rays depletes levels of vitamins C and E. These nutrients are antioxidants; they're essential for protecting your cells from the damage caused by radiation and other toxins. Fortunately, you can easily restock your body's antioxidant supply with foods. For vitamin C, choose oranges, broccoli, kiwifruit, and peppers. Wheat germ and vegetable oils (safflower, corn, and soybean) have generous supplies of vitamin E.

Stay afloat. Remember to drink lots of water. Most experts recommend at least eight eight-ounce glasses a day. If you perspire a lot, you should aim even higher.

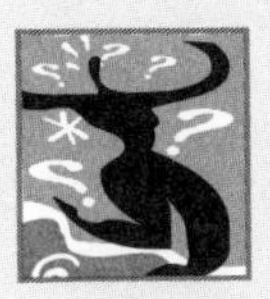

WOMEN ASK WHY

Why do shampoos and conditioners contain vitamins and minerals?

Manufacturers would like you to believe that your hair gets its healthy look from the vitamins and minerals in shampoos and conditioners. The truth is that your hair gets its healthy sheen from the vitamins and minerals you get in food.

The vitamins and minerals these products contain can't be absorbed by your scalp and hair through shampooing. As soon as you rinse your hair, those vitamins and minerals go right down the drain.

Even though vitamins and minerals don't help nurture your hair, they can make it feel softer, and they can help prevent tangles and knots. That's why nutrients like proteins and vitamins B and E are often added to conditioning products.

This isn't to say that vitamins and minerals in your diet aren't important for healthy hair. They're very important. In fact, people who have thinning hair are often advised to get more nutrients like iron in their diet.

So if you're looking for healthy hair in a bottle, reach for the vitamin bottle, not a bottle of shampoo.

Expert Consulted
Diana Bihova, M.D.
Dermatologist in private practice
New York City

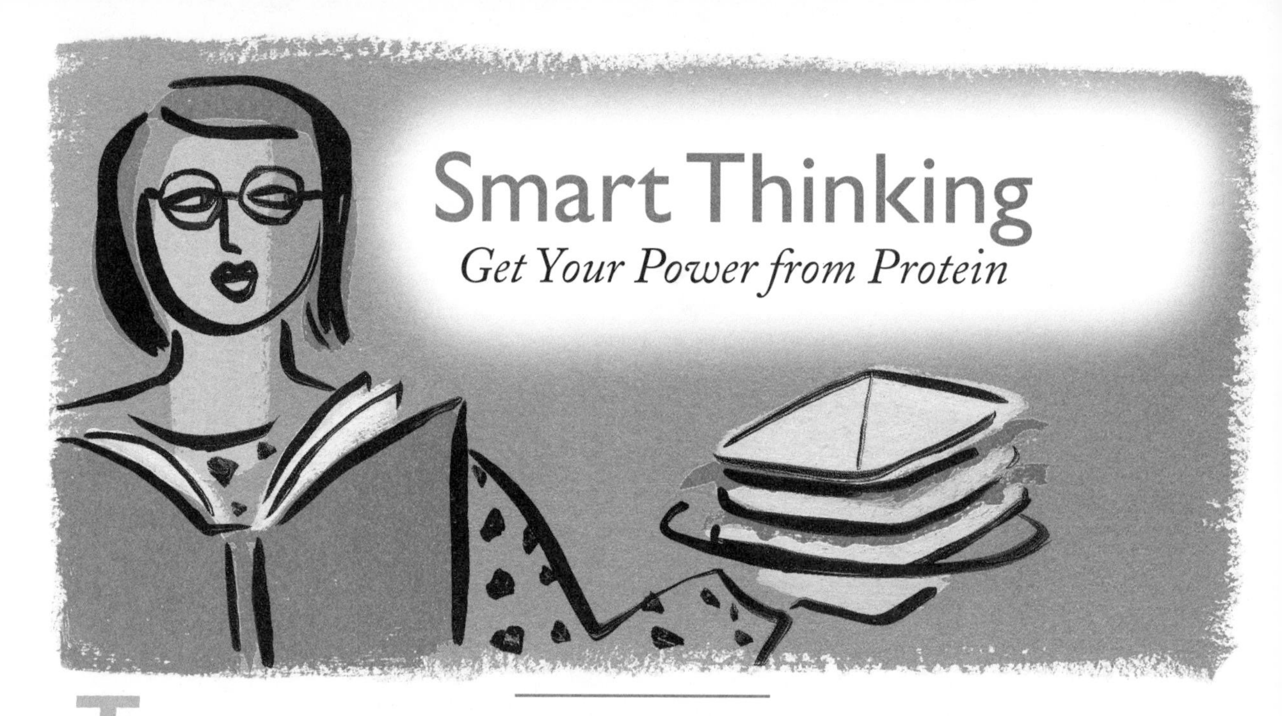

Smart Thinking

Get Your Power from Protein

The Slump—that midafternoon mental malaise that turns two o'clock meetings into group siestas and makes a routine task like balancing a checkbook seem worthy of Einstein. What could possibly cause your usually sharp-as-a-tack mind to become so much oatmeal?

Hunger, for one thing. Like every other organ in your body, your brain requires a steady supply of nutrients over the course of a day to function at its best. Without them, your alertness, concentration, and memory can all become impaired.

The good news is that you can maintain your mental moxie from breakfast to bedtime. All it takes is a little strategic eating—the right foods in the right combinations and at the right times.

A Quick Chemistry Lesson

Whenever you eat a food, your brain uses some of the nutrients it supplies to manufacture neurotransmitters, chemicals that enable the nerve cells in your brain to communicate with each other. How you feel, how you behave, and how well you perform tasks all depends on which type of neurotransmitter is being fired from one nerve cell to the next.

Your mental acuity depends on two particular neurotransmitters: dopamine and norepinephrine. This dynamic duo works to keep you thinking clearly and quickly. At times when you need maximum brainpower, whether for a presentation at work or for a bill-paying marathon at home, you want to ensure high levels of dopamine and norepinephrine in your brain. A little bit of low-fat protein will do the trick.

Protein is rich in tyrosine, an amino acid that your brain converts to dopamine and norepinephrine. These neurotransmitters then leap among nerve cells as you engage in thought.

"Thinking skills, word retrieval, and mental quickness depend on protein," says Judith Wurtman, Ph.D., nutrition research scientist at the Massachusetts Institute of Technology in Cambridge and author of *Managing Your Mind and Mood through Food*. It can counteract midday mental mushiness and extend your brain's high-energy time by as much as three hours.

Now this doesn't give you license to chow down on a steak every day to boost your brainpower. You need to select your protein sources wisely and pay attention to your other eating habits, too. Here's what experts recommend.

Think fin. Fish has a well-deserved reputation as brain food. For one thing, low-fat varieties like haddock, flounder, and cod can be excellent low-fat protein sources. For another, fish supplies B vitamins, which fortify cognitive skills and memory. Other prize high-protein picks include nonfat or low-fat ricotta cheese and turkey breast.

Create a carbo combo. A carbohydrate-only meal can dull your brainpower. That's because carbs give your brain the raw material it needs to manufacture serotonin, the neurotransmitter that leaves you feeling relaxed and even sleepy.

To stay sharp, pair a carbohydrate-rich food with a protein-rich food—for example, a bagel with nonfat cream cheese or pasta with lean meat sauce. The protein slows the digestion of the carbohydrates, so they release their energy at a slow, steady pace. In fact, research suggests that a protein-carbohydrate combination can keep you more alert than either alone.

Save dessert for later. Rather than ending your meal with a sweet treat, save it until about a half-hour before you go to bed, says Carol E. Greenwood, Ph.D., associate professor in the department of nutritional sciences at the University of Toronto Faculty of Medicine. The extra hit of carbohydrates before you hit the sack may quiet your mind and ensure restful slumber.

Smart Eaters, Smart Thinkers

All of us have to think on our feet from time to time. But we met some women whose high-octane professions demand that they be alert, focused, and clear-thinking every minute that they're on the job. We asked them what eating strategies they use to keep their minds in top form all day long. Here's what they had to say.

"I never eat big meals—they make me feel like I need a nap. I stick with small meals all the time. Also, I try to avoid foods that upset my stomach, like chili. They distract my thinking."

Leigh Neumayer, M.D.
Chief of surgery at the Salt Lake Veterans Administration Medical Center in Salt Lake City, Utah

"I never miss breakfast, which usually consists of Egg Beaters, wheat toast, and orange juice. If I go out for lunch, I order fish whenever possible. And I try not to go more than four hours without a light meal or a snack."

Linda Costa
President and CEO of Wordwise, a marketing communications and public relations company in Winter Park, Florida

"In this job, it's really convenient to grab fast food. But I'm learning that heavy, fatty stuff like hamburgers and french fries really slows me down. Salads and vegetables are what keep me going—I eat six small meals a day. And I'm trying to cut back on caffeine and to drink a lot of water instead."

Lieutenant Sonya Domingues
San Antonio Police Department

"I exercise during my lunch hour, so I don't really have time to eat anything. I usually have some low-fat yogurt while I work, then later in the afternoon I snack on baby carrots or a McIntosh apple. And I definitely avoid chocolate—after the initial caffeine-and-sugar jolt wears off, I get really tired."

Lieutenant Colonel Pamela Hale Senterfitt
U.S. Army equal opportunity/sexual harassment officer at the Pentagon in Washington, D.C.

No More Diet Daze

An Eating Strategy That Works

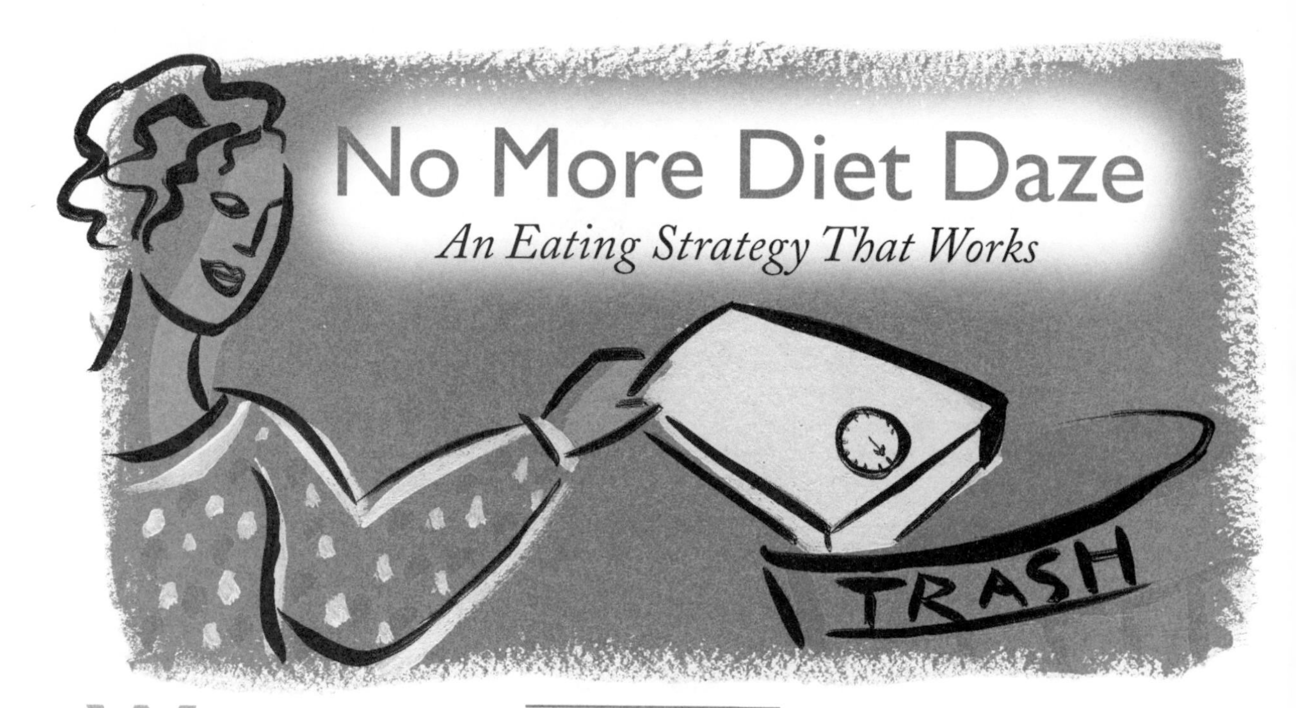

We live in a country that honors hot dogs and apple pie as its national cuisine. Is it any wonder, then, that dieting now rivals baseball as America's favorite pastime?

At this very moment, one out of three women in America is waging her very own battle of the bulge. In fact, the average woman tries at least 10 diets in her lifetime—cutting calories, popping pills, slurping shakes, and even forgoing food completely. Often the pounds do disappear. But, for most women, some or all eventually creep back.

Yet plenty of women manage to achieve and maintain a healthy weight. How do they do it? Simple: They stop dieting.

Many experts agree that you should do the same. "We don't use the word *diet*," says Maria Simonson, Sc.D., Ph.D., professor emeritus and director of the health, weight, and stress clinic at the Johns Hopkins Medical Institutions in Baltimore. "It sends a shiver down people's spines. We say *eating program*."

Why the trade-off in terminology? Because most of us associate "diet" with giving up favorite foods and going hungry. That's why dieting doesn't work.

Never Say Diet

If you are carrying some extra pounds—and according to the latest statistics, at least one in three of us weighs 20 percent more than we should—you have a very good reason for wanting to send them packing.

You see, being overweight puts you at risk for some serious health problems. Research shows that even a relatively modest weight gain—say, 20 pounds between your twenties and forties—can double your risk of a heart attack. Other studies have linked overweight to gallstones, gout, high blood pressure, high cholesterol, diabetes, stroke, and cancers of the endometrium (uterine lining) and possibly the breast.

So unloading the excess baggage is a good thing. It's the way we usually go about it that sets us up for failure. Many of us skip meals, and when we do eat, we skimp on portions. Sure, you lose weight, but you also end up with a body that craves sustenance.

When you don't feed your body enough, it slips into famine mode and starts hoarding the fat that you're trying so hard to get rid of. You don't burn as many calories as usual, as your metabolism shifts into low gear.

Restrict your food intake often enough, and you also become more susceptible to episodes of binge eating. Scientists theorize that as you train yourself to ignore your internal hunger cues, you more easily respond to external cues, which could be anything from a rough day to a television commercial for your favorite fast food.

In short, you simply can't starve yourself slim. If you try, you're likely to end up carrying more pounds, not less.

Fat and Figures

If eating less food doesn't help you to lose weight, try eating less fat. By sticking with nonfat and low-fat foods, you can actually eat more and still drop those persistent pounds.

To prove this point, researchers at Cornell University in Ithaca, New York, had a group of women alternate between a low-fat and a "regular," full-fat eating plan. Except for fat content, the foods were identical in both plans. The women ended up losing ½ pound per week when they ate low-fat. Just as important, the women reported that they didn't even feel as though they were dieting.

As a weight-loss strategy, cutting fat intake works for a couple of reasons. First of all, fat packs a lot of calories: You get nine calories in a gram of fat, compared with four in a gram of carbohydrate or protein. What's more, your body loves to store fat because the process demands so little energy. Just 3 percent of fat calories get burned as they're moved into storage, compared with 23 percent of carbohydrate or protein calories.

How Much Do You Need?

No matter how hard you might try, you couldn't possibly eliminate all the fat from your eating plan. Nor would you want to, says Joanne Curran-Celentano, R.D., Ph.D., associate professor of nutritional sciences at the University of New Hampshire in Durham. Your body needs some fat just to keep itself running. Besides, a certain amount of fat makes food taste good. If you cut back on fat too much, you aren't going to enjoy your food, which means that you'll probably abandon your good intentions at the first opportunity.

The problem is that most of us consume more fat than we need to—a lot more. The average intake in this country stands at about 35 percent of calories. By comparison, many experts consider 25 percent of calories the standard for good health. Some believe that you should aim even lower—say, 20 percent of calories—to lose weight.

Let's suppose that you're consuming 1,800 calories a day. Applying the 20 percent guideline, no more than 360 of those calories should come from fat. Since 1 gram of fat has 9 calories, you should eat no more than 40 grams of fat a day.

Of course, this raises another question: Just how many calories do you need every day? Here's a simple formula: First determine your activity level. (Your activity level is important because exercise burns calories, which means they don't get stored as fat.) Give yourself a 12 if your lifestyle involves light walking at most and you exercise only occasionally; a 15 if your job requires light walking or you get 30 to 60 minutes of aerobic exercise three times a week; or an 18 if you are very active and exercise for at least 60 minutes four or more times a week.

Determine your calorie needs by multiplying your activity level score by your weight in pounds. (If you're overweight, multiply your activity level score by your goal weight. A healthy weight-loss goal is ½ to 1 pound per week.)

Livin' Lean

Shifting the focus of your weight-loss efforts to dietary fat can take some getting used to—especially if you've resorted to the old starve-and-slim routine in the past. But don't think for a minute that sacrifice is the price to be paid for becoming slender and shapely. Simply reducing your daily intake of butter, margarine, or oil by one tablespoon will leave you 10 pounds lighter in a year—even if you do nothing else to lose weight.

To further trim the fat from your eating habits, try these tips.

Document the details. You can't begin cutting back on fat until you know where it's coming from. That's why many experts recommend keeping a food diary for at least a few days. It doesn't have to be anything fancy—just write down what you've eaten immediately after each meal or snack.

A food diary serves two purposes. First, it helps you to spot the "hidden" fat in the course of a day's worth of eating—like the handful of peanuts you grab in the break room or the glass of whole milk you drink at bedtime. Second, it shows you at a glance which foods you might be most comfortable deleting from your menu, says Ronette Kolotkin, Ph.D., director of behavioral programs at the Duke University Diet and Fitness Center in Durham, North Carolina.

REAL-LIFE SCENARIO

There's Help for This Diet Junkie

A year ago, Jane was determined to lose 25 pounds for her 20th high school reunion, now just two months away. A veteran dieter, she first went on a strict low-fat, low-calorie diet and lost 15 pounds fast. But her willpower evaporated as quickly as the weight, and she gained 10 of the pounds back. Then she tried Weight Watchers, and little by little the pounds dropped. But that got boring, too. So she started on diet pills even though they made her feel ill, and suddenly, willpower was no problem. Now she's a perfect size eight. But what can she do to stay there—for at least two months?

As long as Jane remains a "diet junkie," she will always be prone to regaining her weight. Right now, she's just an overweight woman hiding inside a size-eight body. Even though she's now at a healthy weight, she has to work at maintaining her weight just like a recovering alcoholic has to work at staying away from booze.

Here's Jane's problem in a nutshell. As a diet junkie, Jane has trained her body to burn calories inefficiently. Each time she crash-dieted, Jane lost precious, calorie-hungry muscle. But each time she gained the weight back, she gained fat, not muscle. This cycle of loss, gain, loss, gain changed Jane's body composition. Now, even though she may be the size she desires, her body is still mostly made up of fat. Thus, she's a fat

Go slowly. Once you've identified each food that is inflating your fat budget, you have several options: You can look for a nonfat or low-fat version, you can eat less of it, or you can eliminate it from your menu altogether. Whichever option you choose, focus on just one or two foods at a time. If you try to overhaul your eating habits in one fell swoop, you're just setting yourself up for problems.

Remember, too, that it takes at least 13 weeks to become acclimated to low-fat eating. Patience is the key to your success.

woman hiding inside a thin woman's body.

If Jane wants to still be thin at reunion-time—and more important, forever thereafter—she must give up the crash diets and take up a sensible eating program and begin exercising. Exercise is important because muscle burns many more calories than fat does. So whenever Jane lost muscle, she began burning fewer calories. The last thing a woman wants to do is lose muscle. Because of our hormones, it's difficult for women to build muscle quickly. So Jane needs to start an exercise program that includes aerobic conditioning as well as weight lifting to make sure that she builds back some of that lost muscle. Otherwise, she'll gain weight.

With exercise, Jane probably can eat a normal breakfast, lunch, dinner, and even snacks and maintain her current weight. But she needs to give up the muscle-destroying crash diets. Jane needs to keep in mind that it takes a long time to change her body composition from fat to lean. So she must be patient while she eats sensibly and exercises.

This is the only way she stands a chance to be a size eight by the time her next reunion rolls around.

Expert Consulted
Kristine Clark, R.D., Ph.D.
Director of sports nutrition
Pennsylvania State University
University Park

Learn label lingo. The label on a packaged food can be your greatest ally in the battle of the bulge—if you know how to interpret all those numbers. They don't necessarily mean what you think.

Take, for example, the percentage of calories from fat. You'd probably assume—quite reasonably—that this figure is based on the number of calories in the food. But it's not. Instead, it's based on 2,000 calories—an entire day's intake. Depending on your size and activity level, you may need less or more.

For more accurate indicators of a food's fat content, check out the number of fat grams and the number of calories from fat per serving. These figures can help you assess the food's impact on your daily fat allowance.

Roll up the welcome mat. If your goal is to eat less fat, you can do yourself a big favor by banning fat-laden goodies from your kitchen. In fact, now is the ideal time to do a little housecleaning: Go through your refrigerator, cupboards, and pantry, getting rid of all the bad stuff to make room for the good stuff.

Tip the Scale in Your Favor

Bringing your fat intake to a healthy level can work wonders for your waistline. But there's a lot more you can do to peel off those extra pounds and keep them off for good. The following strategies will help you whip your eating habits into shape and make you a weight-loss winner.

Consider calories. This is absolutely critical. "Many people think that they can eat as much low-fat food as they want, but these foods contain a significant number of calories," says Simone French, Ph.D., assistant professor of epidemiology at the University of Minnesota in Minneapolis. "And if you take in a lot more calories than you need—even if they're fat-free calories—you gain weight."

For every 3,500 "unused" calories that you consume, you gain 1 pound. On the other hand, if you cut your calorie intake by 100 calories a day, you can lose 10 pounds over the course of a year—even if you make no other changes in your eating habits.

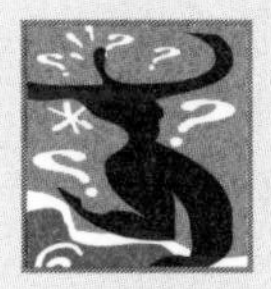

WOMEN ASK WHY

Why do men lose weight faster and more easily than women?

Numerous differences between men and women contribute to this inequality. The most obvious is that men are usually larger than women, so even if a man and a woman lose the same percentage of weight, a man will show a bigger drop in sheer numbers.

Because of hormonal differences, men also have more lean body mass, which includes bone, muscle, water, blood, and organs. Women, on the other hand, have more body fat. This gives men the leading edge because muscle burns calories faster than fat. Hormones also play a key role: The female hormone estrogen thrives on fat, so it likes keeping it around. The male hormone testosterone puts its strength in muscle.

All of those differences add up to one result: Men have much faster metabolisms than women. So a man can eat the same amount of calories as a woman and lose weight faster because his body is burning more of those calories faster.

Also, women tend to diet by restricting food and not exercising. Men tend to diet by exercising more. Although the effect of exercise on metabolic rate is controversial, exercise does "protect" against and minimize the slower body metabolism associated with dieting. Research shows that exercise reverses a decrease in metabolism associated with extreme caloric reduction (less than 800 calories a day).

This doesn't mean, however, that a woman can't beat a man at weight loss—she just shouldn't make a race out of it. By following a low-fat eating plan and taking up a regular aerobic exercise program, plus resistance training to build up muscle mass, any woman should be able to lose weight gradually—and keep it off. In order to keep it off permanently, she has to keep on exercising and stick with her eating plan.

Expert Consulted
Judith Stern, R.D., Sc.D.
Professor of nutrition and internal medicine
University of California
Davis

Keep those carbs coming. Complex carbohydrates—foods such as pasta, bread, beans, rice, and potatoes—always had a reputation for going straight to your hips. But the truth is that your body would much rather burn carbohydrate calories than attempt to store them as fat. Indeed, research has shown that people who achieve and maintain a healthy weight consume an abundance of complex carbohydrates.

What makes complex carbohydrates so figure-friendly? For starters, they have low energy densities—that is, they weigh a lot, but they contain relatively few calories, according to Barbara Rolls, Ph.D., professor of nutrition at Pennsylvania State University in University Park. Foods that have low energy densities can fill you up without filling you out, she explains.

Complex carbohydrates also switch off hunger by triggering certain nerve endings to alert your brain that you're full. With high-fat foods, this message never gets delivered, and you end up eating more than you should.

Of course, not all complex carbohydrates are created equal. Go easy on foods such as packaged baked goods, which are usually made with refined flour and pack a lot of fat and sugar to boot. Stick with whole grains, fruits, and vegetables, Dr. Rolls suggests. "They're virtually fat-free, they contain a lot of nutrients, and they fill you up."

Become a fan of fiber. Foods that are high in fiber create a feeling of fullness, so you tend to eat less of them. "It's a good idea to select high-fiber foods as your carbohydrates," Dr. Curran-Celentano says. "You'll get more nutrients and avoid dips in blood sugar, which can cause food cravings and hunger pangs." Many experts recommend consuming up to 35 grams of fiber a day. Choose whole-grain cereals, beans, fruits, and vegetables.

Drown your hunger. Many experts agree that plain old H_2O is the best appetite suppressant around. When you give your body water, it thinks it has been fed and so stops bugging you for food. In fact, often what you perceive as hunger is really thirst in disguise. To stay well-hydrated and stave off a grumbly stomach, try to drink at least eight eight-ounce glasses of water a day.

Fire Up Your Metabolism

To burn calories, why not add a little fire to your food? Seasoning your meals with sizzling spices can actually boost your metabolic rate and melt away the pounds.

In a study at Oxford-Brooks University in England, researchers had people eat two meals—one bland, the other spiked with hot mustard and chili sauce. While both meals boosted metabolism (your body expends energy to digest all types of food), the spicy cuisine sent it soaring 25 percent higher. And it stayed elevated for about three hours after the last fiery bite.

Chili powder, chili peppers, horseradish, and hot-pepper sauce can rev up your metabolic engine, too. You can tell that they're working when you start to perspire.

While you're at it, you might want to dampen those flames with some ice-cold water. Your body has to expend energy to heat the H_2O to 98.6°F, your normal temperature. Drinking eight eight-ounce glasses a day burns 123 calories. And all you have to do is swallow.

Go easy on the alcohol. You get 106 calories in 5 ounces of wine and 150 calories in 12 ounces of beer. If you have more than one of either beverage, you can really pack in the calories—and eventually, you'll pack on the pounds. There's also evidence that alcohol interferes with your body's fat-burning process, which makes it harder to lose weight. Try not to exceed three drinks a week.

Mind your mealtimes. Warning: Skipping meals can be hazardous to your waistline. Besides leaving you famished and vulnerable to overeating, it also slows down your metabolism. In fact, research has shown that people who bypass breakfast burn about 5 percent fewer calories than people who eat at least three meals a day.

Divide and conquer. Instead of sticking with the standard three squares, make the switch to mini-meals—five or six small meals spread over the course of a day. This style of eating has a couple of advantages, weight loss–wise. For one thing, you never get too hungry, since you're feeding your body every few hours. For another, you avoid taking in too many calories in one sitting. That's important, says Debra Waterhouse, R.D., author of *Outsmarting the Female Fat Cell*, because your body can use only a certain number of calories at a time to function.

Linger over dinner. When you eat something, your brain doesn't get the message for about 20 minutes, says Susan Olson, Ph.D., a clinical psychologist and weight management consultant in Seattle and author of *Keeping It Off: Winning at Weight Loss*. This delay means that you can get full before you actually *feel* full. Taking the time to savor every morsel of your meal can prevent you from overeating.

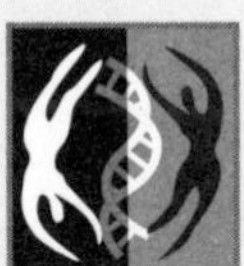

Woman to Woman

A Diet Dropout, She Lost 100 Pounds

Beth Smith, a freelance writer in Tigard, Oregon, lost 100 pounds in two years by going off her diet. Here's her story.

Diets don't work. I've tried them all—the weigh-ins, the packaged meals, the diet drinks, the pills, the eat-a-dozen-eggs-a-day-and-tons-of-fruit plan. Nothing worked.

It's hard carrying an extra 100 pounds around. Everything I did was a chore. I'd get winded going *down* stairs. Instead of walking my children to school, I'd wave from the window.

I had no energy at all, and by the time I hit my mid-thirties, I realized I had no life either. I decided I had to do something about my weight—for myself and for my family.

Since I'm a writer, I do a lot of reading. I decided I had to find out why my diets weren't working. I finally realized that diets don't work because they're temporary. What I needed was a lifestyle change—a lifestyle that centered around eating, but eating healthy foods.

I studied the Food Guide Pyramid—the one with the fat foods at the small end and the fruits and vegetables at the big end. It became my model for good nutrition. I started making small changes, each a step forward. Maybe today I'll eat an extra serving of vegetables; maybe tomorrow I'll cut out some fat. I didn't punish myself. I made changes gradually. And the weight came off gradually.

I found the magic that I was looking for—moderation.

Now I understand that if I have a cookie, I don't need to eat 10 more. There's always tomorrow.

It took two years, but now I'm 100 pounds lighter. I feel younger and look so much better—it's amazing. Now I can ride a bike, go hiking, get out with my kids and run on the beach. I can walk to the mailbox and not have to worry about people staring at me.

I want people to know that if I can do it, anybody can, and I mean that from the bottom of my heart.

Know the source. Here's another little trick of the weight-loss trade: Be careful to distinguish between hunger and appetite. Hunger is driven by a genuine physical need for food. Appetite, on the other hand, often grows from your emotions. Weight-loss experts call it head hunger: You eat because you want to, not because you have to.

To help sharpen your hunger awareness, try this exercise at your next meal. Before you start eating, rate your hunger on a scale of zero to five (zero being the least hungry, five being the most). Eat one-quarter of the food on your plate, then rate your hunger. Wait five minutes, then rate your hunger again. Repeat the sequence. As you concentrate on the process of eating, you just may discover that you're satisfied before you even clean your plate.

Choose foods that satisfy. Researchers at the University of Sydney in Australia put together a list of "bargain foods" that, calorie for calorie, have the greatest potential to satisfy your hunger. The highest-scoring food? The baked potato. It gives you the most bang for your caloric buck, filling you up faster and on fewer calories than any other food tested. Rounding out the top five are fish, oatmeal, oranges, and apples. At the bottom of the satiety barrel: croissants, cake, doughnuts, candy bars, and peanuts.

Part Four

Home Alone with the Refrigerator

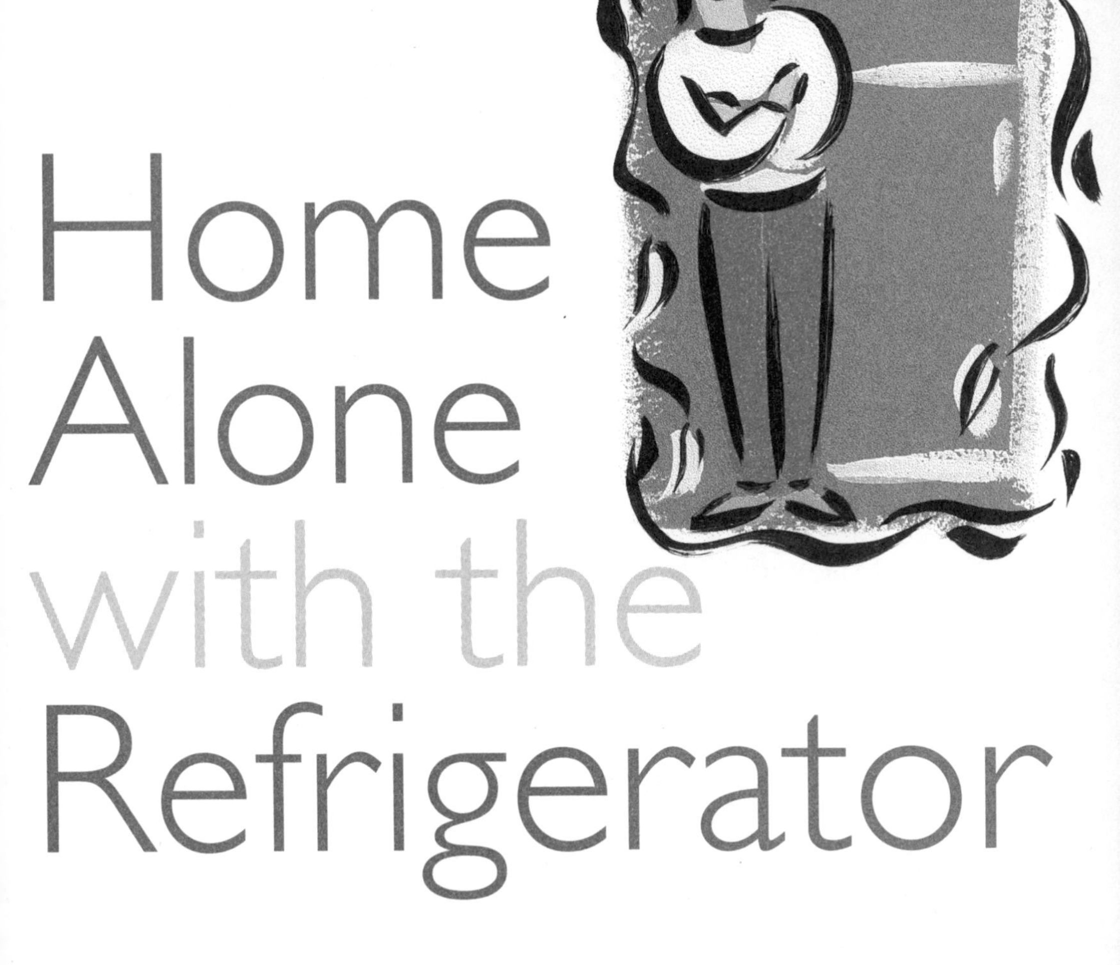

Your Food,
Your Mood
When Emotions, Not Hunger,
Make You Eat

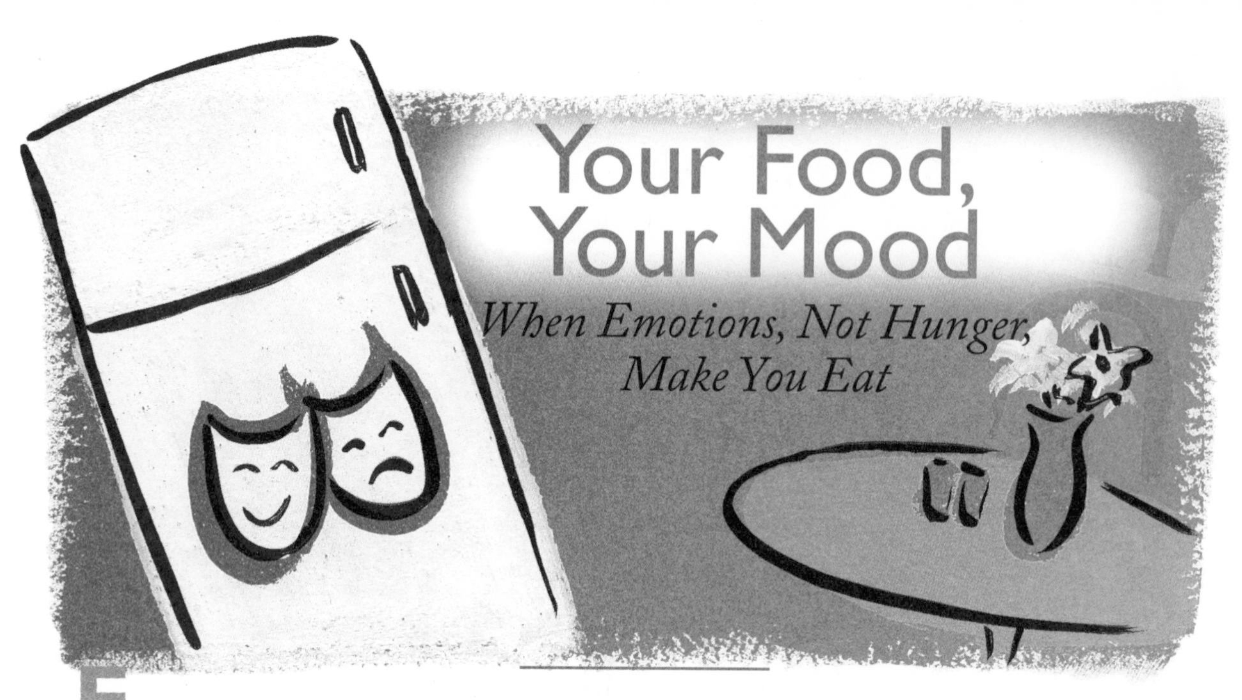

For most of us, it all began sometime in childhood. We'd fall and scrape a knee, and our moms would console us with a big bowl of ice cream. Or we wouldn't get invited to a classmate's birthday party, so Grandma would bake us her special apple pie to cheer us up.

Experiences like these taught us an indelible lesson: Eating makes us feel good. We learned early on to use food as salve for our emotional wounds.

So even though we're all grown up now, we still turn to food to soothe bad feelings. It's not that our stomachs are growling. We're attempting to fulfill a different kind of hunger—what Sandra Campbell, Psy.D., clinical director of the eating disorders program at the Brattleboro Retreat in Vermont, calls a hunger of the soul.

We may eat because we're angry, depressed, anxious, or sad. Or because we have low self-esteem. Or even because we're trying to avoid intimacy.

When we allow our emotions to dictate our food choices, our internal hunger cues—the ones driven by a genuine physical need for sustenance—get thrown off track. The brain chemicals that switch hunger on and off become confused. We end up eating more than we should, which ultimately sinks us into an even deeper funk. "It becomes a vicious circle," says Elizabeth Somer, R.D., author of *Nutrition for Women* and *Food and Mood.*

Tuning in to our internal hunger cues can help us head off emotion-driven bingeing. Even better, it can help us choose foods that moderate our moods in a positive, healthful way.

It's All in Your Head

You already know how what you eat affects your physical health. Essentially, your body breaks down foods and then retains nutrients to fuel its various systems. In much the same way, your brain uses certain substances from foods to produce chemicals that regulate mental functions, including mood, alertness, and memory.

Scientists have identified at least 40 of these chemicals, called neurotransmitters. They fire back and forth between the nerve cells in your brain, enabling the cells to communicate with

How Happy Is Your Diet?

Many of us use food to make us feel good. Unfortunately, we don't always realize that we're doing it. There's double danger in "dining blind." It leads to weight gain because we're overriding our internal hunger cues, but it does nothing to resolve the underlying problem.

The following quiz, developed at the Duke University Medical Center in Durham, North Carolina, can help you determine whether you're an emotional eater. Simply read each question and answer true or false, then tally up your score as noted at the end.

T F If someone hurts me or makes me angry, I feel better if I eat something.
T F When I feel that my family or friends are disappointed in me, I turn to food for comfort.
T F When I have a lot of work pressure, I find myself eating.
T F I often find myself eating because I don't have anything else to do.
T F I eat fattening food only when I'm alone and others can't see me.
T F I overeat when I'm feeling lonely.
T F I overeat after an argument with my mate or my boss.
T F Sometimes I don't stop eating even though I feel nauseous or I can't breathe.
T F I feel very guilty and ashamed when I overeat.
T F I become panicky if food is not available when I want it.
T F I'm always thinking about food.
T F Once I start eating, I can't stop until I finish whatever is in front of me.
T F My eating is always extreme—I'm either perfectly in control or completely out of control.

What Your Score Means

To determine your score, count up the number of items that you answered "true." Then find the appropriate category below.

0 to 2: For the most part, your eating patterns are unrelated to your emotional state.

3 to 6: You have some emotional-eating tendencies that need to be addressed. Begin to pay attention to the relationship between your emotional needs and your eating patterns.

7 to 13: Food plays a central role in your emotional life. There is a strong relationship between how you feel and how much or what kinds of food you eat. You must learn to better recognize your feelings, separate feelings from food, and find other coping mechanisms besides eating.

one another. Having too little or too much of a particular neurotransmitter can alter these signals, paving the way for changes in the way you feel, think, and act. Neurotransmitter deficits and overloads are linked to serious conditions such as depression, mania, and memory loss.

Three of these brain chemicals—serotonin, dopamine, and norepinephrine—influence mood and appetite. "What you eat can dramatically affect the levels of these neurotransmitters—and, therefore, how you feel," Somer says.

Serotonin: Nature's Mood Medicine

Of the three neurotransmitters Somer mentions, serotonin appears to have the strongest effects on mood. "Without enough of it, you can experience symptoms such as food cravings, depression, and insomnia," Somer notes. "How much serotonin you have is often directly related to your diet."

Your brain manufactures serotonin from an amino acid called tryptophan, found in protein-rich foods such as chicken, tuna, and tofu. Ironically, though, eating these foods actually lowers the level of tryptophan—and serotonin—in your brain, Somer says.

Why? Because protein foods have more than two dozen different amino acids, and every one of them makes a beeline for your brain. Tryptophan is the pokiest of the bunch. Invariably, it ends up getting stuck in your bloodstream.

For tryptophan to complete the journey to your brain, you have to get the other amino acids out of the way. You can do that simply by eating a carbohydrate-rich meal. The carbohydrates trigger the release of the hormone insulin, which escorts the other amino acids into your body's cells. Tryptophan then has the all-clear.

Once it reaches its destination, tryptophan completes its mission by serving as the catalyst to increase serotonin levels. Serotonin has a calming, even tranquilizing effect on your mood. If you're stressed, for instance, serotonin makes you feel relaxed. And if you're already relaxed, serotonin sends you off to Dreamland.

Dopamine and Norepinephrine: Primed for Action

The other two players in the brain game, dopamine and norepinephrine, have an impact on your mental sharpness. They influence your alertness, your thinking skills, and your memory. Still, if levels of these neurotransmitters run low, you may feel depressed or experience other changes in your mood. And if they're too high, they can actually stimulate stress.

To manufacture dopamine and norepinephrine, your brain needs an amino acid called tyrosine—which, coincidentally, is also found in protein-rich foods. Compared to tryptophan, which travels more slowly, tyrosine is a speed demon. It routinely beats out other amino acids in the race for your brain, Somer explains.

Of course, this means that when tyrosine is present, tryptophan—being the slowpoke that it is—doesn't stand a chance in the race. You'll have lots of dopamine and norepinephrine but not so much serotonin. As a result, you'll feel more energized than relaxed.

Are You Really Hungry?

You can see how food choices might cause changes in mood over the course of the day. But this still doesn't explain what drives us to binge on particular foods when we're blue. Why do tough times make us want to bury our noses in the fridge instead of a good book?

Sometimes the urge to eat comes from within. As mentioned earlier, hunger—specifically, cravings for certain foods—may be your body's way of tipping you off that it needs something.

Typically, neurotransmitters—the same ones that govern your mood—work with hormones and your stomach to monitor your body's nutrient status. They're like your own personal pit crew, whose job is to ensure that your body is properly fueled at all times. When something runs low, they'll pull you in for a pit stop. You'll recognize their signal as that familiar grumbling and gnawing in the pit of your stomach.

This is what the experts consider true hunger—an honest-to-goodness, biological need for food. It's a basic tool for survival, as instinctive and natural as breathing.

Then there's another type of hunger—what

some weight-loss experts call head hunger. You eat because you want to, not because you have to.

Your emotions can fuel head hunger. You may turn to food to elicit good feelings or to wipe out bad feelings. You may even notice a pattern to your head hunger. Over a period of months or even years, you may repeatedly eat the same food in response to a specific negative emotion or circumstance, says Susan Olson, Ph.D., a clinical psychologist in Seattle.

Emotions à la Mode

Mastering emotional eating, then, starts with recognizing the difference between physical hunger and head hunger. This takes a little practice, but it's worth the effort. You can stop yourself from bingeing—and learn constructive ways to deal with the problems that are causing your emotional distress.

Understanding how food influences your mood is important, too. When you find yourself facing tough times, you can plan your meals to include foods that leave you feeling calm and relaxed rather than uptight and jittery.

The following strategies can help you identify emotion-driven eating patterns and establish more mood-friendly eating habits.

Document your diet. Start to carry a small notebook or a three- by five-inch index card in your pocket or purse. Then each time you eat something when you are not physi-

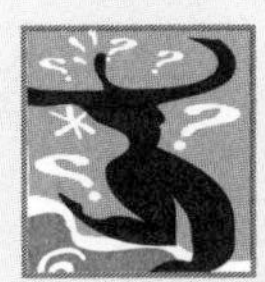

WOMEN ASK WHY

Why can't I stop myself from eating even though my stomach is telling me it's full?

It may be that you're eating to fill up something other than your stomach. Many women eat because of an emotion—like anger, boredom, or frustration—or to put off something they really don't want to do—like vacuuming, filing taxes, or working out a conflict at work. In a way, as long as you're eating, you don't have to deal with what's bothering you or with something else you should be doing. What's more, you know that as soon as you stop eating, you'll feel guilty. So you keep eating and eating.

When women overeat, they tend to choose carbohydrates, which have a relaxing, soothing effect. Eating a lot of carbs causes your brain to produce serotonin, a chemical that makes you feel relaxed or even sleepy. But eating carbohydrates also results in increased blood sugar levels. Your body responds by releasing insulin, which lowers blood sugar. That decrease may cause cravings. Women may also develop an emotional need for carbohydrates.

The trick is to stop your binge before it starts by facing what's prompting you to overeat in the first place. And there are as many reasons for overeating as there are emotions. So first, monitor how you're feeling when you get the urge to eat, then do something to deal with the emotion (besides eating). If you're feeling lonely, call a friend. If you're tired, take a quick nap. If you're feeling stressed or overwhelmed, a warm bubble bath just might do the trick.

In our fast-paced society, however, many women choose food to cope: It has become a drug for dealing with our stressful lives. With a little self-reflection, though, you can learn to monitor your emotions when you have the urge to binge and find healthier ways to cope.

Expert Consulted
Susan Olson, Ph.D.
Clinical psychologist
Seattle

cally hungry, make a note of what it is and how you're feeling. Include information about where you are and who, if anyone, is with you.

"We call this monitoring," says Katherine Halmi, M.D., professor of psychiatry at Cornell University Medical College in New York City and director of the eating disorder program at New York Hospital, Westchester Division, in White Plains. "You write it all down and look for a pattern."

After a week or so, you may notice that you consistently eat when you're depressed, anxious, angry, bored, or lonely. Or you may use food as a substitute for sex and intimacy.

Consider the reason. Once you've identified an emotional-eating pattern, you can dig a little deeper to disclose the "automatic thoughts" that prompt you to reach for food because you need comfort or a quick escape.

Suppose, for instance, that you're hosting a party on Saturday night. You worry that you won't have enough food, that no one will talk to each other, that no one will come. Thoughts like these can make you feel anxious or stressed—and they can drive you to binge.

Stick with a schedule. You can also uncover emotional eating patterns by planning your meals and snacks for regular times, say experts. If you eat on a schedule, then find yourself wanting food an hour after lunch, you can say, "Wait. This isn't necessary. What's going on here?"

Choose high-carbohydrate cuisine. During emotionally trying times, your brain quickly uses up its supply of

FIND YOUR FOOD PERSONALITY

If someone asked you to describe your personality, you might use adjectives like "outgoing" or "reserved," "flamboyant" or "shy." But how would you describe your food personality?

Yes, you do have one. Every one of us does. It's shaped by your eating routine, your favorite foods, your beliefs about what constitutes good nutrition, and a host of other factors.

What's more, your food personality may have very little in common with your "regular" personality. It all depends on you.

In her work with clients, Susan Olson, Ph.D., a clinical psychologist in Seattle, has identified seven basic food personalities, which are profiled below. Read through them to determine which one—or ones—best describes you. (You may find that you have a multiple food personality—but don't panic. It's not as bad as it sounds.) Then read Dr. Olson's advice for developing a nutrition strategy that accommodates your attitude toward food.

Feeler. "I often eat in response to my emotions, both positive and negative. Turning to food when I feel happy, depressed, bored, or angry is a very comfortable and common reaction."

Your strategy: Focus on recognizing and expressing your feelings in more healthful ways, such as hitting a pillow, listening to music, or calling a friend. Also, try to control your eating environment as much as possible. Keep high-fat foods out of your home, for instance.

Human doer. "I eat on the go, and frequently I eat without thinking. When I'm asked to stick with a strict eating routine, I usually have difficulty following through."

Your strategy: You must make sure that your eating style fits into your lifestyle. Grazing is okay, as long as it's healthy. Learn the nutritious choices and stop feeling guilty if you don't eat the way others do. Simplicity works well for you, too. Keep simple "finger foods"—such as bagels, cut-up carrots, and fruit—on hand.

Thinker. "I'm highly critical of myself, and I can be compulsive in my behavior. I tend to think in all-or-nothing terms, so if I believe I've made an eating mistake, it will often turn into an all-out binge."

Your strategy: Your goal is to be gentler on yourself and to keep your life balanced. Be sure to plan fun things so that you don't get too obsessive about eating or anything else. Take 10 to 20 minutes out of your day to listen to a meditation tape, or buy a coloring book and color outside the lines.

Food hedonist. "For me, food is very sensual. I love the look, the smell, and especially the taste of food. I enjoy reading food magazines and trying recipes the way some people get into music or art."

Your strategy: Rechannel your passion for food into other areas, such as reading, crafts, music—even a relationship. If you love to cook, try your hand at creating your own low-fat recipes.

Dreamer. "I want to reach my ideal weight or eat the perfect diet for me. But I'm easily discouraged, and I tend to fall back into counterproductive eating habits."

Your strategy: Work on improving your self-image by focusing on your uniqueness and your positive attributes. Picture whatever makes you feel good—wearing an attractive dress or managing a diet-related health problem—and mentally focus on that goal.

"People" person. "Friends and family mean the world to me. I love nothing better than going to a party or having lunch with a friend in a nice restaurant. But I'm always afraid I'll lose control of sensible eating in social situations."

Your strategy: You're most successful when you focus on the human connection and make food secondary. Brush up on the basics of good nutrition so you can make healthful choices in restaurants and other social situations.

Fitness fan. "My body and my health are very important to me—I'll do anything to learn how to feel and look better. You'll never catch me looking for an excuse to not exercise or eat right. In fact, sometimes I can be too compulsive about eating and/or exercising."

Your strategy: You have a definite advantage. You exercise to burn calories and to relieve tension, and you wouldn't deliberately eat something that would harm your health. The trick is to not become overly obsessive about calories and exercise, to the point where you ignore other parts of your life.

mood-boosting serotonin. And when serotonin is in short supply, negative feelings tend to increase.

Eating foods that are high in complex carbohydrates, including pasta, bagels, and baked potatoes, can raise a low serotonin level, so you feel less stressed and more relaxed. You get a bonus, too: As serotonin increases, appetite usually decreases, which means that you're less likely to eat your way through tough times.

Steer clear of sweets. Eating chocolate, cookies, and other sugary treats can make you feel better pretty quickly, but the effects won't last. In some people, these foods cause blood sugar levels to shoot way up. In response, your pancreas dumps insulin into your bloodstream, which in turn ushers the sugar out of your bloodstream and into cells. Your blood sugar level quickly plummets. This sudden drop can leave you feeling tired and irritable, and it may even trigger a craving, Somer explains.

Trim the fat. Most of us yearn for sweet and fatty or salty and fatty foods. Unfortunately, eating fatty foods seems to prompt cravings for even more fatty foods, according to Sarah Leibowitz, Ph.D., a behavioral neurobiologist at Rockefeller University in New York City.

In animal studies, Dr. Leibowitz found that a high-fat diet prompted the production of a neurochemical that stimulates an appetite for fat.

For a variety of health-related reasons, many experts advise limiting your daily fat intake to no more than 25 percent of calories.

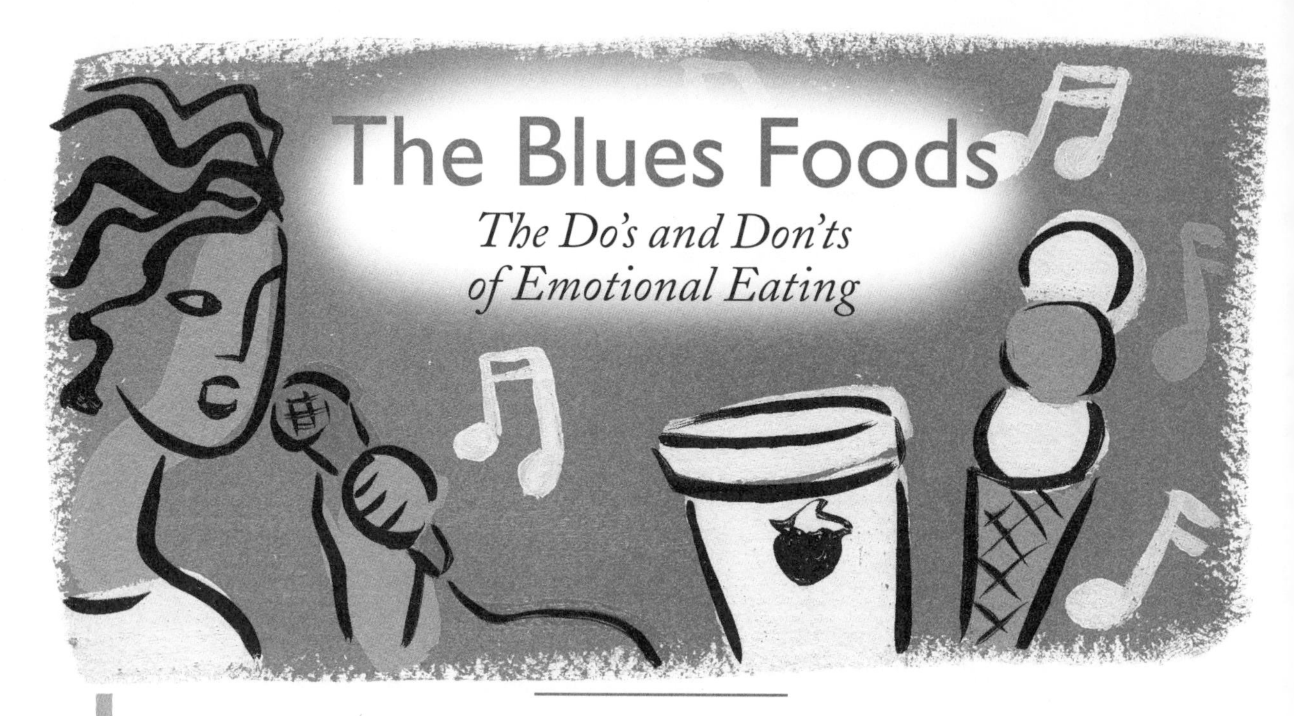

The Blues Foods

The Do's and Don'ts of Emotional Eating

In the movie *Sleepless in Seattle*, actress Meg Ryan pretty much eats her way from one scene to the next. She realizes that she's engaged to the wrong man and devours a bag of potato chips. She falls head over heels for inaccessible Tom Hanks and downs a pint of ice cream. She wallows in her sorrow by watching the classic tearjerker *An Affair to Remember* while shoveling fistfuls of popcorn into her mouth.

"I love that movie," says Elizabeth Somer, R.D., author of *Nutrition for Women* and *Food and Mood*. "Meg Ryan is doing what all of us do—she's using food for comfort. And she manages to look cute while she's doing it."

Of course, there's a big difference between the "reel" world and the real world. When we routinely eat like that, we can pack on pounds. And we deprive our bodies of vital nutrients because we're replacing healthful foods with so-called comfort foods like chocolate, cookies, and ice cream.

Now there's nothing wrong with an occasional indulgence to brighten a blue mood. The key word here is *occasional*. When we habitually use food as emotional anesthesia—when we depend on Ben & Jerry's, or Sara Lee, or Mrs. Smith to ease our inner turmoil—we're headed for trouble, says Linda Smolak, Ph.D., professor of psychology at Kenyon College in Gambier, Ohio. Although emotional eating can temporarily numb our woes, in the long run it makes us not only less healthy but less happy, too.

The Need to Feed

Women naturally turn to food to ease emotional distress or fill an emotional void. Even men do it, although they seldom feel as guilty about it as we do. We tend to be much more conscious of what we consume and much more concerned about how it affects our appearance. So for us, emotional eating is a much bigger issue.

But why do we do it? Well, sometimes the need to feed is biologically driven. You may have noticed, for instance, that when you feel stressed, you crave sweets like candy and cake. Scientists believe there's a reason for that: These foods are rich in carbohydrates, and carbohydrates supply the raw materials that the brain uses to produce serotonin.

Serotonin is the "feel-good" brain chemical that boosts your sense of well-being, explains Dianne Lindewall, Ph.D., supervising behavioral psychologist for the George Washington University Obesity Management Program in Washington, D.C. Because stress rapidly drains your serotonin supply, a craving may be your body's way of recouping its losses.

Often, though, emotional eating is a response to external rather than internal cues. In other words, rather than eating because our bodies tell us to, we eat because we're anxious, or worried, or frustrated, or blue.

How Sweet It Isn't

Nothing boosts a sour mood like a sweet treat. Maybe that's why sugar consumption continues to rise faster than a bundt cake in a hot oven, with the average American woman downing over 100 pounds each year.

But the lift you get from sugary foods doesn't last, explains Maria Simonson, Sc.D., Ph.D., professor emeritus and director of the health, weight, and stress clinic at the Johns Hopkins Medical Institutions in Baltimore. You feel better for an hour, maybe even two. But then the mood-boosting buzz wears off. You may become tired and irritable—and you may want more sugar.

What causes this emotional roller-coaster ride? Your blood sugar level is partly to blame. When you eat sweets, your blood sugar skyrockets. Your pancreas responds by dumping a load of the hormone insulin into your bloodstream. Insulin is responsible for ushering the sugar out of your bloodstream and into cells. As it does its job, your blood sugar level plummets.

Researchers also suspect that eating too much sugar causes your brain to step up its production of feel-good chemical compounds, including the morphinelike endorphins. As they sink back to normal levels, you may experience wild fluctuations in mood and energy.

Besides sending your body into overdrive, too much sugar saps your nutrient stores. For starters, sweets have a tendency to replace nutritious foods in your diet. On top of that, your body has to use up vitamins and minerals in order to process the sugary stuff.

When you're feeling blue, you're better off bypassing sweet treats and choosing baked potatoes, pasta, or bread instead. These foods are rich in complex carbohydrates, which provide vitamins, minerals, and some fiber along with their carbohydrate.

A Match Made in...the Refrigerator?

There's no real harm in finding comfort in a pint of double fudge brownie ice cream—as long as you do it only once in a blue moon. But when you eat to buffer strong negative emotions, to escape reality, or to experience emotional fulfillment, then it begins to disrupt your eating habits.

Emotional eating is cyclical in nature. Suppose you're upset over an argument with your spouse. You turn to food for solace, and you may even feel better for a time. But then guilt, anger, and frustration set in. You're disappointed in yourself for bingeing, and your self-esteem drops. This leads you to isolate yourself from others—and when you do, you feel lonely, bored, and empty. So what do you do? That's right: You eat some more.

FEEL-GOOD FOODS

Sweets and other high-fat foods provide a quick fix for a foul mood. Unfortunately, while their effects don't last, the pounds they pack on do.

You're better off choosing low-fat, less sugary foods—for a couple of reasons. For starters, they're more nutritious, so they fit right in to a healthy diet. What's more, they improve your mood more consistently, without negative aftereffects.

The following chart can help you choose the right food to counterbalance your mood, according to Cheryl Hartsough, R.D., director of wellness and health programs at The Aspen Club in Colorado.

When You Feel...	Avoid...	Eat...
Depressed	Cake, ice cream, pastries	Whole-grain entrées such as pasta primavera and rice and beans
Sleepy and lethargic	Sweets, pizza, high-fat foods	Low-fat, high-protein foods such as broiled or baked fish, veal, poultry, nonfat or low-fat cheese, and egg-white omelets
Tense, anxious, or stressed	Chocolate, cake, ice cream	Fresh fruit, dried fruit, pasta, whole-grain bread, baked potato, rice, vegetables

This "blue mood, more food" cycle can go on forever. There is one way to stop it, though: Identify and resolve the problem that's driving you to binge in the first place.

Yes, eating is a much easier way to cope. But look at it this way: Breaking patterns of emotional eating will leave you free to experience your true feelings, to more easily reach and maintain a healthy weight, and to truly enjoy food—even an occasional goody—to its fullest.

Food without Guilt

This brings up a very important point: Food is a good thing. After all, you couldn't live without it. You can—and should—find pleasure in it.

"Eating can be a wonderful experience," says Connie Roberts, R.D., manager of nutrition consultation services and wellness programs at Brigham and Women's Hospital in Boston. "Some women think that their food troubles stem from enjoying food too much. The key is to learn to have fun with food, without guilt."

That means—you guessed it—reining in emotion-driven eating. Really, it's much easier than you may think. The following strategies will help you do it.

Take 10. When you get the urge to eat, wait 10 minutes before you head for the fridge. This gives you a little time to regroup and to figure out what may have caused the craving, explains Sandra Campbell, Psy.D., clinical director of the eating disorders program at the Brattleboro Retreat in Vermont. Take the opportunity to tune in to your body. Is this real, honest-to-goodness hunger talking? Or has something happened that's making you want to eat?

Create a diversion. Waiting 10 minutes has another advantage. When the time is up, you may realize that you no longer want to eat. If so...good for you!

But if visions of a sweet treat still dance in your head, shift your attention to another, non-food-related activity. At work, read your mail or flip through the newspaper. At home, polish a pair of shoes or repot your favorite fern. Do one small thing—but make it an activity that can compete with eating. (In other words, cleaning the oven probably won't cut it.)

You may even want to invest a few minutes of your time in coming up with an advance list of alternative activities. Post it on your refrigerator at home or tack it to your calendar at work. Then when you're in the mood for food, check your list and see what you could do instead.

Select your snack. You've delayed, you've distracted, and you still feel the need to eat. Then go ahead—but rather than grabbing whatever food is within reach, think about what you really want, suggests Susan Moore, R.D., program manager and senior nutritionist in the George Washington University Obesity Management Program. Are you after a specific taste? Or are you looking for a food that can fill you up? Besides helping you to make more healthful choices, this tactic reminds you that you—not your craving—are controlling the situation.

Do what feels good. From a nutrition standpoint, it's better to tame your craving with, say, a bagel rather than a candy bar. But sometimes a bagel just won't do. On those occasions when you absolutely, positively have to have a goody, help yourself—but watch the portion size.

"I have patients practice buying just one chocolate truffle and enjoying it to the utmost," Roberts says. The point is to not deny yourself the one food that you really want. If you do, you may end up consuming more fat and calories by trying to satisfy your craving with something else.

Take your time. These days, many of us eat with a fork in one hand and a pen, a newspaper, or a remote control in the other. We pay little attention to the process of eating—and we eat too much as a result.

Consume your food slowly and mindfully. Focus on each forkful. By "tuning in" in this way, you're less likely to overeat, explains Barbara Dickinson, R.D., director of nutrition at the weight-management center at Loma Linda University in California and co-leader of the women and food support group.

Conserve calories. So you've indulged a craving. That doesn't mean you've ditched your diet for the entire day. All you have to do is figure out how many extra calories you consumed, then perform a little nip-and-tuck on the rest of your meals to compensate. Suppose you ate a 250-calorie candy bar in the afternoon. You may decide to forgo the dressing on your salad and the butter on your bread when dinnertime rolls around.

Actually, Moore says, if you do a little calorie comparison before you eat, the food you crave may have a little less appeal. You'll be more inclined to reach for something healthful, like a piece of fruit or cut-up vegetables.

Re-engineer your eating environment. If you have easy access to high-fat, high-calorie foods, you're bound to eat them. On the other hand, "if the only thing available to you is air-popped popcorn, you can eat all you want and still take in far fewer calories than you'd get from, say, premium ice cream or a bag of cookies," Dr. Lindewall says.

So go through your refrigerator, kitchen cupboards, desk drawers—anyplace where you store food—and trade in the high-fat, high-calorie fare for more wholesome selections, suggests Chris Rosenbloom, R.D., Ph.D., associate professor in the department of nutrition and dietetics at Georgia State University in Atlanta and a spokesperson for the American Dietetic Association. "If you open the refrigerator and see a bowl of sliced peaches, chances are you'll try them," she says.

Lean toward lean. As you restock, keep your eye on the fat content of the foods you choose. Besides the fact that low-fat foods are healthier for you, they can actually help you beat the blues.

When 555 women reduced their dietary fat

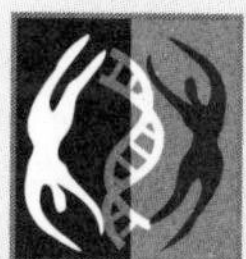

WOMAN TO WOMAN

She's an Emotional Eater No More

As an executive editor at a successful magazine based in New York City, Mary Bolster has a stress-filled job. Not too long ago she learned how to stop that stress (and other emotions) from putting extra pounds on her.

Like most girls in America, I lost my perspective on food and eating when I went through puberty and dieting became the thing to do. I was always either on a diet or overeating and thinking about the day when I would get back on track.

I ate because I was lonely, insecure, bored, frustrated, uncertain...you name it. And I ate anything I considered forbidden, such as chocolate, ice cream, and chips. I didn't eat when I was hungry. I ate when I wanted to feel good.

Then one day I picked up a self-help book about overeating. I guess I was really ready to make a change because the book made perfect sense to me. I began work on my problem immediately.

I started viewing each episode of overeating with curiosity instead of judgment. What was going on in my life that was making me eat? I realized that food wasn't going to solve the problem. But it was a good excuse to eat!

Now instead of eating, I address the emotion rather than ignoring or denying it by eating. If I'm bored, I do something to entertain myself. If I'm sad, sometimes I just stay sad. My real problems, not food, have taken center stage.

I don't obsess about food anymore. In fact, I rarely think about it. I've become more assertive about saying that I'm not hungry when I'm not. I'm also much better at asking for a doggie bag instead of eating more than I should at one sitting. And I've lost weight!

I know that stopping emotional eating is difficult for many women, but I've actually never made an easier change in my life. I think it's a matter of recognizing that you're eating out of emotion, not hunger. Once you get that straight in your head, you'll find that you think less about food and more about how to work on what's really bothering you.

intakes to 20 percent of calories for a year, they reported feeling less depressed and anxious and more vigorous than they did in the days when they thought chocolate chip cookie dough was a viable dinner option. Should you aim that low? That depends on your individual health status. Generally, though, it's a good idea to limit your dietary fat intake to 25 percent of calories.

Listen to the buzz on Bs. Also lay in a plentiful supply of foods rich in the B-complex vitamins, particularly vitamin B_6, folate, and vitamin B_{12}. This trio is crucial for sound mental health, Somer says. "Surveys show that many women consume less than the two milligrams of vitamin B_6 they need each day," she points out. This may help explain why women experience depression more frequently than men, she adds.

Choose baked potatoes, bananas, and chickpeas for vitamin B_6 and lentils, pinto beans, and spinach for folate. Steamed clams and oysters are among the top sources of vitamin B_{12}.

Keep an eye on omega-3's. Nearly 30 percent of certain membranes in nerve cells are made from a type of omega-3 fatty acid. Researchers theorize that when the membranes run low on this fatty acid, they interfere with nerve transmissions and contribute to emotional distress.

Research suggests that maintaining an adequate supply of omega-3's in your system can help steady your emotions. In one small study of patients with clinical depression, those with the most serious cases also had the lowest levels of omega-3's. In a separate study, Japanese students who took fish-oil supplements—a source of omega-3's—were less likely to exhibit hostility toward others during the pressure-cooker atmosphere at the end of the semester.

To get a healthy dose of omega-3's, eat one or two three-ounce servings of omega-3–rich fish every week. Among the best sources are salmon, herring, bluefin tuna, and mackerel.

Eat at intervals. Skipping breakfast and skimping on lunch can leave you hungry, grouchy, and vulnerable to emotional eating. To keep your mood—and your energy level—on a more even keel, plan to eat a small meal at least every four hours, Dickinson advises.

Eating on a schedule has another advantage, too. If you find yourself feeling hungry at "odd" times, you can fairly safely assume that your emotions are doing the talking—not your stomach. Then you can dig a little deeper to discover what's really behind your urge to eat.

Get your snacks in sync. If you tend to eat because you're bored, plan low-fat, low-calorie, fun snacks for between 3:00 and 4:00 P.M. and 8:00 and 9:00 P.M. According to Roberts, research has shown these to be the times of day when "recreational eating" is most likely to take place.

Anticipate emotional eating. If you know you're going to be in a situation where emotional eating is likely, do what you can to prepare for it. You may, for instance, want to cut back your calorie intake a bit to give yourself a little breathing room. (Just remember: Don't skip meals!)

Consider the alternatives. As a long-term goal, you may want to explore other coping techniques that don't involve food, says Maria Simonson, Sc.D., Ph.D., professor emeritus and director of the health, weight, and stress clinic at the Johns Hopkins Medical Institutions in Baltimore. Aromatherapy, meditation, yoga, and scores of other self-care options can help you feel better—and perhaps, in turn, eat less.

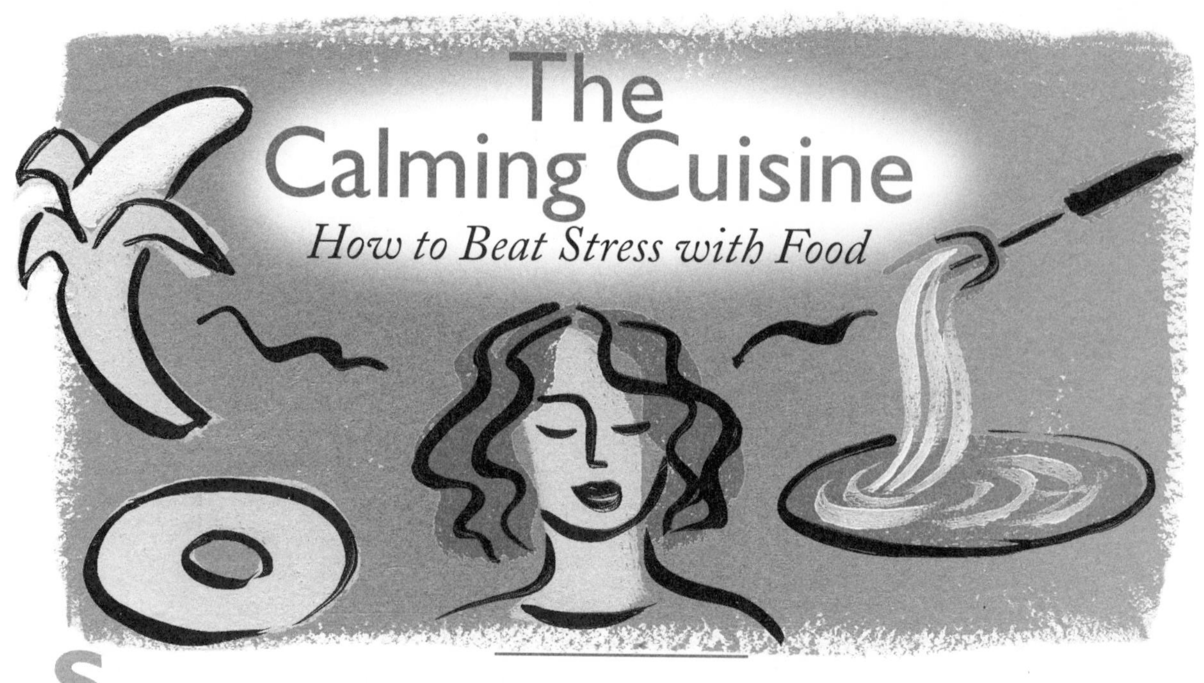

The Calming Cuisine

How to Beat Stress with Food

Stress? No one has to tell you what it feels like. Heck, you're convinced that if you looked up the word in a dictionary, you'd find a photo of yourself.

No doubt about it. We live in jaw-clenching, muscle-knotting, stomach-churning times. And few of us are left unscathed. In a National Center for Health Statistics survey, 75 percent of women between the ages of 25 and 44 reported experiencing moderate to severe stress.

And when stress sets up shop in our lives, our eating habits suffer—big-time. We tend to skip meals, and when we do eat, we make some less-than-admirable food choices. "People grab whatever they can get their hands on; often that's junk food," says Carla Wolper, R.D., a nutritionist for the obesity research center at St. Luke's–Roosevelt Hospital Center and the center for women's health at Columbia-Presbyterian Medical Center, both in New York City.

The bad part is that this downslide into dietary dereliction happens just as our bodies really need us to feed them well. Stress not only interferes with the absorption of nutrients, it also accelerates their excretion. When its nutrient stores are depleted, it's hard for your body to keep up with the demands that stress places on it. Over time, this can take a toll on your health.

But it doesn't have to be that way. In fact, the latest research shows that eating more of some foods and less of others can actually stymie the effects of stress. Adjusting your diet can produce chemical changes in your brain and body that leave you feeling calmer, more relaxed, and ready to face whatever the world throws your way.

Nutritional Antidotes for Stress

To keep your energy and emotions on an even keel and to safeguard your health in the process, give these de-stressing dietary strategies a try.

Calm with carbs. Complex carbohydrates—found in abundance in foods such as pasta, bagels, and baked potatoes—stimulate production of a brain chemical called serotonin. Serotonin mellows your mood, so you feel less tense and anxious and more calm and relaxed. Even better, research has shown that serotonin acts as

EAT AWAY AT STRESS

Now you know why they call it the daily grind: It sure has made mincemeat out of you. You just can't wait to slip into your comfiest sweats and curl up on the sofa with a nice big bowl of...grapes?

Okay, so maybe you had something a little less wholesome in mind. Like ice cream. Or mashed potatoes with butter. Or macaroni and cheese. These are classic comfort foods that many women turn to in times of stress.

While they sure taste good going down, they're not exactly nutrient-dense—with the exception of fat, of course. And because stress depletes your body of key vitamins and minerals to begin with, you run the risk of putting yourself in the red, nutrition-wise.

There are healthier alternatives. Take the aforementioned grapes as an example. The European varieties (like the green Thompson seedless and red Tokay) offer modest amounts of vitamin C and fiber—which help protect your body against the effects of stress—with hardly any fat to speak of. They make great finger food, too, so they're perfect for nervous nibblers.

For more of these new-fashioned comfort foods, take a look at the following chart. Each food supplies at least one key nutrient (listed on the right) known to counteract your body's stress response. Some are also good sources of fiber. And since stress can really do a number on your digestive system, keeping your fiber intake high is critical. Best of all, they'll satisfy even the most severe case of the munchies without expanding your waistline.

Food	Portion	Nutrients
Apple (with skin)	1 (5 oz.)	Vitamin C, fiber
Apricots	3 (3.5 oz. total)	Beta-carotene, vitamin C
Banana	1 (4 oz.)	Vitamin B_6, vitamin C, fiber
Beet greens, boiled	½ cup	Beta-carotene, vitamin C, riboflavin, magnesium
Cabbage, Chinese, shredded, boiled	½ cup	Beta-carotene, vitamin B_6, vitamin C
Cantaloupe, cubed	1 cup	Beta-carotene, vitamin C
Carrot	1 (2½ oz.)	Beta-carotene, vitamin C, fiber
Cauliflower	3 florets (2 oz. total)	Vitamin C
Nectarine	1 (5 oz.)	Beta-carotene, vitamin C, fiber
Peas, green, boiled	½ cup	Thiamin, folate, vitamin C, fiber
Pineapple, cubed	1 cup	Vitamin C, fiber
Potato, boiled	1 (5 oz.)	Vitamin B_6, vitamin C, fiber
Sweet potato, baked	1 (4 oz.)	Beta-carotene, vitamin B_6, vitamin C, fiber
Swiss chard, chopped, boiled	½ cup	Beta-carotene, vitamin C, fiber, magnesium, iron
Tomato	1 (4 oz.)	Beta-carotene, vitamin C, fiber

something of a natural appetite suppressant. The higher your level of serotonin, the less you'll be tempted to overeat.

You can use complex carbohydrates to your advantage when you know you're going to be faced with a stressful task. Suppose you have

REAL-LIFE SCENARIO

Healthful Hints for the Harried

From the moment she rolls out of bed, Sandi is on the go. She gets breakfast for the kids, then gets ready for work while they're eating. She's out the door by 7:00 A.M., dropping them off at day care on her way to the office. There she finally has her own breakfast: a doughnut and a cup of coffee. Errands take up her lunch hour, so she hits the fast-food drive-up window. After work, she picks up the kids and heads for home. The kids are clamoring for pizza, and she's too exhausted to argue. She'll just ask her husband to pick it up on his way home. Life is too hectic to cook ahead. Besides, Sandi hates to cook anyway. But she knows her family needs to eat better. What can she do?

Sandi is just fooling herself by saying that she doesn't have time to cook. In fact, her fast-food lifestyle is actually stealing time. Fast food and takeout aren't fast or soothing. She'd feel a lot less stressed and harried if she relaxed at work while munching on something savory and nutritious that she brought from home.

To get in the habit of making more healthful meals at home, Sandi can try getting up 15 minutes earlier each morning. She can use that time to eat a healthful breakfast—cereal or oatmeal—and pack her lunch. Or she can try packing her lunch the night before. Also, her mornings will go more smoothly if she does some organizing the night before.

For dinners, Sandi can try preparing food for the week on weekends. For instance, each weekend she can make a huge pot of chili, stew, or some other dish. She can store family-size servings in containers and freeze them. Before she knows it, she'll have an arsenal of homemade frozen dinners to choose from each night of the week.

By getting herself organized and her family on a healthy eating plan, Sandi will take a whole lot of stress out of her life. She'll feel happy instead of harried at the end of the day.

Expert Consulted
Nancy Cohen, R.D., Ph.D.
Associate professor of nutrition
University of Massachusetts
Amherst

to make a major presentation at work. Help yourself to some complex carbs about a half-hour before showtime, suggests Judith Wurtman, Ph.D., nutrition research scientist at the Massachusetts Institute of Technology in Cambridge and author of *Managing Your Mind and Mood through Food*. You'll need to eat about 1½ ounces of carbohydrates—or two cups of Cheerios—in order to experience the tranquilizing effects, Dr. Wurtman says.

Be sugar-free. Don't let sugar's status as a simple carbohydrate fool you. It doesn't affect your body in the same way that some of its complex cousins do. Sugar gets absorbed from your bloodstream into cells quite quickly, giving you an almost instantaneous energy boost. Consequently, your blood sugar level can go for a roller-coaster ride, rising and then falling. And that can leave you moody and miserable.

Befriend B_6. In a study at the Jean Mayer USDA Human Nutrition Research Center on Aging at Tufts University in Boston, a group of volunteers experienced increases in irritability and tension when their diets ran low on vitamin B_6. Researchers suspect that there's a link between B_6 and dopamine, a brain chemical that at moderate levels is associated with feeling good. When you don't get enough B_6, your dopamine supply is depleted, and you end up being even more susceptible to the effects of stress.

You can boost your intake of the

vitamin by choosing foods such as bananas, potatoes, and prunes. One banana, for instance, supplies about 0.7 milligram of B_6. If that seems low, keep in mind that the Daily Value for B_6 is just 2 milligrams, which means that one banana gives you 34 percent of the amount of B_6 you should be getting every day.

Arm yourself with antioxidants. Research has proven that stress causes your body to step up its production of free radicals, destructive molecules that damage healthy tissue and weaken the immune system. This, in turn, can pave the way for serious ailments such as heart disease and some cancers.

The antioxidant nutrients—beta-carotene and vitamins C and E—intervene in that process, neutralizing the free radicals and pulling the plug on their dirty work. In times of stress, you can do your health a favor by eating lots of antioxidant-rich foods as well as by taking an antioxidant-rich multivitamin/mineral supplement, says Elizabeth Somer, R.D., author of *Nutrition for Women* and *Food and Mood.* Carrots, broccoli, and sweet potatoes offer abundant supplies of beta-carotene. For vitamin C, choose oranges, kiwifruit, tomatoes, and sweet red peppers. Vitamin E is plentiful in wheat germ and vegetable oils. (Just be sure to avoid oils that contain high amounts of saturated fat, such as coconut and palm.)

The Right Food at the Right Time

Anti-stress eating is as much a matter of when you eat as what you eat. Read on.

Fuel up first thing. You should make a point of eating breakfast every day. But on high-stress days, your morning meal takes on special significance. The right mix of foods can give you an energy boost that will sustain you at least until noon. The following tempting A.M. menu is recommended by Georgia Hodgkin, R.D., Ed.D., associate professor in the department of nutrition and dietetics at Loma Linda University in California: high-fiber, low-sugar cereal with skim milk; a bagel, an English muffin, or a slice of toast with a tablespoon of peanut butter or nonfat cream cheese; and fruit or fruit juice.

Choose a light lunch. A heavy, high-fat noontime meal can leave you fatigued and lethargic—not what you want when you have an audience with the boss or a bank loan officer at 2:00 P.M. Eating that way at dinner is no better. Fat takes a long time to digest, and that can prevent you from getting a good night's sleep just when you need it most.

Stick with leaner, lighter fare for your midday and evening repasts. In fact, some experts recommend limiting your total daily fat intake to no more than 25 percent of calories.

Downsize your meals. Some experts believe that in times of stress, we're better off consuming mini-meals instead of the standard three squares. This is because eating small portions more often keeps blood sugar levels on a more even keel. In fact, research has shown that when you go for more than four hours without eating, your blood sugar level drops low enough to cause fatigue. And while a big meal can leave you feeling sluggish, a mini-meal won't, says Tammy Baker, R.D., a nutritionist in Scottsdale, Arizona, and a spokesperson for the American Dietetic Association.

How do you make the switch to mini-meals? Perhaps the easiest way, according to Elizabeth A. Brown, R.D., nutritionist and weight-control specialist at the Lehigh Valley Hospital Center for Health Promotion and Disease Prevention in Allentown, Pennsylvania, is to divide each of your usual big meals into two smaller ones, then spread them out so that you're eating every three to four hours.

Chocoholics Anonymous

What Women Crave and Why

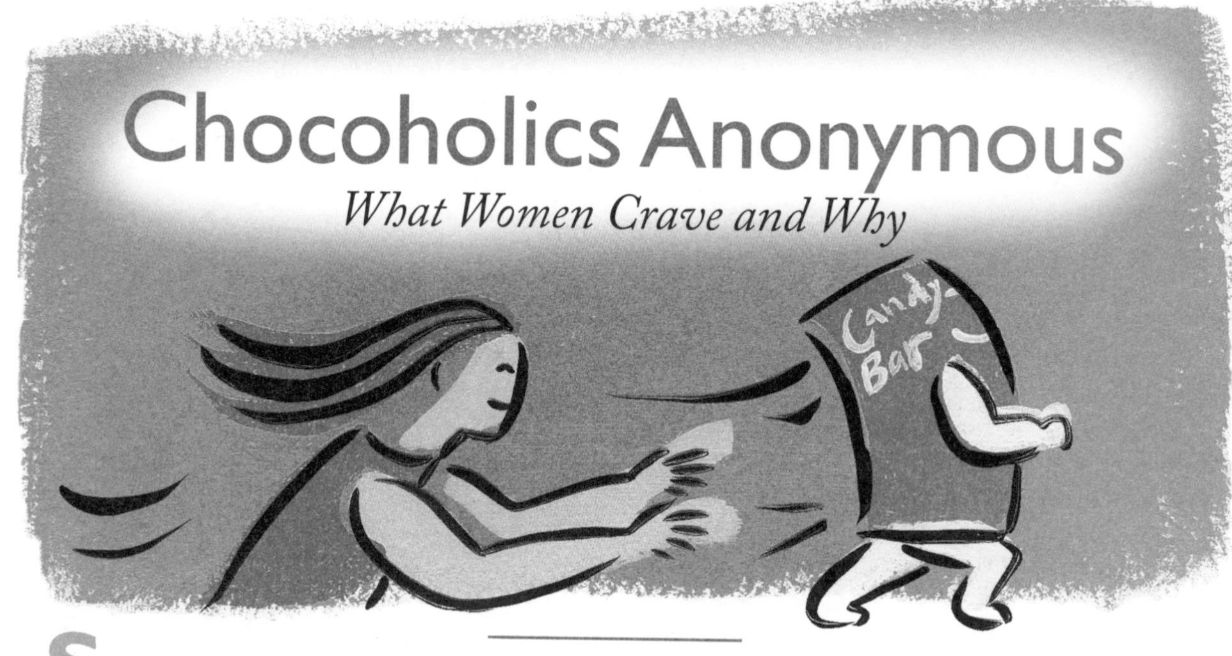

So just how serious is the love affair between women and chocolate?

Well, in one survey, half of the women said that they would prefer eating chocolate to having sex—which should give their amorous spouses something to think about the next time Valentine's Day rolls around.

In fact, while both genders experience cravings for particular foods, chocolate appears to have an almost exclusively female fan club. Sure, other sweets flirt with our senses, but chocolate has the power to make so many of us swoon. "Often women tell me that chocolate is the one thing they can count on to give them pleasure whenever they want it," says Anne Kearney-Cooke, Ph.D., director of the Cincinnati Psychotherapy Institute. By one estimate, chocolate accounts for 68 percent of cravings among women.

For all its sweetness, chocolate has its dark side—nutritionally speaking, anyway. It doesn't offer much in the way of nutrients: It has lots of calories and saturated fat and few vitamins and minerals. Every health-conscious bone in your body may tell you to avoid the stuff. Still, when the urge to indulge strikes, you may find it almost impossible to resist.

You can conquer that craving without blowing your healthy eating habits. And you don't necessarily have to break off your relationship with chocolate to do it.

Sweet Emotions

Cravings are a virtually universal phenomenon among women. One survey found that 97 percent of us get a yen for some food or another from time to time. What could possibly make you want a food so badly that you would walk a mile uphill in a raging snowstorm to get it?

Craving may be your body's way of persuading you to replenish its supply of certain substances. Women sometimes yearn for sweet, fatty foods such as chocolate when we're running low on endorphins, "feel-good" brain chemicals that boost mood, according to Debra Waterhouse, R.D., author of *Why Women Need Chocolate*. Feed the craving, and your endorphins bounce back, improving your mood, she explains.

Other scientific explanations for chocolate cravings abound. Some experts say that chocolate elevates levels of a soothing brain chemical called serotonin. Others contend that it compensates for a magnesium deficit.

Then again, maybe we want chocolate simply because it tastes so darn good. Maybe we just can't get enough of its melt-in-your-mouth richness and creaminess. That's what researchers at the University of Pennsylvania in Philadelphia concluded after an experiment in which they gave one group of chocophiles real chocolate and another group a gelatin capsule containing chocolate's active ingredients. Only the people who ate the real thing said that they felt satisfied.

Ride the Crave Wave

Chocolate, in itself, really isn't all bad. In fact, there is tantalizing evidence that it may actually have some health *benefits*. Scientists at the University of California, Davis, discovered that chocolate contains flavonoids—the same compounds that give red wine its heart disease–defying punch.

Problems arise when chocolate becomes a dietary staple, crowding out other, more nutritious foods. That's when the fat and calories start adding up.

So how do you balance your healthy eating habits with the over-

Woman to Woman

She Gets Her Daily Dose of Chocolate

Fran Seligson, R.D., Ph.D., loves chocolate, so when she started working as associate director of nutrition at Hershey Foods in 1987, she knew she had to find a way to indulge in her favorite confection without gaining weight. Fortunately, Fran found a way to balance her overall diet and lifestyle to include her favorite chocolate treats.

Chocolate is central to my job, and I eat my fair share of it. At Hershey, no matter where you turn, chocolate is there, and I can't resist.

It isn't unusual that come 10:00 A.M., I'm out at the candy basket eating my way through three to five Hershey's Miniatures or Hershey Nuggets. That might sound like a lot, but it takes that many to keep me satisfied until lunch. If I'm still hungry after lunch, I'll treat myself to one or two more.

When I came to work for Hershey, I knew I had to find a way to indulge in chocolate and not feel guilty at the end of the day. I like the taste of chocolate—it's a really pleasurable eating experience, and I won't deny myself that pleasure.

Over the years, I've learned to structure my diet and lifestyle to accommodate chocolate goodies. I make sure that I eat healthy, low-fat foods throughout the rest of the day: fruit, bagels, salads with oil and vinegar, and chicken (without the skin) and rice for dinner. I try to use low-fat substitutions when I cook, such as skim milk instead of cream.

I've also learned to control portion sizes, and I can recognize when I am satisfied instead of letting the taste of foods run away with me. I'm always aware of calories and fat, even when I'm eating five Hershey's Miniatures!

Aside from my healthy, nonsweet eating choices, my other saving grace is exercise. I run three times a week, lift weights twice a week, swim once a week, and walk a lot in between.

Right now, this diet and exercise plan works for me. I can eat chocolate and maintain my weight. On the days when I eat more chocolate than usual, I'll cut back at lunch or dinner or make sure that I'm more physically active.

Healthy choices and exercise for the sake of chocolate—it's a great trade-off!

whelming urge to splurge? Score a craving coup with these smart strategies.

Tune in to your cues. This may be the most important piece of advice, not just for managing your cravings but for managing your entire diet. You need to distinguish between a real, physical need for a food and a desire to eat that's triggered by some external factor—perhaps the sight or smell of a food.

Count on your stomach, your hormones, and your brain chemicals to steer you in the right direction. They'll lay low as long as your body is properly fed. And when it's not, they'll speak up. Your stomach will growl, and your hormones and brain chemicals will place the order: "Send us something sweet!"

But if the smell of freshly baked brownies makes you crave chocolate, watch out. That's an external cue, and it's just itching for you to overindulge.

Wait it out. When a craving strikes, don't give in to it right away. Instead, try to put off eating for 10 minutes or so. That's about how long it takes for a craving to run its course.

Now we know that 10 minutes can seem like an eternity when you're convinced that a certain candy bar is calling your name. So distract yourself by taking a walk. That way, if you beat your craving, you've done two good things for yourself.

Fool it with fruit. If you have a hankering for something sweet, a piece of fresh fruit just might fill the bill, says Maria Simonson, Sc.D., Ph.D., professor emeritus and director of the health, weight, and stress clinic at the Johns Hopkins Medical Institutions in Baltimore. And it won't send your blood sugar on a roller-coaster ride like chocolate and other sweets can. When that happens, your craving may be intensified.

Stay low. A low-fat or nonfat treat can tame your craving without guilt. For instance, when nothing but chocolate will do, fix yourself a cup of homemade cocoa made with low-fat (1 percent) milk. Two tablespoons of the cocoa powder supply just one gram of fat. Or enjoy a "cold fondue" recipe suggested by Elizabeth Somer, R.D., author of *Nutrition for Women* and *Food and Mood*: Serve up 2 cups of cut fresh fruit and 1/4 cup of chocolate syrup.

Other saintly skinny selections that may satisfy your chocolate craving include the following:

- Entenmann's Light Fudge Brownie—zero grams of fat, 120 calories
- Alba Dairy Shake Mix made with skim milk—zero grams of fat, 70 calories
- Quaker Chewy Low-Fat Chocolate Chunk Granola Bar—two grams of fat, 110 calories
- SnackWell's Devil's Food Cookie Cakes (2 cookies)—zero grams of fat, 100 calories

With all of these, of course, you need to pay attention to the serving size. Eat too much, and you'll defeat the purpose of choosing low-fat or nonfat fare in the first place.

Have a little something. Sometimes you can't quiet a chocolate craving with anything less than the real, full-fat, full-calorie thing. When that's the case, do what you have to do. Just keep the portion small, Somer says. One-half ounce—about equal to three chocolate kisses—should do the trick. You'll get about 75 calories and almost five grams of fat.

If you can, eat your chocolate with a meal, Somer adds. That way, you're less likely to overdo than if you would have a candy bar and nothing else.

Don't count on carob. Carob has gotten a reputation as a healthy alternative to chocolate. In fact, a carob bar and a chocolate bar supply equal amounts of fat and calories.

Part Five

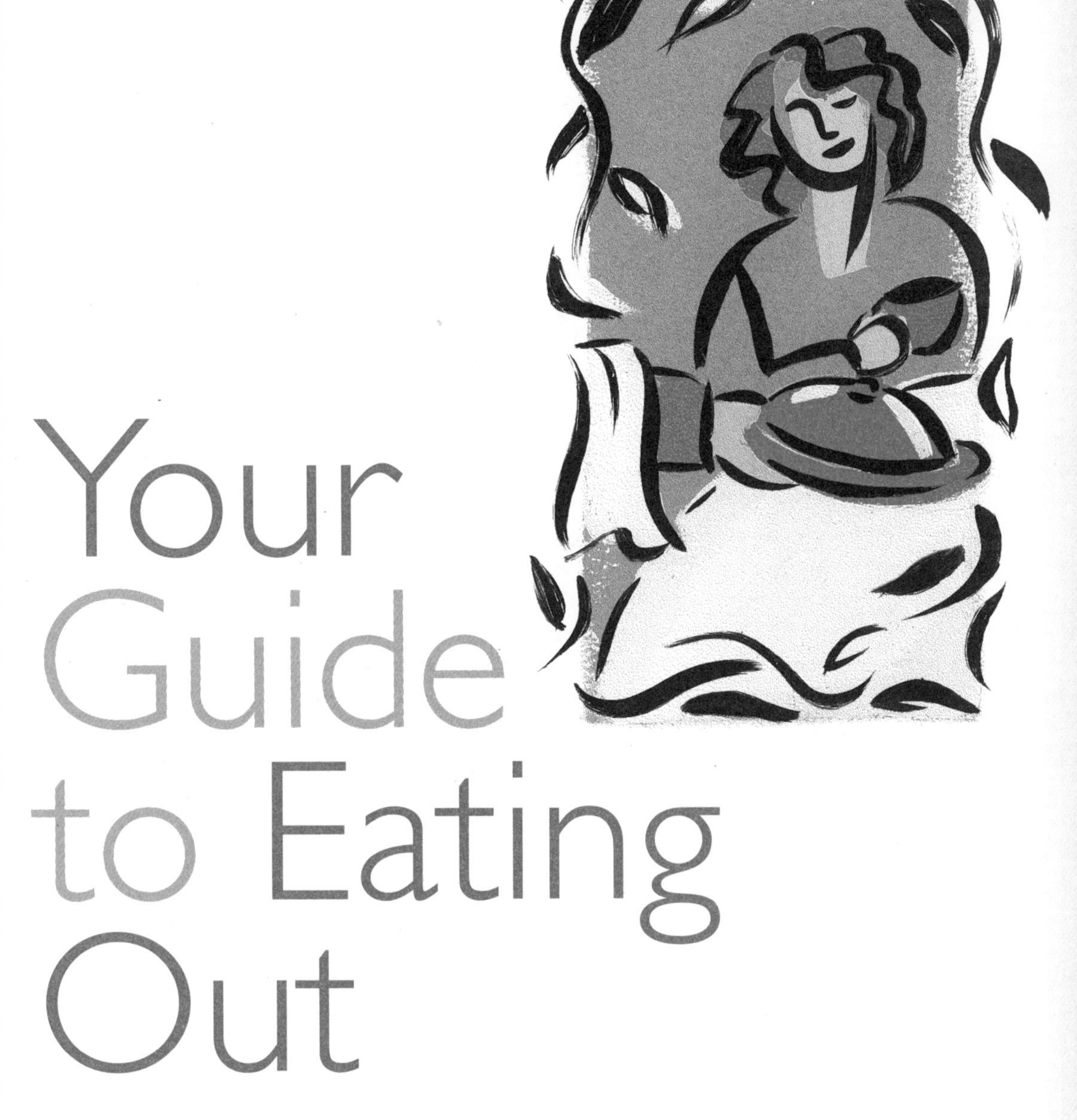

Your Guide to Eating Out

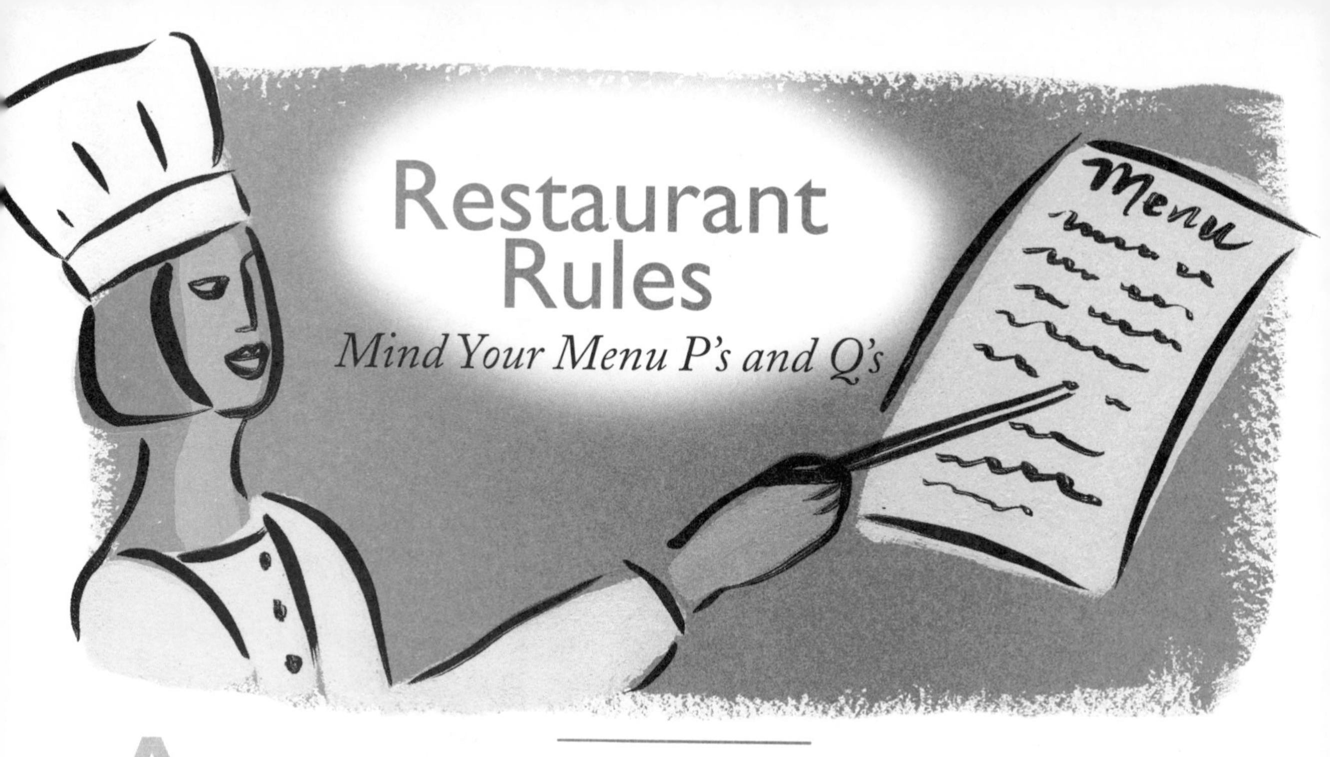

Restaurant Rules

Mind Your Menu P's and Q's

According to a National Restaurant Association survey, the average American woman eats out about four times a week. That's 208 times a year—208 meals in which you put your healthy eating habits on the line.

At home, you control what goes into a dish, how it's prepared, and how much of it you put on your plate. Restaurants, though, are a whole other ball game. You find yourself at the mercy of whoever is wielding the pots and pans in the kitchen. What's more, everything from the menu to the decor entices you with the same subliminal message: "You must be famished. C'mon. Eat up!"

Heeding this call didn't matter so much, say, 20 years ago, when folks dined out once in a blue moon. "But these days, with one-third of our calories coming from foods eaten away from home, what we put in our mouths in restaurants does count," says Jayne Hurley, R.D., senior nutritionist with the Center for Science in the Public Interest, a nonprofit consumer group in Washington, D.C., and a writer for *Nutrition Action Healthletter*.

Unfortunately, while eating out has become at least an every-other-day ritual for many of us, we still tend to think of away-from-home meals as treats. This mind-set leads us to choose foods that have too many calories, too much fat, and too few vitamins and minerals. When we walk into restaurants, it seems, the principles of good nutrition get checked at the door.

Make no mistake: They absolutely do count. But they don't mean that you get to nibble on the cottage-cheese-on-lettuce "diet plate" while watching your dining companions feast on prime rib. On the contrary, you can order a meal that satisfies your appetite but doesn't fill you with guilt in the process. A little strategizing is the key.

Eating Right Made Easy

You can start planning for your meal long before you even set foot in the restaurant. Here's what the experts recommend.

Preview the menu. Stop by your favorite restaurants as well as any new ones you'd like to try and request copies of their menus. Then keep them at home or in your office, so you can decide what you want to order before you venture out to eat. Choosing your meal ahead of time makes you less likely to succumb to the beckoning sight and scent of other, less nutritious foods.

Save up for a splurge. If you're going out for a special occasion—perhaps a co-worker's birthday or your wedding anniversary—and you know you might overindulge, simply "bank" some calories by eating a little bit less at preceding meals, suggests Carole Livingston, author of *I'll Never Be Fat Again*. That way, you can enjoy your food without guilt because you know you haven't blown your calorie budget.

But don't go too far and actually skip meals. It simply doesn't work. When mealtime finally rolls around, you're positively famished, and you end up stuffing yourself.

Use your imagination. As part of her premeal preparation, Hope S. Warshaw, R.D., author of *The Restaurant Companion: A Guide to Healthier Eating Out*, says that she does a mental run-through of what she's going to order. She says it helps her to eat healthfully in restaurants, and she recommends that you do the same.

"Mental imagery is very powerful. When you envision yourself succeeding, it's more likely that you will," agrees Susan Olson, Ph.D., a clinical psychologist and weight-management consultant in Seattle and author of *Keeping It Off: Winning at Weight Loss*.

Woman to Woman

She's Paid to Eat, and She's Slim, Too

Patricia Unterman gets paid to eat—and eat she does. She is a restaurant reviewer and restaurant owner in San Francisco and author of Patricia Unterman's Food Lover's Guide to San Francisco. *Here's how she manages to maintain a healthy lifestyle despite her occupational hazards.*

My jobs require me to be around food all day. As a restaurant owner and reviewer, I start eating at 7:00 A.M. and keep on eating all day long. I've been doing this since 1972, so I've learned a lot of tricks.

Restaurant reviewing is my biggest challenge because I can't order only lean foods like fish or pasta. I have to sample everything possible, and that includes high-fat foods—fried dishes, cream sauces, and butter sauces, which, by the way, I love. *Sample* is the magic word. There are usually four of us ordering a variety of foods. I *taste* it all. I never eat everything that I order. If I did, I physically wouldn't be able to taste the other foods.

To avoid temptation, I nibble all day at my restaurant, so I'm never ravenous when I go out to do a review. That way I don't stuff myself.

What really keeps me thin, though, is exercise. I'm adamant about exercising regularly. I'm an avid tennis player, and I try to hit the courts three or four times a week. If I can't squeeze in a game, I'll go to the gym and hop on the treadmill or Stair-Master for 50 minutes.

It's difficult to eat healthy when you dine out, especially for me because I have to sample a wide array of courses: appetizers, salads, meats, pastas, and desserts. Plus, restaurant portions can be so huge! I have to constantly remind myself that the most important diet strategy in restaurant dining is controlling portion sizes.

Sup solo. Researchers at Georgia State University in Atlanta found that people tend to eat more in the presence of others. In fact, the more dining partners you have, the more food you consume. In the study, eating with one person increased food consumption by 28 percent; with two people, by 41 percent; and with six or more people, by 76 percent. The researchers theorize that having company at mealtime causes you to linger over your food. So eating by yourself may not be a bad idea.

Make the first move. If you do eat with others, try to place your order first. That way, you won't be swayed by everyone else's meal choices.

Be nosy. Don't shy away from grilling your server about various menu items. You have a right to know exactly what it is that you're eating and whether it meets your nutrition standards.

Design your own dish. If you can't find something on the menu that suits you, ask whether the chef can "customize" a meal for you. For instance, you may notice that the restaurant serves pasta as well as a steamed vegetable side dish. Perhaps the chef can combine the two. "Don't be afraid to make special requests," Livingston says. "Often, the better the restaurant, the easier it is to make alternate choices."

Start with soup. In a study at Johns Hopkins University in Baltimore, people who began a meal with a soup appetizer consumed 25 percent fewer calories over the course of the meal than people who had a cheese-and-crackers appetizer. The researchers theorize that soup fills you up, so you don't feel like eating as much. Just remember to steer clear of any concoctions that begin with the words *cream of*.

Favor fish. If you can't make up your mind, fish is almost always a smart choice. Besides being low in fat, many varieties—including salmon, mackerel, tuna, and herring—have an abundance of omega-3 fatty acids. Research has shown that omega-3's can improve your cholesterol profile and lower your risk of heart disease.

Of course, fish loses its nutritional value when it's fried or coated with butter, cheese, or tartar sauce. Ask to have yours grilled, broiled, steamed, baked, or blackened, Hurley suggests.

Put side dishes in the spotlight. Who says you have to order an entrée? You can create a perfectly acceptable meal by picking and choosing among side dishes and appetizers. This

RED LIGHT, GREEN LIGHT

Those fancy-schmancy words and phrases in restaurant menus often reveal a great deal about what's in a dish or how it's prepared. You just have to know how to interpret them.

The following glossary features some key terms that you're likely to come across when you eat out, along with a brief definition of each. Keep in mind that recipes can vary from one restaurant to the next, so it's still a good idea to ask the server about ingredients and cooking methods.

✘ ***Alfredo.*** A rich sauce made from a combination of butter, Parmesan cheese, and heavy cream.

✘ ***Au fromage.*** The French term for "with cheese."

✘ ***Au gratin.*** Refers to a dish that is topped with either cheese or a mixture of bread crumbs and butter, then baked until brown.

✘ ***Au lait.*** The French term for "with milk."

✘ ***Bearnaise.*** A thick sauce that includes white wine, egg yolks, and butter among its ingredients.

✘ ***Bisque.*** A rich soup usually made from pureed seafood and cream.

✘ ***Bolognese.*** A sauce that's prepared by sautéing meat (usually ground beef, ham, and/or pork) and vegetables in butter, then adding wine and milk or cream for flavor.

✔ ***Braised.*** Indicates that a food is cooked in liquid.

✘ ***Carbonara.*** A sauce that lists cream, eggs, Parmesan cheese, and bacon bits among its ingredients.

- ✔ ***Florentine.*** A term used to refer to a dish that is served or dressed with spinach.
- ✔ ***Grilled.*** Indicates that the food is cooked by setting it on a rack directly over a heat source, allowing the fat to drain away.
- ✘ ***Hollandaise.*** A creamy, rich sauce made from butter, egg yolks, and lemon juice.
- ✔ ***Marinara.*** A tomato-based sauce seasoned with basil, garlic, oregano, and onions.
- ✔ ***Poached.*** Indicates that the food is gently cooked in liquid just below the boiling point.
- ✔ ***Primavera.*** Refers to the use of fresh vegetables in a dish. (Just make sure that they're not coated with a cream sauce.)
- ✔ ***Steamed.*** Indicates that the food is placed on a rack or in a steamer basket over boiling or simmering water in a covered pan.
- ✔ ***Stir-fried.*** Indicates that the food is rapidly cooked in a pan or wok; should use little or no oil.
- ✔ ***Sweet-and-sour.*** A sauce that includes sugar and vinegar among its ingredients for a balance of flavors.
- ✘ ***Tempura.*** Indicates that the dish contains fish or vegetables that have been batter-dipped and deep-fried.
- ✔ ***Vinaigrette.*** An oil-and-vinegar combination used to flavor salads and other cold dishes.

is an excellent way to increase your intake of grains, vegetables, and fruits, notes Evelyn Tribole, R.D., author of *Healthy Homestyle Cooking* and *Eating on the Run*. Plus, you get to sample a little bit of everything, which makes for a more interesting meal.

Dress yourself. Request that any sauce or salad dressing be served on the side. This allows you to control how much goop goes on your food. In fact, instead of pouring it on, leave it in the container. Lightly dip your fork in the sauce or dressing, then pick up a forkful of food. You get the flavor without a huge dose of fat and calories.

Drown your appetite. Drinking lots of water throughout a meal can fill you up, so you feel less hungry. Ask your server to bring a bottle of mineral water or a pitcher of tap water to your table, then sip constantly.

Bypass the bar. Drinking and dining don't mix. Besides supplying empty calories, alcoholic beverages also enhance your appetite, causing you to overeat. If you want something bubbly, have a glass of club soda with a twist instead.

Take half home. Ask your server to put half of your meal in a doggie bag before bringing the rest to your table. Then have him keep the bag in the kitchen until you're ready to leave. This tactic should reduce the temptation to try to scarf down the whole thing in one sitting. Even better, you'll have a nice lunch or dinner for the next day.

Finish last. Women who have weight problems tend to eat faster than women who don't. So take your time. Eat a portion of your meal, then lay down your fork and wait 10 minutes or so before taking another bite. This technique enables you to savor the entire dining experience—the food and the conversation. And at the end of 10 minutes, you may just find that you're not hungry anymore. If you are, then help yourself to a few more forkfuls.

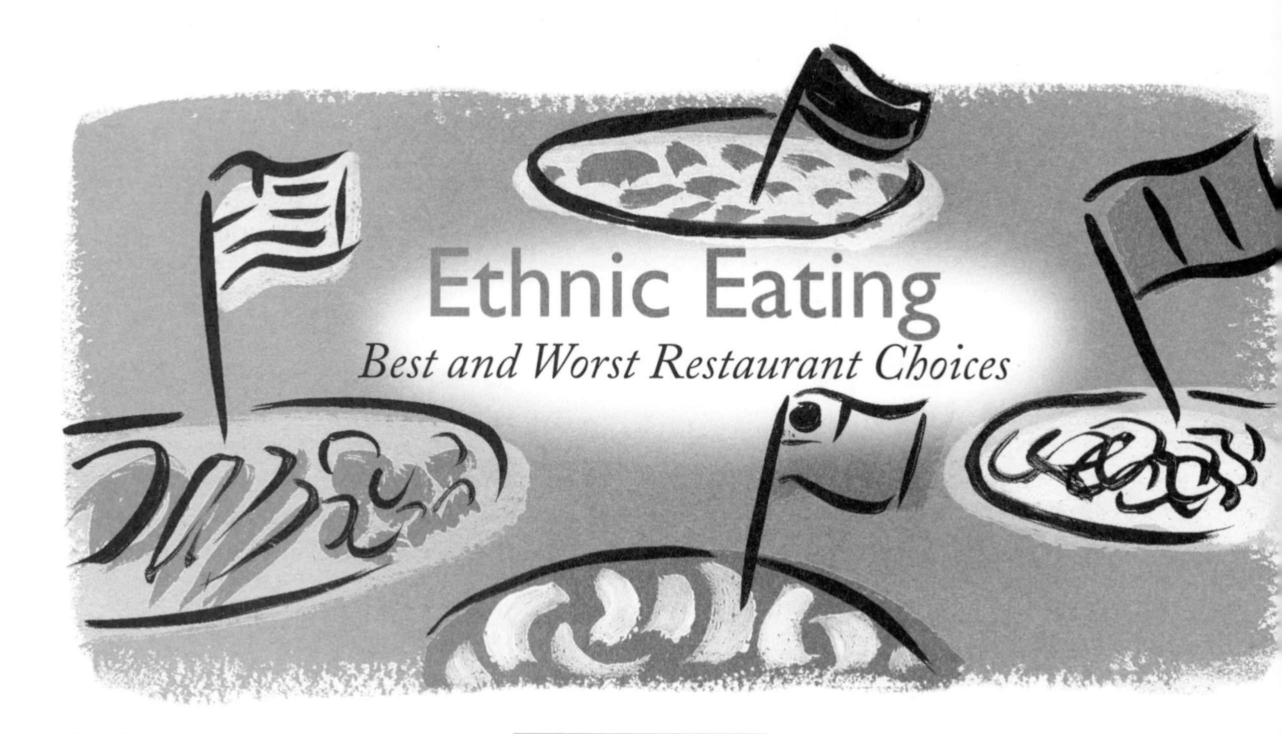

Ethnic Eating

Best and Worst Restaurant Choices

Where in the world should you go for dinner?

Thanks to the proliferation of ethnic eateries in this country, you can treat your tastebuds to authentic Greek souvlakia, Japanese yakitori, or Indian chapati without traveling too far from home. In fact, according to a survey conducted by the National Restaurant Association, 98 percent of restaurants have some sort of ethnic dishes on their menus.

The popularity of ethnic cuisine in the United States shouldn't come as a big surprise. After all, our nation's status as the world's melting pot has bestowed us with a wonderfully diverse culinary heritage. And with a growing public awareness of the link between good nutrition and good health, many folks view ethnic foods as healthful alternatives to hamburgers, hot dogs, and other all-American fare.

"In most ethnic places, you can get a lot more vegetables and grains as well as lighter sauces," notes Aliza Green, a restaurant food consultant in Elkins Park, Pennsylvania, and former chef. "And the more authentic the restaurant, the better."

Still, that doesn't mean that all ethnic dishes are automatically good for you. Intermingled with those veggies and grains may lurk a fair amount of butter, cream, or oil. So you need to exercise some caution when placing your order. Take fettuccine Alfredo, for example, Green says. In some Italian restaurants, it's the most frequently ordered entrée. But it's loaded with cream and butter. (The fat content of the dish is so high that some nutritionists darkly dub it "heart attack on a plate.")

You can easily avoid nutrition traps. You just have to know what to look for. Join us as we take you on a culinary world tour, exploring 11 of the best-known and best-loved ethnic cuisines. We asked a number of nutrition authorities to point out which foods to choose and which to avoid, so you can put together a meal that satisfies your nutrition sense and pleases your palate. Consider what follows your passport to healthy ethnic eating.

Welcome to the World's Fare

First, familiarize yourself with the following ethnic-eating ground rules. They apply to any cuisine, from French to Mexican.

Speak up. Even the most detailed menu descriptions don't always tell the whole story. Don't hesitate to ask questions about the ingredients and cooking methods used to prepare a particular dish. Otherwise, you may end up getting more fat and calories than you bargained for.

Also, if an ingredient or the cooking method doesn't quite suit you, find out if it can be changed. Most chefs are willing to do what it takes to make their patrons happy.

Show the entrée the exit. Order a couple of appetizers rather than a single entrée. This strategy is especially good with Indian, Thai, and Chinese foods. It saves you from huge main-dish portions and allows you to experience the different tastes and textures characteristic of the cuisine.

Be careful, though: Since appetizers are often "finger foods," you can easily eat too much by picking and nibbling your way through the meal.

Pack your (doggie) bag. If you do order an entrée, tell your server right up front that you want to wrap half of it to take home, suggests Jayne Hurley, R.D., senior nutritionist with the Center for Science in the Public Interest, a nonprofit consumer group in Washington, D.C., and a writer for *Nutrition Action Healthletter*. That way, you won't be tempted to eat the whole thing.

In a Chinese restaurant, for example, you may get three to four cups of food in a typical serving, Hurley notes. The same may hold true for Mexican and Italian eateries. That means you could take in 1,000 calories or more in one sitting.

Order for two. You can also trim down an oversize portion by splitting an entrée with a companion, says Hope S. Warshaw, R.D., author of *The Restaurant Companion: A Guide to Healthier Eating Out*. "In Asian restaurants, you typically split things," Warshaw points out. "I do this all the time. At one typical restaurant meal, for example, three of us shared two different dishes."

Italian: Pasta Perfect

You don't have to travel to Rome to do as the Romans do—at least not when it comes to eating. By one estimate, as many as two-thirds of all restaurants in the United States include Italian dishes on their menus. Indeed, more people order Italian than any other type of food, making it the most popular ethnic cuisine in this country.

For the nutrition-conscious woman, a plate of pasta makes a delicious meal, without a lot of fat. The vast majority of pasta dishes get no more than 30 percent of calories from fat and no more than 10 percent of calories from saturated fat.

But authentic Italian cuisine is much more than just pasta. Vegetable and bean dishes are quite common, too. In fact, the people of southern Italy follow what many nutritionists consider to be the healthiest diet in the world: the Mediterranean diet, which is characterized by lots of grains and produce, little meat, and olive oil instead of butter.

Travel to the northern part of the country, and you'll discover an entirely different version of Italian cuisine. There, the more beef, butter, and cream in a dish, the better folks seem to like it.

This, unfortunately, is the cooking style that most restaurants on this side of the Atlantic emulate. We favor fettuccine Alfredo, lasagna, and anything parmigiana—which, naturally, are loaded with calories and fat.

"Italian food is really simple. The secret is the pasta," Hurley says. "As long as you get a plate of spaghetti or linguine, you can top it with tomato sauce, marinara sauce, red or white clam sauce, meat sauce, even meatballs, and you're practically guaranteed a lower-fat meal."

Become a bean counter. Beans figure prominently in authentic Italian cuisine. Pasta e fagioli, for instance, is a hearty soup that combines pasta and white beans (or *fagioli*, in Italian). Minestrone is similar, except that the cook throws vegetables into the mix. Take advantage of these delicious dishes to increase your daily fiber intake.

Order goodness by the slice. And you thought pizza was junk food? Consider this: The crust supplies carbohydrates; the cheese, protein and calcium; and the sauce and vegetables, vitamins A and C. Skip the meat toppings, and you have a healthful food that gets a respectable 25 to 30 percent of its calories from fat.

Bag the garlic bread. Yes, it's bread, and you're supposed to eat bread. But toasted garlic bread is soaked in oil or butter. Request plain Italian bread instead, and if you must have something on it, spread your slice with just the thinnest smear of butter.

Be anti-antipasto. Beware the antipasto dishes that include olives, cheeses, and smoked meats. Besides supplying fat and sodium that you don't need, these foods jack up the calorie content of your meal. If you want something to nibble on, order a vegetable antipasto with grilled mushrooms, roasted peppers, zucchini, and caponata (a Sicilian relish).

Help Yourself to...

- Any dish described as marsala (broth-based and cooked with wine)
- Chicken cacciatore
- Cioppino (a fish stew)
- Marinara, pizzaola, and other meatless, tomato-based sauces
- Pasta primavera (as long as it doesn't have a cream or butter sauce)

Hands Off...

- Any cheese-filled pasta such as cannelloni, lasagna, and ravioli
- Any sauce labeled "crema" or "fritto"
- Fettuccine Alfredo
- Risotto (a rice dish made with butter and cheese)
- Veal piccata or saltimbocca

Greek: More Than Just Gyros

Greek cuisine has found its niche in, of all places, the shopping mall food court. Should you visit one of these culinary kiosks, you'll most likely find a selection of popular specialties such as gyros, moussaka, and baklava. Unfortunately, these foods tend to be less healthy than most Greek dishes. They don't do justice to this Mediterranean cuisine, yet another variation of what nutritionists now recognize as one of the healthiest cuisines in the world.

Like other people who live in countries of the Mediterranean region, Greeks eat an abundance of grains and vegetables. In fact, most of their meals have bread as the centerpiece. Meat—lamb is a favorite—makes an appearance only on special occasions, and fruit is the dessert of choice.

Greek cooking also uses generous amounts of olive oil. While it is pure fat, it's mostly monounsaturated—the kind that can actually lower your cholesterol and reduce your risk of heart disease.

To enjoy a healthful Greek meal, of course, you may have to stray from the dishes that are most familiar to you—the higher-fat offerings that tend to most pleasing to the American palate. So as you peruse the menu, keep these pointers in mind.

Go for grilled. Grilling is among the healthiest cooking methods, and Greek chefs tend to do a lot of it. So scan the menu for dishes that feature grilled seafood, poultry, meat, or vegetables. Among the favorites are souvlakia, which is skewered chunks of marinated lamb, sometimes with green peppers, onions, or other vegetables; and shish kebab, which is skewered chunks of marinated meat or fish and vegetables.

Slim down your salad. A Greek salad makes a great accompaniment to a meal—or a meal in itself. But you may want to order yours without fatty, salty ingredients such as anchovies and kal-amata olives. As always, request your dressing on the side.

Be cautious with cheese. Feta, a classic Greek cheese, has a lot of fat and a lot of salt—mainly because it's preserved in brine. And the popular appetizer saganaki is actually fried kasseri cheese that some restaurants soak in brandy, then serve flambéed. Go easy on both.

Help Yourself to...

- Fish baked with plaki sauce (garlic and tomato sauce)
- Shish kebab
- Souvlakia
- Tabbouleh (bulgur mixed with chopped tomatoes, parsley, mint, olive oil, and lemon juice)
- Torato (a cold soup made with eggplant, peppers, and yogurt)
- Tzatziki (a dip or dressing made from yogurt, garlic, and cucumbers)

Hands Off...

- Avgolemono (a soup or sauce made with chicken broth, egg yolks, and lemon juice)
- Baba ghanoush (served as a spread or dip)
- Baklava and other rich desserts
- Falafel (a dish made with deep-fried chickpea croquettes)
- Moussaka (a dish made of meat and eggplant, often covered with egg- or cheese-enriched béchamel sauce)
- Spanakopita (a vegetable pie made with feta cheese and eggs)

French: Ooh-La-Lunch

Mention French cuisine, and most people envision rich sauces and to-die-for desserts. If this includes you, then you're in for a healthful surprise. French cooking has undergone a makeover of sorts. Cream and butter, once mainstays of French recipes, have all but slipped from view. In their place are fruits, veggies, and other wholesome, garden-fresh ingredients.

In its high-fat heyday, French cuisine had all the makings of a heart attack waiting to happen. In fact, the French still eat about as much saturated fat as we do. So why do they have the second-lowest rate of heart disease in the world?

Experts believe that the answer lies with the red wine they savor with almost every meal. Red wine has an abundant supply of flavonoids, chemical compounds that help keep the heart healthy.

Don't think, though, that washing down your cassoulet with a glass of Beaujolais will somehow neutralize your meal's artery-clogging effects. The best way to make your dining experience a healthful one is to seek out a dish that features low-fat ingredients and is prepared in a low-fat way. As you scan the menu, keep these tips in mind.

Show a sense of style. French cooking consists of several different styles, and some are fattier than others. When a restaurant says it serves haute cuisine or cuisine bourgeois, that's your cue to be on the lookout for dishes prepared with butter, cream, eggs, and other high-fat ingredients. Nouvelle cuisine, on the other hand, favors fresh ingredients and smaller portions. Even healthier is cuisine minceur, a relatively new style that avoids fats and cream. In fact, its name literally means "cuisine of slenderness."

Select skinny sauce. If you're having a dish with a sauce, look for one that is wine-based rather than cream- or butter-based. If you want to try a dish with a heavy sauce, ask the server if you can get an appetizer-size portion.

Help Yourself to...

- Bouillabaisse (a seafood stew)
- Consommé (meat or fish broth)
- French bread
- Ratatouille (a vegetable dish cooked in olive oil)
- Sauces labeled coulis, puree, reduction, or vegetable
- Seafood that is poached or steamed

Hands Off...

- Cassoulet (a classic meat-and-beans dish featuring sausage, pork, and duck or goose)
- Dairy-based sauces such as béarnaise and beurre blanc
- Pâté
- Quiches
- Soufflés
- Sweetbreads (which are not bread at all, but organ meats)

Chinese: For Healthy Eating, Look to the East

Nutritionists continue to heap praise on the traditional Chinese diet as one of the healthiest in the world. By eating generous portions of rice and vegetables and only the smallest amounts of meat, native Chinese manage to keep their daily fat intakes to about 15 percent of calories. In the United States, our daily fat intake is more than double that amount.

Come to think of it, that may explain why Chinese cuisine puts on a little weight when it crosses the Pacific to our shores. The Americanized version features mounds of meat, deep-fried appetizers, and pools of sodium-charged soy sauce, while rice is relegated to practically garnish status.

Actually, Chinese cooking varies from region to region, and some styles are healthier than others. Most restaurants in this country specialize in Cantonese dishes, which feature roasted and grilled meat, steamed dishes, and mild flavors. Szechuan cooking, on the other hand, features many fried foods and tends to be hot and spicy. And then there are dishes from Shanghai, the coastal regions of the country, where seafood is a staple ingredient.

Generally, authentic Chinese cuisine favors healthful cooking methods, such as stir-frying and steaming. In fact, rather than ordering an entrée off the restaurant menu, you may want to request a simple dish of chicken or shrimp with steamed vegetables. From a nutrition standpoint, it's one of your best bets, and just about any Chinese chef can do a top-notch job of preparing it.

Here are some more strategies to help you enjoy Chinese cuisine at its healthiest.

Broaden your horizons. Traditional Chinese cooking relies heavily on vegetables. You'll get your fair share of the familiar, like broccoli, cabbage, and peppers. But be sure to introduce yourself to some more exotic selections, too—native favorites such as bamboo shoots, lily pods, lotus root, and water chestnuts.

Sample soy foods. Soy has earned superfood status, and for good reason. Research so far has shown that it may not only minimize the physical effects of menopause but may also reduce the risk of breast cancer. If you want to get more soy foods in your diet, here's your opportunity. Soy is a staple in Chinese cooking. In fact, it supplies most of the protein in the Chinese diet. Look for dishes that have a soy product, such as tofu or miso, as an ingredient.

Sip soup. Chinese restaurant menus usually feature a selection of low-fat, flavorful soups. They're perfect to start your meal or as a main dish. What about the eggs in egg drop soup?

They do raise the cholesterol content, but not by much. Incidentally, hot-and-sour soup also has an egg base.

Pick up sticks. If you're having Chinese food (or Thai food), try your hand at chopsticks. You say you're not good at using them? That's even better! They slow you down, so you eat less.

Be sodium-sensitive. One item to watch in Chinese cuisine is sodium. Soy sauce, for instance, supplies 343 milligrams per teaspoon. Monosodium glutamate (MSG) also supplies a generous amount of sodium, although it still has one-third as much as table salt. But MSG has yet another downside: It has been linked to headaches.

Eschew cashews. Nuts are fat pills. One large, oil-coated cashew carries about one gram of fat. Imagine how that adds up when you pour ½ cup of them into an entrée. So tell your server to hold the nuts—or at least cut the amount to two to three tablespoons, max.

Don't miss teatime. Most Chinese restaurants serve green tea with their meals. By all means, drink up. Green tea is loaded with compounds called polyphenols, which act like disease-fighting antioxidants. In fact, early research suggests that green tea may help protect against certain types of cancer and heart disease. (Be aware, though, that black tea doesn't have the same therapeutic properties.)

Find your fortune. A fortune cookie has just 30 calories and absolutely no fat. When you compare that with other desserts, your future looks healthier already!

Help Yourself to...

- Hot-and-sour or wonton soup
- Rice (brown is best, but white is okay)
- Shrimp with garlic sauce
- Szechuan shrimp (stir-fried in hot sauce)
- Steamed vegetable dumplings
- Stir-fried vegetables

Hands Off...

- Anything crispy or batter-coated (both terms indicate the food has been fried)
- Egg foo yong
- Egg rolls
- Fried rice
- Kung pao chicken
- Moo shu pork

Japanese: The *Other* Asian Cuisine

After years in the shadow of Chinese food, Japanese food has at last come into its own in this country. While Japanese restaurants have yet to match the proliferation of their Chinese counterparts, you'll have a much easier time finding one these days.

All we can say is...it's about time! Japanese cooking has much to offer, flavor-wise and nutrition-wise. For starters, it can claim one of the lowest fat contents among ethnic cuisines. Most dishes get less than 20 percent of their calories from fat. Grains and vegetables are dietary mainstays, as are seafood and soy. Meat, however, is not. When it is served, the portion is kept small.

The Japanese favor low-fat cooking methods, too, such as broiling, grilling, and steaming. And they use as little oil as possible.

Not sure what to look for on a Japanese menu? Let these tips serve as your guide.

Use your noodles. Rice is a staple of Japanese cuisine. But if you'd like to try something a little different, order a dish made with buckwheat noodles (soba) or wheat noodles (udon). You'll most likely find them in soups or as "beds" on which other foods are served.

Sample sushi. There's more to sushi than just raw fish. It can take many forms. The main ingredient is actually boiled rice flavored with rice vinegar. The rice may be garnished with fish, tofu, or vegetables, then wrapped in thin sheets of seaweed.

Sushi made with raw fish—especially mackerel and tuna—offers a generous dose of heart-healthy omega-3 fatty acids. And since it's uncooked, it has no added fat. (For more information on eating this Japanese delicacy safely, see "Sushi Savvy.")

Try your pot luck. Nabemono—which literally means "things in a pot"—is the Japanese version of a one-dish meal. Yosenabe is one kind of nabemono, featuring chicken, seafood, and vegetables in seasoned broth.

Get wise to sodium. Soy sauce, teriyaki sauce, and miso sauce all have very high sodium contents. They're also quite common in Japanese cooking. If you're concerned about your sodium intake, request that the chef prepare the dish without the sauce and ask for low-sodium soy sauce on the side.

Help Yourself to...

- Any dish described as nimono (simmered), yaki (broiled), or yakimono (grilled)
- Chirinabe (a one-dish meal made with fish, tofu, and vegetables)
- Shabu-shabu (meats and vegetables cooked in broth)
- Tofu and other soy foods
- Yakitori (either grilled or broiled chicken)

Hands Off...

- Any dish described as agemono (deep-fried) or tempura (batter-dipped and deep-fried)
- Fish that has been salted, smoked, or pickled
- Sukiyaki

SUSHI SAVVY

Time was when people—okay, college frat boys—would swallow live goldfish only on a dare. Now we're *paying* to sit at sushi bars and eat raw fish. Dead fish, yes, but raw just the same.

Of course, there's more to sushi bars than raw fish. The word *sushi* actually refers to vinegared rice. Traditionally, the rice is topped with a wide variety of garnishes, such as cooked egg, raw or cooked fish and shellfish, and cucumbers, avocados, and other vegetables. Technically, sliced raw fish is known as sashimi. Some eateries may mistakenly call sashimi sushi or sashimi sushi.

Salmon and tuna are the most popular choices at sushi bars, followed by mackerel, shrimp, rockfish, snapper, abalone, and scallops, among others. But not everyone is gaga over raw fish. For many, their reluctance has little to do with taste and more to do with safety. Like raw beef, pork, or chicken, raw fish may contain harmful bacteria, such as *Listeria monocytogenes*. To prevent contamination, it's important that raw fish be properly handled. And fish sometimes have parasitic worms. To kill these parasites, raw fish needs to be frozen.

Aside from disease-causing bacteria, certain large tropical fish could harbor hazardous and potentially life-threatening toxins. Be aware that if illegally or recreationally harvested, fish like barracuda, red snapper, and Australian coral trout may harbor what is called a ciguatoxin. This problem, however, does not usually occur with commercial products because their distribution is regulated by the industry.

If served in a well-established restaurant and prepared by a qualified, knowledgeable sushi chef who has undergone

Thai: Is It Hot Enough for You?

If you enjoy Chinese or Japanese food, you may want to give Thai a try. Thai cooking stir-fries lots of rice and vegetables, so it can be just as nutritious as the other Asian cuisines. It also makes extensive use of herbs. Recipes often call years of training under a master, sushi can be safe. The chef knows how to buy the right species of fish during the right season and how to prepare it properly. According to Kayo Io, manager of the Fuki-Sushi Restaurant in Palo Alto, California, word of mouth is the best way to find restaurants with top-notch sushi chefs. But for the very best flavor and freshness, it's important that the fish be eaten within 10 to 20 minutes of preparation.

"If you still have a concern about safety, ask the chef if he freezes the fish or buys it frozen," suggests Ann Adams, Ph.D., a research parasitologist specializing in seafood products at the Food and Drug Administration's seafood products research center in Seattle.

Whatever you do, never eat raw salmon that has never been frozen. There's a higher risk that salmon may be infected with parasites than other fish, says Dr. Adams, who tested almost 500 samples of sushi for parasites.

"In fact, if you're pregnant, you may want to avoid raw fish and go with cooked fish," says Dr. Adams. During pregnancy, infection from *Listeria* bacteria can cause abortion, stillbirth, or premature birth.

As for benefits, sushi can play a potential role in a healthy diet. Fish in general is low in fat and a good source of minerals. And fish like salmon, mackerel, and tuna supply healthy omega-3 fatty acids. Although sushi is expensive, fans extol its flavors and textures.

If you want to try sushi, you should start out with a light-tasting fish that's not high in oil, such as halibut or snapper, and shellfish such as abalone, shrimp, or scallops before moving on to oilier fish such as yellowtail, tuna, and mackerel.

for tantalizing, aromatic seasonings such as lemongrass, lime leaves, and Thai basil.

Thai food can be a real adventure for your tastebuds. To make sure it's a healthful one, keep these tips in mind.

Keep an eye on coconut. Coconut milk is a staple of Thai cooking. Unfortunately, it can turn an otherwise healthful dish into a fat-laden fiasco. When added to a curry, for example, it can increase the fat content to more than 40 percent of calories. Be sure to ask your server how various dishes are prepared. The use of coconut milk or cream may not be obvious.

Feel the heat. If you've never tried Thai food, be forewarned: Many dishes are *very* hot.

Help Yourself to...

- Forest salad
- Pad thai (a stir-fried noodle dish)
- Sautéed ginger beef or chicken (but request minimal oil)
- Soups made with lemongrass
- Yum neua (broiled beef with onions)

Hands Off...

- Anything served with peanut sauce
- Hae Kuen (deep-fried prawn cakes)
- Hot Thai catfish (fried)
- Royal tofu (fried)
- Yum koon chaing (a sausage-and-pepper dish)

Indian: A Complex Treat

Traditional Indian recipes bombard the palate with a unique blend of sweet and spicy. Yogurt often shows up in the same ingredients list as curry powder and other smoldering seasonings.

Perhaps the best-known Indian specialty is curry, which actually is a catch-all term for hot, spicy, gravy-based dishes that get their heat from—appropriately enough—curry powder. Curry powder, in turn, is a blend of up to 20 herbs, spices, and seeds, which may include cardamom, cloves, coriander, cumin, and mace. Curried food is often accompanied by chutney, a spicy condiment that combines fruit, vinegar, sugar, and spices.

The traditional Indian diet includes an abundance of grains, beans, and vegetables. Meat and fish are served not as entrées but as ingredients in entrées.

By all accounts, Indian cuisine has the makings of a healthful diet. But it's not without its nutritional danger zones. Use the following strategies to get through the menu maze.

Try tandoori. Tandoori is a cooking method in which foods are baked in a brick-and-clay oven (called a tandoor). Indian chefs often prepare fish and chicken in this way. When you choose a tandoori dish, you can be confident that you're getting something healthy.

Love those loaves. Don't miss the opportunity to try one of the astounding array of Indian breads. Just make sure that it has been baked rather than fried. Among the names to look for are chapati, kulcha, and naan.

Give up ghee. Many Indian dishes are soaked in ghee, which is clarified butter. When used in the preparation of a food, it can raise the fat content to 50 percent of calories.

Coconut oil, another staple, also has a mean streak. It contains mostly saturated fat—the unhealthy kind.

So ask your server how the dish you'd like to order is prepared. If he mentions either of these ingredients, request that the chef use a lighter cooking oil.

Help Yourself to...

- Any dish marinated in yogurt
- Dal (a spicy dish made with lentils)
- Karhi (chickpea soup)
- Khur (a dessert made with milk and rice)
- Mulligatawny (a kind of lentil soup)

Hands Off...

- Any dish referred to as kandhari, korma, or malai (indicating that coconut or cream is an ingredient)
- Fried breads such as paratha and poori
- Pakora (deep-fried breads and vegetables)
- Samosa (a fried pastry sometimes stuffed with vegetables or meat)

Cajun: Nice and Spicy

Red-hot spices are the cornerstone of this style of cooking, which got its start on the Louisiana coast. Chefs describe it as a hybrid of French and Creole cuisines.

You'll find a lot of seafood on Cajun restaurant menus. It often shows up as an ingredient in a classic Cajun specialty, jambalaya.

But Cajun cooking has other traditions that aren't quite so healthy. As you peruse the menu, keep the following in mind.

Find out about fat. With its generous use of seafood, vegetables, and rice, Cajun cooking seems like the nutrition-conscious person's dream. But dig a little deeper, and you'll discover that it uses lots of animal fat, especially pork fat. This is why it's so important to ask your server how a dish is prepared before ordering.

Help Yourself to...

- Blackened fish or chicken (heavily seasoned and cooked quickly with little oil)
- Greens, such as kale and okra
- Jambalaya, made without high-fat ingredients such as pork and sausage
- Seafood gumbo
- Shrimp Creole

Hands Off...

- Andouille, boudin, and other sausage dishes
- Dirty rice (fried rice mixed with fatty meats)

- Etouffée, a crawfish-and-vegetable stew with a roux base (roux is a combination of flour and fat)
- Hush puppies (deep-fried dumplings)
- Mud pie

Caribbean: Paradise for the Palate

Envision yourself on a tropical island. Then look around. By the roadside, the trees burst with bananas, papayas, avocados, mangoes, oranges, and pineapples—all staples of the Caribbean. And chili bushes stand laden with their pungent fruit—the secret to the special spiciness of many of the islands' best-loved dishes.

In many ways, Caribbean cooking defies categorization. It boasts an array of ethnic influences because people from all over the world—France, Spain, England, Africa, China, India, and Portugal—settled on the islands and brought their native cuisines with them. "Then as people moved around the islands and cultures intermingled, new dishes emerged," explains Donna Morton de Souza, R.D., a nutritionist in Miami and former corporate dietitian for Royal Caribbean International.

Still, de Souza says, there is common ground in Caribbean cooking. Exotic fruits and chili peppers are staple ingredients, as are nutmeg, ginger, and curry spices. You'll notice some bean dishes on menus, too—in fact, black bean soup is considered an island specialty.

Because Caribbean cuisine has such a diverse heritage, you may find that restaurants differ in the dishes they serve. But these general guidelines can help you know what to look for.

Try something new. Take advantage of the opportunity to sample some of the Caribbean's exotic native produce. Look for dishes prepared with callaloo, a leafy green that's similar to kale; chayote, a fruit that looks something like an overgrown pear; or breadfruit, a versatile fruit distinguished by its bumpy green skin.

Be careful with coconut. Many Caribbean recipes call for either the meat or the milk of the coconut, or (like Indian or Thai cuisine) they're cooked in coconut oil, de Souza says. But like any other nut, coconut has an abundance of fat—most of it the heart-unhealthy saturated kind. Try to steer clear of dishes that have any form of coconut as an ingredient. If you aren't sure, ask.

Forget fried fare. Frying seems to be the cooking method of choice for many Caribbean dishes. "Take fritters, which are a popular appetizer," de Souza says. "They're made with healthy ingredients, like chickpeas or fish, but then they're deep-fried." Other common deep-fried specialties include codfish cakes, plantain chips, and shrimp with anchovy stuffing.

Pare the portion. "A restaurant may serve a meal a little differently, but when I ate on the islands, I remember getting a heaping plate of food," de Souza says. "It had a little bit of everything." Since most restaurants are given to oversize portions to begin with, you may want to consider sharing a meal with your dining companion—or if not, just take home the extra.

Help Yourself to...

- Black bean soup
- Broiled or grilled seafood
- Jerk chicken ("jerk" refers to a seasoning blend usually made from chili peppers, garlic, onions, thyme, and spices)

Hands Off...

- Anything fried
- Anything made with coconut, coconut milk, or coconut oil
- Baked papaya with meat filling
- Blood sausage
- Pepper pot

Mexican: Better Run for the Border

Authentic Mexican cuisine bears little resemblance, nutrition-wise, to the Americanized stuff served in most restaurants. The Mexican people tend to follow a healthy high-carbohydrate, low-fat diet with lots of grains and beans and moderate amounts of meat. They use generous amounts of spices to flavor their foods and seldom cook in oil.

When the cuisine migrated across the border, something definitely got lost in the translation of the recipes. Our version of Mexican features gobs of high-fat cheese and sour cream, which you'd be hard-pressed to find south of the border. Everything, it seems, gets soaked in oil and deep-fried. And shredded iceberg lettuce doesn't really count as a nutritious vegetable.

In fact, when the *Nutrition Action Healthletter* analyzed 15 popular dishes at 19 midpriced Mexican restaurants, only one—chicken fajitas—got less than 30 percent of calories from fat. Most of the meals, which came with accompaniments such as refried beans and guacamole, provided an entire day's allotment of fat in one sitting.

Thankfully, some Mexican restaurants have begun overhauling their menus to offer healthier, more authentic selections. For instance, two of the country's largest Mexican restaurant chains—Chi-Chi's and El Torito—have trimmed the fat from some of their old recipes and developed new, leaner entrées for their health-conscious patrons.

If you can, order à la carte rather than a full dinner. That way, you can bypass all the high-fat, high-calorie trimmings that come on the plate. Here are some more strategies for keeping your Mexican meal nutritious and delicious.

Veg out. Traditional Mexican cooking features an array of exotic, flavorful produce. Look for dishes that contain nopales (cactus leaves), which taste like slightly tart green beans; jícama, a turniplike root vegetable with a nutty flavor; and tomatillos, which look like small green tomatoes but taste like a combination of lemons, apples, and herbs.

Say "si" to salsa. According to the people who keep track of such things, Americans now spend more money on salsa than on ketchup. This condiment—a mix of tomatoes, onions, chilies, and herbs—has practically no fat and supplies generous doses of vitamins A and C to boot. Use it instead of sour cream, cheese, and guacamole to give your meal a burst of flavor.

Skimp on chips. Just 50 chips in that complimentary basket of tortilla chips that the server just set under your nose contain more than three-quarters of your fat allotment for the entire day. If you're not careful, they'll disappear before you even crack open the menu.

To limit your chip consumption, decide up front how many you want to eat. Then take that number out of the basket and move the rest out of reach. Even better, have the server return the basket to the kitchen.

Reject refried beans. Unlike many of the canned refried beans you buy in the supermarket, the restaurant version is usually prepared in lard—sometimes with bacon and cheese added to the mix. A ¾-cup serving supplies a whopping one-third of your daily allotment of saturated fat.

Come out of your shell. If you order a taco salad, resist the temptation to nibble on the tortilla shell that it's served in. And watch out for high-fat toppings, too—black olives, cheese, sour cream, guacamole, and the like.

Help Yourself to...

- Bean enchiladas
- Black bean soup and gazpacho soup
- Chicken soft tacos

- Fajitas
- Seafood prepared Veracruz-style (cooked in an herbed tomato sauce)
- Seviche (fish marinated in lime juice)

Hands Off...

- Chilies rellenos (deep-fried, cheese-stuffed chilies)
- Chimichanga
- Chorizo (a spicy pork sausage)
- Flautas (corn tortillas rolled around a meat or poultry filling, then deep-fried)
- Quesadillas
- Taquitos (fried)

American Steakhouses: Here's the Beef

In no way does the proliferation of ethnic restaurants suggest that typical American food is on the endangered species list for the food chain. Rather, American food has become yet another ethnic cuisine from which to choose. And nothing captures the essence of the typical American diet like the steakhouse does. Everything comes in one size: big. Make that really big. If that slab of red meat isn't the same circumference as your plate, why, it has no right to be calling itself a steak.

"Steakhouses are known for huge, huge servings," agrees Liz Applegate, Ph.D., a nutrition lecturer at the University of California, Davis, and author of *Power Foods*. When you eat a typical steak, you're getting two or three times—if not four or five times—as much protein as you should be getting.

But red meat does have its virtues. Steak, in particular, is a great source of zinc and a good source of iron and other trace minerals that women tend to run low on. "So it's an item that can be had in the diet," Dr. Applegate says. "The motto here is moderation."

The following tips can help you round up a healthy steakhouse feast.

Skimp on size. If you want steak, order the smallest one on the menu, suggests Evelyn Tribole, R.D., author of *Healthy Homestyle Cooking* and *Eating on the Run*. "Believe me, that is still bigger than you might think." According to the *Prevention* Food Pyramid for Women, you don't need more than three ounces of meat a day. A serving of meat the size of a deck of cards is about three ounces. In other words, if you order a six-ounce filet mignon, that counts as your meat quota for two days, not one.

Mull over the menu. You don't have to order steak just because you're at a steakhouse. The restaurant may offer other entrées, such as shish kebabs or stir-fries, that use meat as an ingredient rather than as the centerpiece of the meal.

Leave the fat behind. If you do order a steak, be sure to trim off all the visible fat before you dig in. This reduces the fat content of your meal a little more.

Choose bird over beef. You might also discover a poultry dish or two on the menu. Poultry, of course, generally has less fat than red meat, and even within the poultry section of the menu, you may find that some entrées are healthier than others. Chicken breast, for example, has less saturated fat and cholesterol than chicken legs or wings—especially Buffalo wings. You can spare yourself even more fat grams by removing the skin.

Help Yourself to...

- Sirloin cuts
- Tenderloin cuts, such as filet mignon

Hands Off...

- Anything with "rib" in the name, such as prime rib, rib-eye, and spareribs

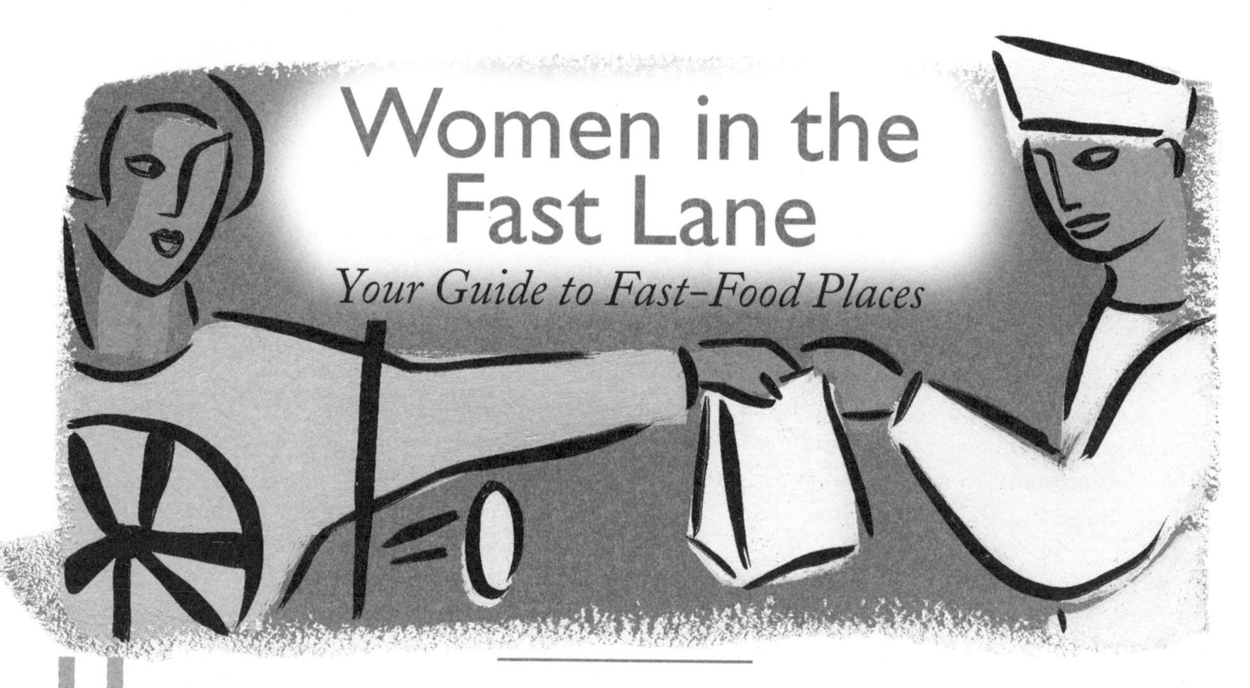

Until about 50 years ago, "fast food" pretty much referred to anything that could outrun a hungry hunter. Then two brothers by the name of McDonald got an idea: Why not run hamburger stands on the same principles of mass production that work so well for manufacturers?

To say their idea caught on is an understatement. Indeed, fast food has become a staple in the typical American diet. At least one survey has shown that 44 percent of women eat in fast-food restaurants at least once a week. We're making a substantial contribution to the estimated $100 billion the fast-food industry rakes in each year.

Why the love affair with no-frills fare? Convenience is a big factor. And of course, the food does come cheap. The trouble is that you may pay for it in terms of your good health. Many menu mainstays have questionable nutritional profiles, supplying way too much of some nutrients and way too little of others. For instance, most fast-food items get between 40 and 50 percent of their calories from fat. And we all know what kind of damage excessive dietary fat can do to our hearts and our waistlines.

Now none of this means that fast food has no place in a healthy diet. The trick is to make it an occasional treat—and to choose your meal wisely.

Menu Moxie

Contemplating a meal at Bubba's Burger Barn? You can pick up something reasonably healthful—if you know what to look for on the menu. Here's what the experts recommend.

Look at the big picture. As you decide what to order, consider what you've eaten earlier in the day and what you plan to eat later on. Try to strike a nutritional balance with your food choices. And don't forget to round out your meal with add-ons that are a little more nutrient-dense—like a side salad, a piece of fruit, or a carton of skim or low-fat (1 percent) milk.

Select the right size. Sure, those oversize sandwiches, fries, and drinks can save you a few cents. But boy, oh boy, can they tax you nutrition-wise. "Stay away from anything called jumbo, giant, supersize, or colossal," says Jayne Hurley, R.D., senior nutritionist with the Center for Science in the Public Interest, a nonprofit consumer group in Washington, D.C., and a writer for *Nutrition Action Healthletter*. "That's generally a dead give-away that a food is loaded with calories and fat."

Forget the fried stuff. Stick with sandwiches that are grilled, broiled, or roasted. And while you're at it, tell the person behind the counter to hold the cheese, mayonnaise, "special sauce," and other high-fat goop.

Build a better burger. When you have a hankering for some ground round, select the smallest hamburger on the menu, Hurley suggests. Then dress it up with lettuce, tomatoes, and dollops of ketchup and mustard. Again, try to skip the special sauce—but if you can't bear to taste your burger without it, at least get it on the side, so you have more control over how much you consume, she says.

Make spuds your buds. "People think of french fries as a side dish, but they're really not," Hurley says. "Eating fries is like eating a whole other sandwich." A large order of fries supplies as many calories and as much fat as a McDonald's Quarter Pounder.

Instead, choose a baked potato. It has no fat, no cholesterol, just a smidgen of sodium, and healthy doses of fiber, vitamin C, and other nutrients to boot. For toppings, try broccoli, salsa, or cottage cheese rather than the usual butter or sour cream.

Sip smart. Wash down your meal with juice or skim or low-fat milk. Both supply valuable vitamins and minerals, and their flavors nicely complement just about any food. Soda can be okay, too. Just remember that in terms of nutrition, it doesn't hold a candle to juice or milk.

REAL-LIFE SCENARIO

She Eats on the Run—All the Time

Selene loves to eat but hates to cook, so mealtime usually means eating out or getting takeout. The one exception is breakfast—she has a bowl of whole-grain cereal every day. Lunch is usually pizza or a fast-food burger or chicken sandwich. Selene is as devoted to the gym as she is to staying out of the kitchen, so weight is not her problem. She knows she's getting plenty of vitamins—look at all the foods she's eating! But she wonders: Is her casual attitude toward her diet doing her any harm?

No one is saying that you can't eat a well-balanced diet if you eat out all the time. Most likely, however, Selene's diet falls short of meeting her nutritional requirements, particularly in the grain, dairy, and fruit and vegetable departments.

What Selene's diet seems to offer is plenty of fat. While it may not seem important since she doesn't have a weight problem, she's getting lots of calories with too few nutrients, like vitamins, minerals, complex carbohydrates, and fiber.

One way for Selene to easily correct this is to sneak a few healthy snacks into her day. For example, a cup of yogurt for calcium and an apple for fiber can provide some of the nutrients fast food lacks. In addition, Selene could jazz up her fast-food meals by adding a few vitamin-packed vegetable toppings the next time she calls to order pizza.

If she watches her fat intake, includes healthy snacks in between meals, and adds more fiber-rich grains and fruits and vegetables to her typical take-out menu, Selene *can* eat a well-balanced diet without learning to cook. But she has to make a conscious decision to do it right.

Expert Consulted
Marsha Hudnall, R.D.
Director of nutrition programs
Green Mountain at Fox Run
Ludlow, Vermont

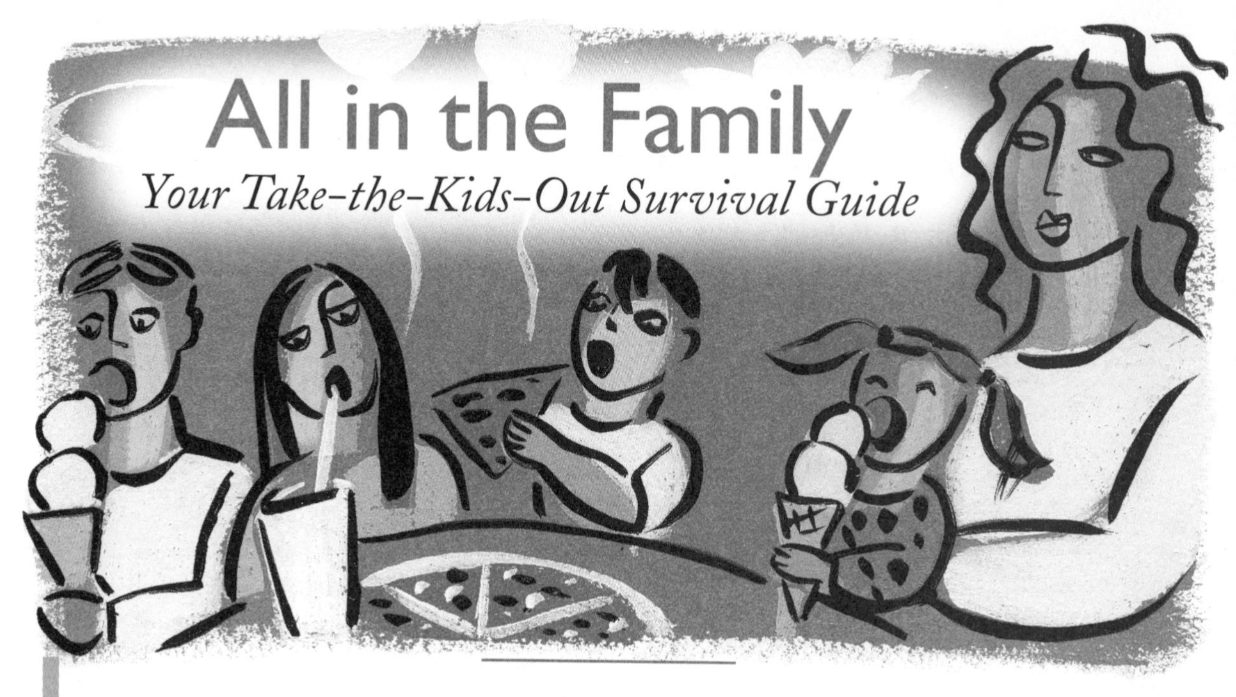

All in the Family

Your Take-the-Kids-Out Survival Guide

It's Friday night at your family's favorite burger palace, and you've just eaten an entire weekend's fat intake in one hour—the proof still shines on your hands.

You leave the restaurant feeling bloated, blaming the kids for insisting on coming here, the waitress for taking so long to clear your plate, and the restaurant for blatantly exposing you to the triple-decker cheeseburger photo in the first place.

How can any woman defend herself against the onslaught of complimentary chips, monster burgers, and mocha mud pies when she takes the kids to the local family restaurant?

Starting It Off Right

You haven't finished scooting into the booth and already you're greeted by a basket of free chips and a list of must-try appetizers. Life is swell. Well, maybe—but you may just blow your fat and calorie budgets before the main course arrives. Here's how to keep seemingly harmless starters from undermining your efforts.

Simplify your drinks. Suddenly you're 10 again, and you just have to have that fruity non-alcoholic umbrella drink. Better not, says Jane Ziegler, R.D., program coordinator for the Allen Center for Nutrition at Cedar Crest College in Allentown, Pennsylvania. "Specialty drinks have lots of sugar, and they may have some cream, whole milk, or ice cream to make them creamy." Let the kids get them and have one sip. Spend your calories elsewhere.

Skip the appetizers. "Appetizers to me are a real danger zone. The meal is usually more than most people can handle anyway, plus appetizers are often high-fat foods," says Ziegler. How high-fat? Well, according to a study by the Center for Science in the Public Interest, which looked at dinner houses across the country, it'll cost you 48 grams of fat for an average order of 12 Buffalo wings, 51 grams of fat for nine fried mozzarella sticks, and a whopping 79 grams of fat for an eight-piece order of potato skins—and that's not including the sour cream.

Start your salad sooner. The kids won, so now you're staring down potato skins. You may have even heard one call your name. Solution? "Ask that your salad be served immediately," suggests Ziegler. "And try to get to the restaurant at a time when the wait for your entrée won't be long."

Can This Spud Be Saved?

Pity the poor potato.

You see, it has—how shall we put this?—a bit of a weight problem. In a matter of seconds, a lean potato can increase its fat content 20-fold. That's like you ballooning to more than a ton by the time you finish reading this sentence. Scary, huh?

It happens to the potato all the time. But it didn't always have this problem, you know. Growing up, it did its best to stay healthy. And by the time it reached adulthood, it had some very impressive vital statistics: just 145 calories and 0.2 gram of fat.

So what went wrong?

Well, for one thing, it started hanging out in bars—potato bars, that is. It developed a fondness for fatty toppings like sour cream and chives or cheese sauce and bacon. Its calorie count tripled instantaneously, and its fat content skyrocketed to more than 20 grams.

Even worse, it discovered the deep fryer. Now to us humans, floating around in a vat of boiling fat doesn't seem like an especially good time. To a potato, it's nirvana. But there's a price to be paid for this little indulgence: The potato, when french-fried, gets almost half of its calories from fat.

And when the potato gets transformed into potato skins, it loses its last shred of nutritional dignity. The once-svelte spud now supplies a whopping 60 percent of its calories as fat.

Of course, you can save the potato from its fat-laden fate. Help it to stay trim and healthy by ordering it baked and plain. Add salsa for fat-free flavor, if you wish.

Your potato will thank you.

Sidestepping Entrée Traps

You know the rule, but you still spend the first half-hour rehearsing it in your head: "Fried—bad; grilled—good." There, that seems easy enough. But as you peruse the menu, the clarity fades. You recognize some "watch-out" words—smothered, covered, loaded, sautéed, rich, creamy, and thick—and a few "good choice" keywords—poached, broiled, roasted, and steamed. Still, there's a lot on the menu to consider.

Familiarize yourself with these common dinner-house traps before the waiter with the two-tone hair sells you on the quesadilla.

Plan ahead. Don't jump headfirst into that New York strip steak. "Find out beforehand what the portion size is, then decide what you're going to eat," says Jody Mortenson, executive director of research and development for Friday's Hospitality Worldwide. "That steak could be 12 to 14 ounces. I know I only need 3 ounces of protein, so I'd ask for an extra plate and share."

Make your own fixings. Your fajita is still sizzling and now you, too, are starting to sweat, faced with enough guacamole, sour cream, and cheese to binge on for a week. Don't let the temptation even get to your table, says Mortenson. "I ask for mine without 'all the good stuff,' which happens to be the expensive stuff, so restaurants are happy to comply. A good substitution in my opinion is pico de gallo, which is tomatoes, onions, cilantro, and jalapeño peppers. Lettuce is also good for that extra crunch and flavor."

Know thy order. Everyone has ordered but

you—and they're all staring. Flustered, you quickly point to the Vegetarian Bandito and turn in your menu. You feel great about your choice; that is, until it arrives, hidden under gobs of cheese.

That's not uncommon, warns Ziegler. "And many vegetarian entrées are made with cream cheese—not nonfat or low-fat cream cheese, but regular—to give them a little more zip." To keep it low-fat, hold the cheese or order a soy entrée, if they have one, like a soy-based meat alternative, she suggests. "Those are typically lower in fat, if they're not adding a special sauce or extra cheese."

Question all that glitters. You can't help but notice how beautiful that grilled chicken breast is—after all, it *is* glistening from that booth across the room. A lot of chains brush butter on otherwise healthy, grilled items, says Mortenson. "It gives the perception to the guest that it's a juicy, moist, flavorful piece of meat," she adds. Just remind your waitress that you're ordering that low-fat entrée for a reason and have them hold the butter.

WHO'S POLICING THE MENU?

You've just finished bragging to your waitress about how great you're going to look in your new swimsuit when suddenly the kitchen door swings open and you get a glimpse of Richie, the tattooed chef, dousing your grilled chicken with butter. So much for "guiltless."

But that's not fair, you say—the grilled chicken in question had a cute little "heart smart" icon next to it on the menu. Can't someone stop Richie?

Yes. The FDA.

As of May 1997, all health-related menu claims became subject to "truth in menu" rules established by the Food and Drug Administration. The menu policing started in an attempt to help consumers get accurate health and nutritional information, says Judy Peters, director of customer relations for Heart Smart Restaurants International, a Scottsdale, Arizona, company that analyzes recipes for restaurants across the country.

The kickoff to the FDA restaurant guidelines came from lawsuits brought by consumer advocacy groups that proved some menus' health claims weren't justifiable. "With these regulations, restaurants that put a heart next to an item and say it's good for you now have to back that up and show that indeed the fat content is really what they say it is," explains Peters.

Shut off autopilot. You yell at the kids when they do it to your home-cooked meals, so be sure that you don't automatically add butter either. "Taste your food first to see what it needs," says Mortenson. "We try to season our food for the masses, and it probably doesn't need any more."

Take your time. Okay, so you feel as if you're in a race: Tommy's finsished licking his plate and big Tom has just unbuckled. Don't let that rush you. "Eat slowly so your body and brain can connect and you know when you're full," says Ziegler.

Drop the fork. You don't have to clean your plate. That's one of your many "mom" perks. Have it boxed. "The sooner you do that, the less likely you are to pick at it when you're not really hungry," says Ziegler.

"The best exercise you can get is pushing away from the table. And if you do choose to take it home, perishable food should not be kept at room temperature for longer than three hours," says Carolyn Raab, R.D., Ph.D., food and nutrition specialist for the Oregon State University Extension Service in Corvallis, who specializes in food safety.

So what's considered a health or nutrient claim?

- "Low"—low sodium (140 milligrams or less per serving), low-calorie (40 calories or less per serving), low-fat (three grams or less per serving), low-cholesterol (20 milligrams or less and two grams or less of saturated fat per serving)
- "High"—an item "high" in a nutrient, as in "high fiber," must contain at least 20 percent of the Daily Value for that nutrient
- "Free"—calorie-free, sugar-free, sodium-free, fat-free
- "Light"—means the item has one-third fewer calories or 50 percent less fat than a similar food (this doesn't apply to terms such as *lightly breaded* or *light cream sauce*)
- Symbols—a heart symbol or skinny typeface indicates that specific health claims are associated with that dish, and the claims should be explained in the menu

Although restaurants were given nine months' notice to comply, Peters warns that change may be slow. "Many of the smaller, single-unit restaurants still have no idea. They just put a heart next to an item and think that's okay."

To be sure that you're getting what you're promised, ask for the proof. Restaurants don't have to include the number of fat grams or calories on their menus, but to make the claim, they must have the nutritional analysis readily available upon request, says Peters.

Ending It Sweetly

Just when you thought the potential for damage was over, the kids start banging their fists on the table and chanting "dessert." Unless you're in the mood to disappear into the bathroom and pick food out of your teeth for 20 minutes, you'll be faced with temptation. Here are some tips for taming your sweet tooth.

Distract yourself. You're stuck at the table for another half-hour while the kids make three trips up to the sundae bar. Enjoy a cup of coffee or some hot spiced tea. "For me, it's a closure to the meal, and it gives me something to do with my hands while someone else is eating," says Dr. Raab. But be careful what you add. After-dinner drinks made with cream or liquor can have as many calories as a slice of cheesecake.

Go fruity. See if maybe that hankering for something sweet can be satisfied by some fruit. "Sometimes there's a fruit dessert like strawberries with cream—just have them hold the cream," suggests Ziegler. "Or get a fruit ice or sorbet, which are usually a small serving size."

Sherbet may be a better choice than the ice cream offered in most restaurants, which is usually top-of-the-line and has more calories and fat, says Dr. Raab. Low-fat frozen yogurt is also a good option, but again, the calorie amounts aren't that different, she adds.

Indulge a little. Truth be told, you won't balloon up if you have just a few bites. If some chocolate will send you out the door a happier person, treat yourself and split a dessert with the family. "That way, you get just enough to be satisfied," says Dr. Raab.

"There's room for all foods in your diet. Moderation is the key," adds Ziegler.

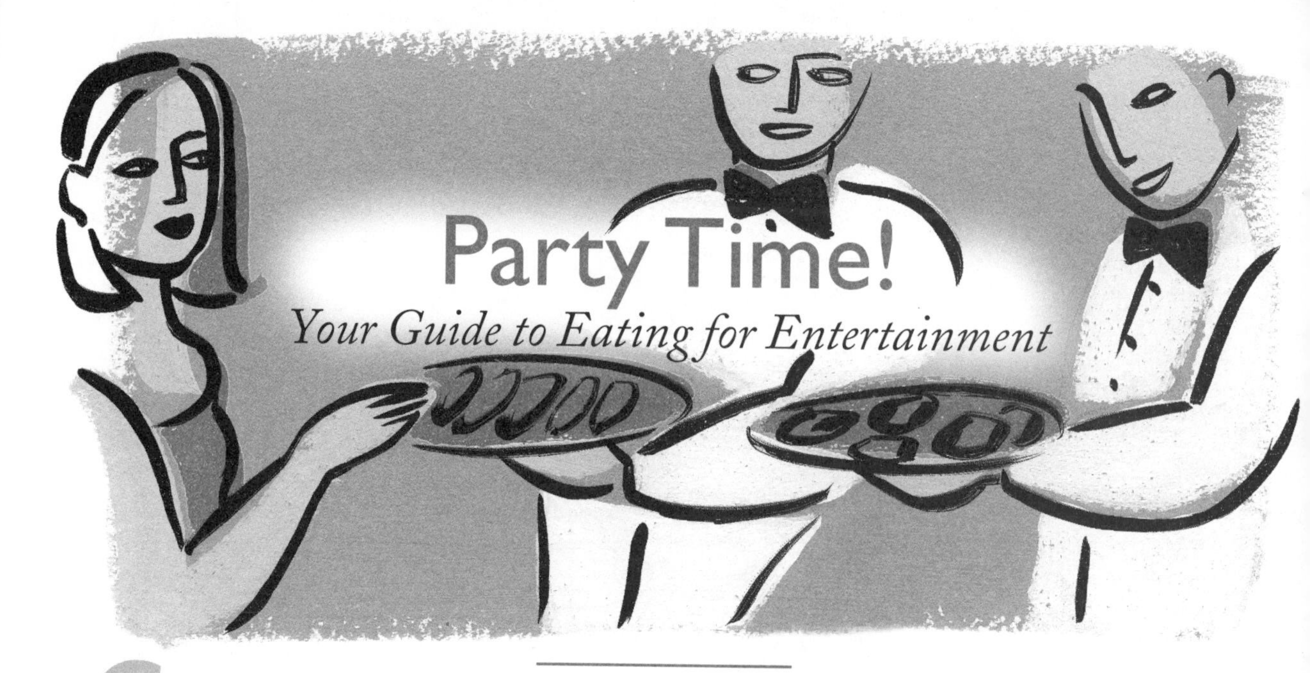

Party Time!

Your Guide to Eating for Entertainment

Call it the Golden Rule of Good Times: Where there's fun, there's food. After all, can you imagine a birthday without cake? The Fourth of July without burgers and hot dogs? The movies without popcorn?

Of course, the Golden Rule of Good Times has led to the Axiom for Amplified Appetites: When you're socializing and you're surrounded by food, you're more inclined to eat too much. So should you throw out your social calendar and turn down all invitations to special events for fear that you might overindulge?

No. Nothing's wrong with treating yourself once in a while. Let's face it: We like eating. We derive pleasure from it. And that's okay, as long as we indulge without *over*indulging.

It is possible to enjoy a holiday dinner, a tailgate party, or a night out on the town without guilt. Just remember the Law of Smart Partying: Eat, drink...and be wary.

Healthy Holidays

From Thanksgiving to New Year's, the five-week winter holiday season can seem like one long, continuous feast. In fact, 69 percent of the people participating in a joint CNN/*Prevention* magazine survey revealed that they pretty much eat whatever they want during the holidays. And 40 percent said that they expect to gain weight as a result of their dietary lassitude.

For the average person, that means packing on five to seven pounds, according to Jo Ann Carson, R.D., program director of clinical dietetics at the School of Allied Health Sciences at the University of Texas Southwestern Medical Center at Dallas. If that seems like a lot for such a short amount of time, think of it this way: To gain five pounds, you have to consume 17,500 extra calories over the 35 days between Thanksgiving and New Year's. That's 500 extra calories a day—a cinch for most of us.

It's not just that food is an ever-present temptation at this time of year. It's also that the holidays are emotionally charged times, especially for women. Even if our emotions don't get the best of us, "we're socializing with our relatives and friends and paying less attention to what we're eating," says Barbara Whedon, R.D., a dietitian and nutrition counselor at Thomas Jefferson University Hospital in Philadelphia. "And there's constant pressure to eat—we don't want to offend the host by not trying her best recipe."

Considering the circumstances, you'd need all the willpower in the world to not give in to the urge to nosh. Relax—and cut yourself some slack. You can get through any holiday with your healthy eating habits intact if you keep these tips in mind, say experts.

Fill up beforehand. Your mom has her usual spread planned for Thanksgiving dinner. So you decide to make room for the impending feast by skipping breakfast—and maybe even lunch. Bad idea. All you're doing is making yourself ravenous. By the time you sit down, you could eat the entire turkey yourself—and maybe even the platter it's sitting on.

A much better option is to eat something before the big event, Whedon says. A carbohydrate-rich snack—a piece of fruit, a slice of bread, even a small plate of pasta—can quiet hunger pangs especially well. With your stomach no longer calling the shots, you can make healthier food choices.

Hit the (water) bottle. Another extremely effective appetite suppressant is good ol' H_2O. In fact, what you perceive as hunger may be thirst in disguise. Experts advise drinking at least eight eight-ounce glasses of water a day. But you may want to slurp down a few more when a big meal is in your future.

Gravitate toward veggies. Holiday meals usually feature a cornucopia of vegetable side dishes. Give these foods star billing on your plate. They'll fill you up, so you won't have a hankering for fattier fare. Just make sure that the ones you choose aren't swimming in butter or dripping with cheese sauce.

Occupy your plate. Leave a little something on your plate at all times. It serves as a tacit signal to your host that you're so full you can't even finish what you have on your plate. That way, she won't try to foist more food on you—and you won't feel guilty for saying no. Just make sure that your decoy dish is something you don't particularly care for, so you don't keep nibbling away at it.

Excuse yourself. When you're finished eating, get up from the table. "Sitting in close proximity to food is much too tempting. It's your cue to eat," explains Susan Olson, Ph.D., a clinical psychologist and weight-management consultant in Seattle and author of *Keeping It Off: Winning at Weight Loss*. Put some distance between yourself and all those goodies. And when you do, occupy yourself with something you enjoy, so you don't wander back to the table out of sheer boredom.

A Party Primer

Mention "party," and what comes to mind? Food and booze. Usually, there's an abundance of both. When everyone around you is mingling bites of cocktail weenies, chicken nuggets, and chips 'n' dip with sips of their favorite alcoholic beverages, it's mighty hard not to join in on the feeding frenzy.

Too often, eating and drinking become the focal point of a party. This is especially true when you don't know many people. You may hover around the buffet or the bar because you feel more comfortable there.

Remember, parties are for socializing and schmoozing. Try to eat less and talk more. And stick with these foolproof strategies suggested by experts to navigate those sumptuous spreads.

Practice preemptive nibbling. "Never go to a party on an empty stomach," says Agnes Kolor, R.D., a Pearl River, New York, nutritionist who consulted for *The Oprah Winfrey Show*. Snack on a banana or pretzels beforehand. That way, you won't feel like making a beeline for the buffet as soon as you arrive.

Make sure the pretzels are salt-free, though. The salty kind just makes you thirsty.

Make a contribution. Give your host a hand by offering to bring a dish. Then choose something that supports your healthy eating habits—maybe salsa and nonfat tortilla chips or a vegetable plate with yogurt dip. That way, you know you have something healthful to nibble on.

Take it all in. When you do hit the buffet, don't just start spooning food onto your plate with abandon. First examine the entire spread, from one end to the other. Look for anything healthful, like cut-up fruits and vegetables, steamed shrimp, and sliced chicken breast. You might even wander into the kitchen to see whether more wholesome selections have been prepared but just haven't made it to the buffet table yet.

Favor fiber. Choosing fiber-rich foods from the buffet has a couple of advantages. For starters, these foods fill you up, so you won't feel like going back for fattier fare. Also, they take a long time to chew. You'll eat more slowly, which gives you better portion control. Besides, experts recommend that you consume 20 to 30 grams of fiber a day, and this is an ideal way to ensure that you meet your quota.

Fruits and veggies like apples, pears, oranges, and carrots have lots of fiber, as do air-popped popcorn and beans of any kind.

Feel the heat. Fiery spices act as appetite suppressants, so you won't eat as much. And as a bonus, they speed up your metabolism, allowing you to burn up the calories from your food a little faster. Look on the buffet for condiments such as hot mustard, cocktail sauce, salsa, and horseradish. Or top a burger with jalapeño peppers.

Seek out special dishes. Bypass those mixed nuts—you can eat those anytime. Instead, sample foods that you get only once in a blue moon. Maybe your host makes out-of-this-world chocolate chip cookies or a guacamole dip that's to die for. Go ahead and give it a try. Just keep a rein on your portion.

Keep your distance. Once you've made your food choices, do your socializing away from the buffet table, advises Edith Howard Hogan, R.D., a dietitian in Washington, D.C., and a spokesperson for the American Dietetic Association. "Fill your plate once, taking small por-

SMART STRATEGIES FOR SOCIAL BUTTERFLIES

For some women, wining and dining is a job requirement. In any given week, they attend not one but several receptions, dinner parties, and other food-focused events. How do they navigate the gustatory gauntlet and come out with their healthful eating habits intact? Here are some of their strategies.

"Depending on the type of event, I usually eat something small but filling about an hour beforehand. I also drink a large glass of water to curb hunger. That way, I can make better, non-hunger-driven food choices.

"At a party, I allow myself two 'bad' foods—maybe a brownie and a high-fat hors d'oeuvre—so I don't feel like they're off-limits. At a dinner, I won't deny myself any course. Instead, I find something healthy offered for each course. If the only desserts available are all rich, I'll take two bites and leave the rest."

Laura Noss
Account supervisor for Hill and Knowlton Public Relations Worldwide in Washington, D.C.

"Veggies keep my eating habits in line. When predinner hors d'oeuvres are served, I stick with veggies and avoid anything fried. Then during dinner, I eat all of my salad and leave at least half of the main course uneaten. And I always ask for salad dressing on the side.

"I love dessert, so I usually order sorbet—it has no fat. As for alcoholic beverages, I prefer red wine and wine spritzers (chardonnay with seltzer water) over cocktails. Even then, I limit my intake, and I make sure to drink at least twice as much water as alcohol."

Juliane M. Snowden
Account executive for the Equity Group in New York City

"To avoid being tempted by the high-fat hors d'oeuvres at parties, I eat a big low-fat salad beforehand. And I make a point not to stand next to the buffet table. If there's dancing or some other physical activity going on, I participate with gusto.

"If drinks are served, I order sweet vermouth with soda and a wedge of lemon. It's a sophisticated, refreshing beverage. When I can, I mix my own drink. That way I can control the amount of alcohol. If there's a bartender, I ask him to go easy on the vermouth."

Amy Watson
Principal of PROfusion Public Relations in Laguna Beach, California

tions. Then walk away. Otherwise, it's too easy to keep nibbling."

"I tell people to never stand right beside the buffet table," agrees Kolor. "When you do, you're constantly eating. Your hand automatically reaches down—it's an unconscious motion. You have more control if you put your food on your plate and then move on."

Stash your plate. Once you've cleaned off your plate, put it aside for the cleanup crew. (Or, if it's disposable, throw it in the trash.) If you stand around holding it, it just becomes a magnet for more food.

Keep your hands full. You may feel more comfortable having something in your hand when you mingle—kind of like a security blanket. If that's the case, make it a glass of mineral water, tomato juice, or diet soda. This strategy has an added advantage: If your host sees that you're holding a drink, she won't try to push liquor and other high-calorie beverages on you.

How to Navigate Bars

It's one of the three great ironies of the entertainment world: Only one of the Beach Boys surfed. The Monkees didn't play guitar on their records. And Sam Malone, bartender for *Cheers*, didn't drink.

In the real world, bellying up to the bar is tricky business, and not just because of the extra calories supplied by alcohol.

Suppose you decide to join your coworkers for happy hour at a nearby pub. You start out with a beer, which gives you the munchies. So you reach for those super-salty nuts or pretzels, which make you thirsty. So you order another beer. And around and around you go, filling up on calories that have nothing to offer you, nutrient-wise.

With a little preparation and a lot of common sense, you won't get caught up in this nutritional vortex. Here's what you need to know before you hoist that first glass.

Don't go empty. You've heard this before, but it bears repeating: If you go out on an empty stomach, you're bound to eat more. And what you're eating won't win any nutrition awards: Buffalo wings, potato skins, corn chips, cheese, and so on.

"If you're heading out right after work, plan to have a snack around four o'clock," says Liz Ap-

TIPS TO KEEP FROM GETTING TIPSY

The number one reason that people drink too much at parties is social awkwardness, according to Katherine P. Prescott, national president of Mothers Against Drunk Driving. You may feel uncomfortable because you don't know anyone—or because everyone else has a glass of something and you don't.

First off, know that you don't have to drink; it's perfectly acceptable to "opt out," so to speak. But if you choose to imbibe, the following strategies suggested by experts can help temper alcohol's intoxicating effects.

Eat first. You should never drink anything on an empty stomach. If you do, the alcohol moves into your bloodstream faster—which means you'll feel it sooner.

Linger over your liquor. Try to limit yourself to one drink per hour. Even better, order a tall glass of your favorite brew, then nurse it all night.

Have a water chaser. You can temper the negative effects of alcohol—not only intoxication but dehydration, too—by working in some water now and then. Between drinks, ask the bartender for mineral water with a twist or a club soda. This strategy can cut your alcohol and calorie consumption in half, according to Evelyn Tribole, R.D., author of *Eating on the Run.*

Dilute your drink. You can also minimize alcohol's effects by watering down your beverage. If you have a cocktail, for instance, get it "on the rocks" or ask the bartender to add more mixer or juice.

Forget the aspirin. A long-standing myth holds that taking aspirin before a night on the town can prevent you from becoming intoxicated or having a hangover the next day. The fact is that aspirin slows the rate at which alcohol passes through your body. Researchers theorize that the drug inhibits a certain stomach enzyme from breaking down alcohol, so it more readily enters into your bloodstream. And since the alcohol lingers in your system longer, you may actually feel its effects longer.

plegate, Ph.D., a nutrition lecturer at the University of California, Davis, and author of *Power Foods.* "Stop by the cafeteria and pick up an apple, a carton of yogurt—something low-fat. Don't set foot in a bar when you're starving."

Skip salty snacks. Pretzels, corn chips, nachos, and other salty selections only make you drink more than you intended. "Bars kind of play you, you know?" Kolor says. "You eat all of their salty foods, so you end up buying more of their drinks."

If you do get hungry, order something that doesn't have a lot of salt, such as cut-up vegetables.

Food and Flicks

A movie just isn't a movie unless you have something to munch on while you're watching it. It's almost as though buying a ticket to the world of film fiction automatically suspends nutrition reality, too.

When you think about it, though, you're usually only in the theater for about two hours. "You can go that long without food," says Sachiko St. Jeor, R.D., Ph.D., professor of clinical nutrition and director of the nutrition education and research program at the University of Nevada School of Medicine in Reno. "Get into watching the movie as a pure experience, without shoveling down food you can't see—or really enjoy."

If you must have food at your fingertips, remember these guidelines for making smart choices for cinema snacking.

Pick the right popcorn. Popcorn is the classic treat to munch on during a movie. But theaters prepare it in a number of different ways, some of which can wallop you with artery-clogging saturated fat or trans-fatty acids.

When one group of researchers analyzed popcorn from six cinema chains across the country, they found that an average large order of unbuttered kernels had two days' worth of heart-damaging fat. Add the mysterious butterlike flavoring, and you may as well eat nine McDonald's Quarter Pounders. No kidding.

Your best bet is the air-popped variety. Order it plain, and you can eat as much as you want. After all, you're getting loads of fiber.

If the theater you frequent makes its popcorn in oil, ask whether it's nonhydrogenated. It still carries a load of fat, but not the nasty trans-fatty acids.

Cotton to candy. Some confections are kinder to your heart—and to your waistline—than others. Choose those that have no or low fat, such as licorice, mints, caramels, hard candy, and jelly beans. Keep in mind, though, that you're still consuming calories—empty calories. These foods have virtually no nutritional value.

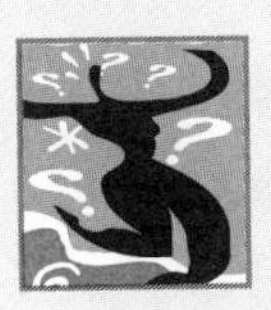

WOMEN ASK WHY

Why can't I seem to stop nibbling whenever I'm within range of a buffet table?

The reason you can't stop after one bite is because food acts as a kind of disinhibitor, meaning that once you take that first mouth-watering bite, it's your cue that taking the second and third bites is okay. It's kind of like opening up a conversation with a stranger at the party. Once the introductions are made, the rest comes easily.

A buffet table spread with hors d'oeuvres and other varieties of delectables is an invitation for indulgence. After all, when you're at a party, you're way too busy socializing and celebrating to notice if you've eaten 5 cheese balls or 25. Plus, when you're sampling a little bit of everything, it's tough to keep tabs on *what* you're eating, let alone how much you're eating. In any kind of social environment where there's food, chances are you're going to eat whether you're hungry or not.

As funny as it may sound, the best way to beat the buffet binge is to eat something healthy *before* you go to the party. That way, you won't have to hide from the buffet, because you won't feel hungry. And, if you do reach for something to eat, you're more likely to reach for something healthy because you're in control of your appetite.

On the other hand, if you show up hungry, you're going to end up nibbling all night. It's just as foolhardy as going food shopping on an empty stomach. So, to keep your eating to a minimum, nibble something healthy before the big bash.

Expert Consulted
Joanne Curran-Celentano, R.D., Ph.D.
Associate professor of nutritional sciences
University of New Hampshire
Durham

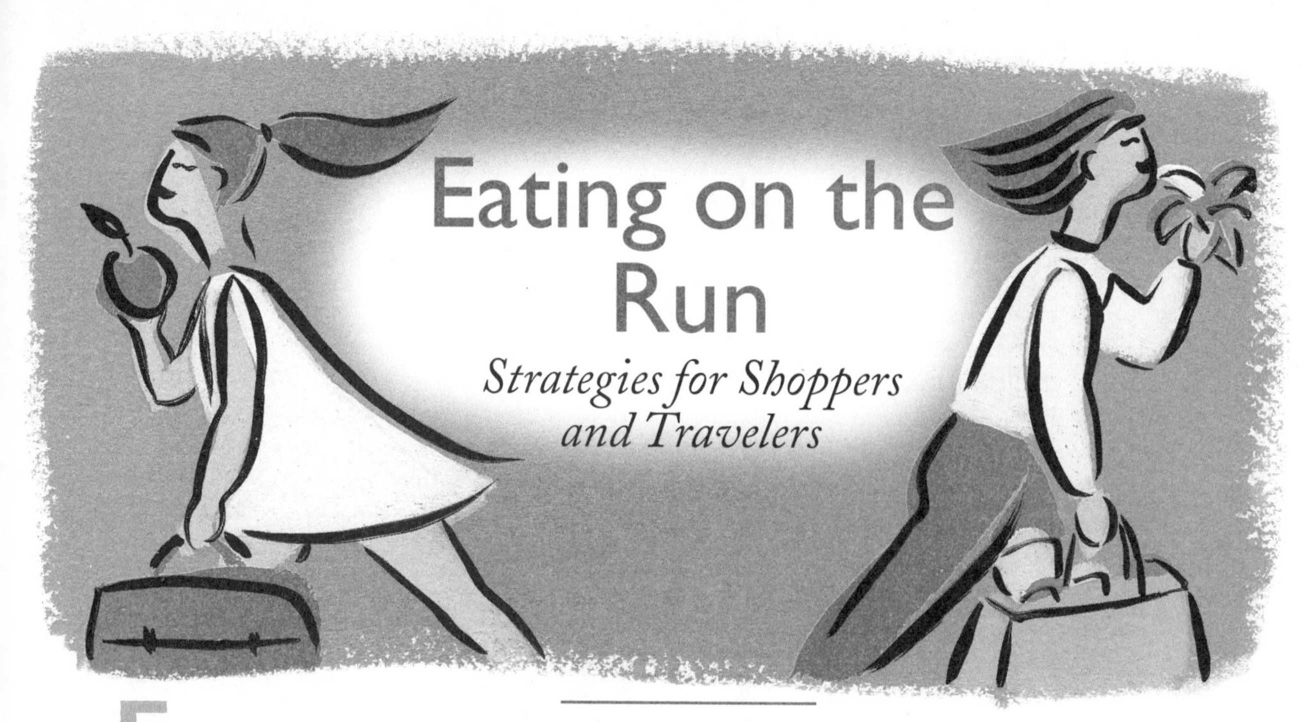

Eating on the Run

Strategies for Shoppers and Travelers

Eating healthfully would be so much easier if temptation weren't lurking around every corner. From the candy bar in the vending machine to the fast-food court at the mall, food beckons you and teases your senses into submission: "C'mon. Aren't you feeling just a teensy-weensy bit hungry? *Hmmm?*"

There are ways to outwit these edible enticements—and you don't have to rely on your willpower to do it. And if you're genuinely hungry, you can find healthful foods amidst the cookies and cappuccinos, the nachos and nuts. You just have to know what to look for.

Vending Machines: Hit the Jackpot

Buying food from a vending machine is kind of like playing a slot machine. Since you can't read the labels, you have no idea what you're getting, nutrition-wise. So you drop in your change, pull the lever, and hope for the best.

"Vending machines are convenient, especially when your stomach starts grumbling at midafternoon," says Edith Howard Hogan, R.D., a dietitian in Washington, D.C., and a spokesperson for the American Dietetic Association. "They do offer better selections these days. But they tend to have their problems, too." If your choice is limited to candy bars and potato chips, for instance, it's not much of a choice at all. Either way, you're going to get between 10 and 25 grams of fat.

Your best bets: Look for fresh fruit, fruit juice, single-serving boxes of cereal, and pop-top single-serving cans of tuna, Hogan says. If none of these is available, then pretzels are a good low-fat, low-calorie option.

Convenience Stores: Good to Go

There are 93,200 convenience stores in the United States. More likely than not, you probably have easy access to one around the clock.

Once considered bastions of nutritionally vacant foods, these mini-supermarkets are turning over a new leaf. Twenty-eight percent of all convenience stores now stock some sort of produce, according to the National Association of Convenience Stores. "I was in a 7-Eleven the other day, and my heart went pitter-patter," says Evelyn Tribole, R.D., author of *Healthy Homestyle Cooking* and *Eating on the Run*. "They had fresh fruit—apples and bananas. They had low-fat muffins, too."

Still, you need to keep your guard up when you start browsing convenience-store aisles. You're going to encounter lots of high-fat, high-calorie grab-and-eat foods, says Liz Applegate, Ph.D., a nutrition lecturer at the University of California, Davis, and author of *Power Foods*.

Your best bets: If you just want a snack, Dr. Applegate suggests picking up pretzels or low-fat fig bars. For something more substantive, like a sandwich or burger, choose the least expensive one on the menu. It usually contains less meat—and less fat. You can wash it down with orange juice or grape juice for an extra dose of vitamin C.

If you're buying something for the road, steer clear of the megabags of snack foods. They make it almost impossible to exercise any portion control.

Woman to Woman

She Stays Healthy on the Road

For Christine Connor, an investment analytics specialist from Medford, Massachusetts, business travel is a way of life and so is healthy eating. But finding healthy choices on the road isn't easy. Here's her secret to success.

I travel a lot for my job, and I can tell you that it's hard to find healthy choices among the fat-laden food options in airports and hotels.

I had always been a healthy eater, so after my first few business trips and the dining options I found on the road, I knew I had to find a way to maintain my normal lifestyle while away from home. I find it takes some effort and good planning, but it's well worth the effort.

First, I always try to eat before I go to the airport so I can avoid those greasy fries and cheeseburgers. And I always carry healthy snacks with me. I bring foods that are easy to pack—apples, bananas, bagels, and rice cakes.

If for whatever reason I have to eat in an airport, I'll search for a salad. If the airport has a Chinese food stand—a lot of them do—I'll order just plain rice. Or I'll opt for a snack; I can usually find a bag of pretzels at the airport bookstore. When I get tempted by all the candy, I'll get a package of Twizzlers. If I order room service at a hotel for dinner, I'll get a plain baked potato and a salad with low-fat dressing.

I also drink plenty of bottled water. When I'm flying, it's the only thing I drink, so I don't get dehydrated. I stay away from soda and alcohol to avoid empty calories.

Also, I don't let travel interfere with my workout routine. I'm a runner, and I run and lift weights at least four times a week.

For someone who travels as often as I do, it's important to stick with your routine diet and exercise program. Believe me, I know it can be difficult, but the payoff is great.

Malls: Nutrition-Wise Selections

Perusing the food court at the local mall, you may think you've entered the land of giants. Who else could possibly eat those humongous soft pretzels, cookies, and hot dogs?

Well, truth be told, those tantalizing aromas

are pretty darn hard to resist. And many of us do eat the whole thing—probably more often than we'd care to admit.

You may already suspect that these "monster foods" also pack monster doses of calories and fat. So here's the bad news: A giant-size order of nachos supplies 1,650 calories and 110 grams of fat. A giant-size muffin antes up 705 calories and almost 30 grams of fat. We could go on, but you get the idea.

To minimize mall munchies, your smartest move may be to eat *before* you shop. It's the same principle that applies to grocery shopping: If you fill your stomach first, you're less likely to succumb to the sight and smell of foods, explains Michele Tuttle, R.D., former director of consumer affairs for the Food Marketing Institute in Washington, D.C.

Your best bets: Some mall café chains offer made-to-order sandwiches, which gives you control over what goes in them. At Au Bon Pain, for instance, you can choose from healthful fixin's such as smoked turkey, romaine lettuce, tomatoes, roasted red peppers, red onions, and whole-grain breads.

If you want something more "snackish," frozen yogurt is a refreshing treat. Both Friendly's and TCBY sell nonfat and low-fat varieties that range from 100 to 134 calories per serving.

Can't resist those cinnamon buns? You'll be happy to know that Cinnabon has introduced the "minibon delight," a reduced-fat cinnamon roll that contains about one-third of the calories (260) and one-quarter of the fat (6.5 grams) of the "classic" cinnamon roll.

Airlines: First-Class Fare

Airplane food has long been the butt of, pardon the pun, tasteless jokes. But consumer demand and competition among airlines is driving a shift toward better, more healthful in-flight meals.

Most airlines now offer their passengers a variety of special meals, including diabetic, kosher, vegetarian, low-sodium, low-fat, low-cholesterol, Hindu, and Muslim, says Tribole. Swissair, for instance, has 24 different variations to choose from, while Delta has 19.

Most airlines require that you request special meals ahead of time. If you can, do it when you book your flight. But don't sweat it if you forget. Even without advance reservations, certain carriers, like American Airlines, can serve Weight Watchers frozen meals on request on its transcontinental flights.

Your best bets: Ask ahead of time if your flight includes a meal. If it doesn't, pack healthy snacks such as bagels, a piece of fruit or dried fruit, single-serving boxes of cereal, and nonfat or low-fat sliced cheese. Or take along a packet of instant soup (bean, lentil, or pea) and request hot water when the beverage cart goes by.

In addition, many hotels will furnish a boxed lunch at a guest's request. Give room service a call to find out if you can get "one for the road."

Just remember to avoid cantaloupe, watermelon, carbonated drinks, and other gas-causing foods before or during a flight, says Maria Simonson, Sc.D., Ph.D., professor emeritus and director of the health, weight, and stress clinic at Johns Hopkins Medical Institutions in Baltimore. Otherwise, you can develop a painful gas bubble in your gastrointestinal tract from the change in altitude.

Remember, too, to drink lots of water—at least one glass for every hour that you're flying, Hogan advises. You can lose more than a pint of water through your skin and through breathing during a three-hour flight. And dehydration can leave you feeling cranky and fatigued. Ditch the alcoholic and caffeinated beverages, though: They dehydrate you even more.

Index

Underscored references indicated boxed text. *Italic* references indicate illustrations.

D

E

F

G

H

M

N

O

P

Q

R

S